NURSING - ISSUES, PROBLEMS AND CHALLENGES

COLLABORATION WITH THE ADVANCED PRACTICE NURSE

ROLE, TEAMWORK AND OUTCOMES

NURSING - ISSUES, PROBLEMS AND CHALLENGES

Additional books in this series can be found on Nova's website under the Series tab.

Additional e-books in this series can be found on Nova's website under the e-book tab.

NURSING - ISSUES, PROBLEMS AND CHALLENGES

COLLABORATION WITH THE ADVANCED PRACTICE NURSE

ROLE, TEAMWORK AND OUTCOMES

EILEEN R. GIARDINO, PH.D.
ROBERT G. HANKS, PH.D
AND
ANGELO P. GIARDINO, M.D., PH.D.
EDITORS

nova publishers
New York

For permission to use material from this book please contact us:
Telephone 631-231-7269; Fax 631-231-8175
Web Site: http://www.novapublishers.com

Library of Congress Cataloging-in-Publication Data

ISBN: 978-1-63321-311-1

Library of Congress Control Number: 2014942814

Published by Nova Science Publishers, Inc. † New York

This book is dedicated to Nancy Busen PhD, RN, FNP-BC, the Margaret A. Barnett/PARTNERS Professor in Nursing and Department Chair of Family Health at the University of Texas Health Science Center-Houston, School of Nursing. A practicing nurse practitioner herself, Dr Busen is best known as an educator of graduate students who aspire to be advanced practice nurses as well as an avid supporter of the faculty who work tirelessly to educate advanced practice nurses. Dr. Busen is a champion for advanced practice nursing.

ERG

This book is dedicated to all the advanced practice registered nurses who provide healthcare to patients, families, and communities.

RGH

This book is dedicated to Ann L O'Sullivan, PhD, FAAN, CRNP, the Dr. Hildagarde Reynolds Endowed Term Professor of Primary Care Nursing at the University of Pennsylvania School of Nursing, who during our three years as collaborative practice partners serving a group of young parents and their children in Philadelphia during the mid-1990s taught me a great deal about patient care, patient empowerment and how interdependent we all are in our effort to provide the best care possible to those we have the privilege of knowing in our professional roles.

APG

CONTENTS

FOREWORD BY PATRICIA L. STARCK

I remember the excitement when Dr. Loretta Ford and Dr. Henry Silverman had a pioneering vision that developed the concept and implemented the advanced nursing practice role that became the pediatric nurse practitioner. Of course, there were those who objected -- both individuals and organizations -- chastised nursing for following a "medical model" and preparing "physician extenders", but history has proven what a brilliant idea this was. One of the reasons I believe the advanced practice role has not only survived but thrived, is that the role was developed based on a need in the community. I am proud that our profession, over the years, has responded many times to assessing the need and being creative and dedicated enough to meet the challenge. APRN programs have emerged and evolved accordingly. The Doctor of Nursing Practice role is another example of the foresight in identifying a societal need and creating a solution.

Now, more than ever, our nation is in need of innovative solutions. Health care leaders as well as other community leaders have recognized the value of promoting the APRN provider as an essential part of addressing the demand for a health care system that provides access, quality, and cost control. Business leaders are looking to our profession for entrepreneurial and alternative models.

One of the benefits of serving in academic leadership in nursing is the great sense of satisfaction in seeing the successes that have occurred in advancing the mission of the nursing profession. It has been most gratifying to be a part of the development of the roles of the Advanced Practice Registered Nurse (APRN). It is remarkable to see the APRN address the needs of the health care system for both individual patients and for organizational systems. To see the contributions that Advanced Practice Registered Nurses make in their leadership responsibilities in a wide variety of organizations and professional settings is equally as remarkable as are their clinical accomplishments. APRN achievements were not earned easily, nor were the well deserved accolades won without a great deal of creativity, scholarly investigation and continual attention and investment in the hard work that occurs at both the bedside and at the system levels. The one constant in the APRN professional development journey has been the consistent emergence of challenges, each being met with a focused, effective resolve to prepare for the inevitable rise of another.

Advanced practice nursing has experienced monumental changes over the past decades. Clinicians in other health care professions as well as the patient consumers see that advanced practice nurses offer clinical and administrative expertise to our nation's health care environment.

But nurses never rest on their laurels and new health care challenges never cease. As soon as the leaders and front line providers in advanced practice nursing achieve one professional accomplishment, there is the next professional challenge ahead. Clearly APRNs are poised to expand their roles and responsibilities in direct patient care, organizational systems, and population health in this 21st century.

The University of Texas Health Science Center at Houston, School of Nursing, has played an instrumental role in the development of advanced practice nurses who now serve Texas, the USA and other countries as well. Our programs prepare advanced practices nurses to meet the challenges of the 21st century. Our faculty are actively engaged on every level of practice and scholarly pursuit. We consider ourselves Pacesetters, helping to create the trends of the future.

This book serves as an informative text to nurses and other health care professionals to detail the education, clinical practice issues and clinical roles of the advanced practice nurse and most specifically of nurse practitioners. The chapters address how nurses are practicing at the advanced practice level and how advanced practice nursing strives to expand the boundaries of nursing practice. The text describes the evolving roles and responsibilities of advanced practice nurses in a variety of clinical settings. The chapters detail the educational background required for the APRN, the licensure and credentialing process, and roles and responsibilities of nurse practitioners in a variety of clinical focus areas such as primary care, acute care, and mental health. Chapters clarify the different educational levels of masters and doctorally prepared advanced practice nurses and how the educational preparation affects clinical and administrative practice. Two chapters address collaborative aspects of advanced practice which are case management and the nursing science officer. The book concludes with the impending workforce challenges our nation faces with regard to health care. It is encouraging to see that advanced practice nurses are regarded as part of any realistic solution to meeting the growing needs of our US population. And, advanced practice nurses are also seen as key professional participants in achieving many of the quality improvements anticipated in the health care system as planned in our on-going health care reform efforts. To that end, it is important that nurses and other health care professionals understand the underlying principles and practice considerations of the advanced practice nurse.

Patricia L. Starck, PhD, RN, FAAN
Dean and John P. McGovern Distinguished Professor
Huffington Foundation Chair for Nursing Education Leadership
Senior Vice President for Interprofessional Education

FOREWORD BY PATTIE BONDURANT

"By virtue of their regular, close proximity to the patients and their scientific understanding of care processes across the continuum of care, nurses have a considerable opportunity to act as full partners with other health professionals and to lead in the improvement and redesign of the health care system and its practice environment." The Future of Nursing: Leading Change, Advancing Health. P23 [emphasis added]

The quote from The Future of Nursing: Leading Change, Advancing Health captures several key elements that are of importance to those of us interested in the development of advanced practice nursing and operational leadership in health care organizations. Advanced practice nurses have:

- Proximity to patients
- Scientific understanding of care process
- Partnerships with other health professionals, and finally
- Leadership in the improvement and redesign of both systems and practice

The four characteristics above are woven into the fabric of what makes an advanced practice nurse such a valuable member of the health care team. Essentially, APNs are nursing professionals whose education and experiences equip them to shoulder sophisticated roles and responsibilities in patient care. APNs: 1) are close to the patient, families and community they serve; 2) rely on their scientific knowledge of evidence-based best practices; 3) foster collaboration and partnerships with a wide range of other colleagues, and 4) lead performance improvement efforts from direct care to the broader systems of care delivery. Advanced practice nurses are ideally suited to leadership responsibilities because of their education that is rooted in the depth and breadth of their clinical experience. APNs are positioned to make valuable contributions to improve clinical performance and outcomes.

The training and experience in my own professional development that lead me to become a doctor of nursing practice (DNP) provided me with an excellent background and set of skills to participate and lead a community wide health care improvement initiative. The Greater Cincinnati Beacon Collaboration (GCBC) was a 30 month, 13.75 million dollar health information technology infrastructure enhancement project that sought to achieve measurable improvements in health care quality, safety, efficiency and population health. The

GCBC brought together a wide array of health care providers including over 200 adult primary care providers, over 300 pediatricians, 21 regional hospital in an effort to improve the system of care for over 35,000 patients with diabetes and another 30,000 patients with pediatric asthma.

The GCBC appointed me along with many collaborators interested in substantial health care transformation to make that lofty goal a reality. Because of our focus on the actual patients, on the science that underpins the processes of care and our commitment to collaboration across all disciplines and stakeholders, the GCBC was successful at transparently assessing the range of problems and issues, considering possible solutions, setting priorities that balanced resources and needs, and putting systems in place to monitor and evaluate the impact of interventions. The entire project in Cincinnati as well as elsewhere can be found on the web at www.healthbridge.org/beacon]

The point of sharing this vignette is to provide a context for the optimism that advanced practice nurses can lead efforts to improve performance in health care systems as well as in direct patient care. Advanced practice nurses have the ability to "get the big picture" and to successfully navigate the details due to the grounding that we have from our close proximity to the patients being served and a firm commitment to the scientific underpinnings of the care process.

This purpose of this book is to clarify the focus of the advanced practice nurse in light of the roles and responsibilities that advanced practice nurses hold, and to articulate the core information of what nurses and other health care professionals should know in order to collaborate with the advanced practice nurse. The role of the advanced practice nurse continues to strengthen as a force in the health care arena and I am proud to be an advanced practice nurse at the forefront of improving the nursing profession, health care systems, and the individual care of the patients I serve.

Pattie Bondurant DNP, RN
Vice President for Nursing, Newborn Center at Texas Children's Hospital
Houston, Texas

FOREWORD BY DEBORAH BECKER

"What nursing brings to the future is a steadfast commitment to patient care, improved safety and quality, and better outcomes." (The Future of Nursing: Leading Change, Advancing Health)

Roles for nurses continue to evolve as nurses find ways to meet the ever-growing and expanding needs of a wide range of patients and communities throughout our population. Nowhere is this more evident in nursing than around the seismic changes occurring in the roles and responsibilities that continue to emerge for advanced practice nurses. The value contributed to the overall health care system by highly skilled advanced practice registered nurses (APRNs) is well documented in the professional literature and the evidence for delivering high quality and safe care along with promoting better outcomes forms the basis for the aspirational 2010 Institute of Medicine report, The Future of Nursing. Nurses are asked to "practice to the fullest extent of their education and training" and in so doing have the potential to fully realize the opportunity to contribute significantly to the patients and communities they steadfastly serve. The authors in this book explore the opportunities from the perspective of advanced practice nursing as it is today and where it could be tomorrow.

A discussion of the contributions of advanced practice nurses, either potential or realized, to the health and well being of their patients and communities ideally begins with a clear definition of the role and responsibilities. The 2008 Consensus Model for APRN Regulation provides a foundational definition that is of particular interest because of its depth and breadth. An Advanced Practice Registered Nurse (APRN) is a nurse who has:

- Completed an accredited graduate-level educational program preparing him/her for one of the four recognized APRN roles;
- Passed a national certification exam that measures APRN role and population-focused competencies and maintains continued competence as evidenced by recertification through the national certification program;
- Acquired advanced clinical knowledge and skills preparing him/her to provide direct care to patients, as well as a component of indirect care; however, the defining factor for all APRNs is that a significant component of the education and practice focuses on direct care of individuals;

- Developed a practice that builds on the competencies of registered nurses (RNs) by demonstrating a greater depth and breadth of knowledge, a greater synthesis of data, increased complexity of skills and interventions, and greater role autonomy;
- Educational preparation to assume responsibility and accountability for health promotion and/or maintenance as well as the assessment, diagnosis, and management of patient problems, including the use and prescription of pharmacologic and non-pharmacologic interventions;
- Clinical experience of sufficient depth and breadth to reflect the intended license and
- Obtained a license to practice as an APRN in one of the four APRN roles: certified registered nurse anesthetist (CRNA), certified nurse-midwife (CNM), clinical nurse specialist (CNS), or certified nurse practitioner (CNP).

The seven elements to the definition above are substantially grounded in the knowledge, skills and attitudes necessary to be clinically competent in patient care. What is clear is that advanced practice nurses, whatever their specific roles, by way of training, experience and professional commitment, bring a great deal of clinical expertise to their roles and responsibilities. As such, the education and training of APRNs is of critical importance since clinical competence is an essential element that highly regarded professionals bring to the table and forms the basis for their contributions. Towards that end, my own work focuses on how best to use a variety of educational modalities to provide and enhance the clinical competency of APRNs.

This book describes the educational requirements of APRNs at the masters and doctoral levels and the many roles in which advanced practice nurses serve. A historical overview of advanced practice nursing is followed by discussions of the advanced practice nurse role in a variety of clinical settings such as acute care, primary care, women's health and specialty care. The book concludes with a look forward towards the health care provider workforce needs for the coming years and discusses the literature examining how advanced practice nurses can help inform as well as be an integral part of the solution to growing patient and community needs. As we look to the future of nursing, it is clear that advanced practice nurses, whatever their specific role, by way of training, experience and professional commitment have a great deal to offer our patients and communities. As the profession of nursing continues to develop, the opportunities for APRNs to serve and contribute will develop as well. Advanced practice nurses truly embrace the full continuum of responsibilities as the IOM report calls for "from the bedside to the boardroom" as well as from the classroom, the simulation lab and the research center.

Deborah Becker PhD, ACNP, BC
Practice Associate Professor of Nursing
Division Chair | Helene Fuld Pavilion for Innovative Learning
Director, Adult Gerontology Acute Care Nurse Practitioner,
University of Pennsylvania |School of Nursing

PREFACE

"Americans should be able to count on receiving care that meets their needs and is based on the best scientific knowledge. Yet there is strong evidence that this frequently is not the case... Quality problems are everywhere, affecting many patients. Between the health care we have and the care we could have lies not just a gap, but a chasm."

Institute of Medicine (IOM). 2001.
Crossing the Quality Chasm: A New Health System for the 21st Century.
Washington, D.C: National Academy Press. (pg 1)

This book is firmly rooted in our collective understanding that advanced practice nurses are essential clinicians and leaders in the health care delivery system. It takes a team effort for our nation to narrow and ultimately fill the quality chasm as identified the IOM's 2001 report of the Committee on the Quality of Health Care in America. Ten years later, the IOM issued another report entitled The Future of Nursing: Leading Change, Advancing Quality that provided a framework for how nursing in general and advanced practice nursing specifically, can help the health care system traverse the chasm.

The number of advanced practice registered nurses (APRN) has grown over the past forty years to now be recognized as a critical provider of care in today's healthcare delivery system. The spectrum of increasing health care needs across all age ranges has created new opportunities for advanced practice nurses to apply their expertise in a multitude of practice settings.

There have been at least two waves of growth in advanced practice nursing - the initial occurred in the mid-1960s when nurses started to formally expand their practice roles to meet the needs of the growing population in primary and acute care settings, and then again from the 1980s to the present time. As advanced practice nurses, we incorporate our educational preparation, in-depth knowledge and clinical expertise to address the health needs of individuals, families, communities and populations. We apply theory, knowledge, and research to advance the nursing profession and provide evidence based research to improve patient care. APRNs provide health care services in a wide range of clinical settings and specialty areas. APRNs provide quality care to all people nationally and even internationally, including cutting-edge healthcare technology settings to providing basic services to underserved communities.

The authors who have contributed chapters for this book on the roles of advanced practice nursing come from a variety of advanced practice backgrounds, and prepared at the masters and doctoral levels of education. It is an exciting time to be part of the health care system owing to the magnitude of the potential impact for the changes and reforms that are emerging. As an APRN, we approach the health care system and patient care with a focus on team work, collaborative practice, and a holistic approach to meeting the needs of patients and our communities. It is particularly rewarding to see how health care professionals, policy makers, and those we serve see advanced practice nursing as "part of the solution" to what ails our current fragmented health care.

Reflecting on what Loretta Ford, the co-founder of the nurse practitioner movement, we can all be gratified that what makes sense is actually coming to pass with regard to the full use of advanced practice nurses in our complex health care systems and processes. Put simply, Dr. Ford "realized that more nurses should be able to have specialized training so they could make basic decisions on their own about the health status of patients…[and]…in large part to her efforts, there are more that 140,000 nurse practitioners working in the United States today. Many can prescribe and diagnose as doctors can, but their nursing background emphasizes health promotion and patient empowerment" (Landau, 2011). Dr Ford's legacy is now carried on by many advanced practice nurses and the potential and expectation is that in the next decade the roles and responsibilities will continue to develop around the needs of patients, communities and the actual health care system as well.

APRNs are at the forefront of the transformation changes that are occurring in the health care system changes. We practice side by side with other members of the health care team including nurses, physicians, physician assistants, social workers, and other healthcare workers as a collaborative effort. This practice of collaborating with our health care partners was the initial impetus for this book. We realize that many of our colleagues, including those in the nursing profession, do not fully understand the basic underpinnings of advanced practice nursing, what an advanced practice nurse is, what the roles of advanced practice nursing are, and what the educational background of the APRN is. To that end, we decided to write a book that describes the basic tenets of advanced practice nursing. The audience of this text is all of our colleagues in nursing and other health professions who interface with advanced practice nurses, but may not truly understand the different roles within advanced practice nursing and the variations in practice of APRNs.

The chapters in this book synthesize available literature on this journey to improve care and foster necessary reforms and changes in the delivery of health care we have so that it reflects what our patients not only could have but what we know they ought to have.

The book, *Collaboration with the Advanced Practice Nurse: Role, Teamwork, and Outcomes* describes many specifics of advanced practice nursing pertaining to the four specific roles. This text describes the basic underpinnings of advanced practice nursing, including educational requirements, licensure and credentialing, and how APRNs work independently or collaboratively with physicians dependent on the state and the site in which an APRN practices. The chapter on the Doctor of Nursing Practice describes the DNP and how the degree transforms the APRN from a provider of services to a transformational leader in the health care arena.

Section Two focuses primarily on nurse practitioner practice. Chapters describes the practice of the primary care, acute care the psychiatric mental health nurse practitioners.

Section Three covers some specialty roles of the nurse practitioner, including the burgeoning role of nurse practitioners in convenience care clinics. The chapter on the certified nurse midwife (CNM) describes a separate advanced practice nursing role that focuses on the care of women through the pregnancy and birth process. There is a chapter on the administrative aspects of the nurse practitioner and how the DNP degree strengthens the focus of practice to include going from a provider of care to an evaluator and change agent of clinical care.

We hope that *Collaboration with the Advanced Practice Nurse: Role, Teamwork, and Outcomes* provides the reader a greater understanding of the educational preparation, clinical roles, and practice considerations of the APRN and how then the APRN can work collaboratively with other health care professionals to care for the health needs in the health care system.

Pulling together a project such as this requires a great deal of voluntary effort on the part of the chapter contributors who take time and care to review the relevant literature to explain the details that are of importance to advanced practice nursing. We like to express our appreciation to the many contributors who readily agreed to take on extra work to author the chapters contained in the book. In addition, the academic institutions where the authors teach and work also deserve special thanks for providing the scholarly environment and encouragement so that projects such as this can be conceived and brought through to completion. A book like this only comes together with meticulous editorial help from administrative professionals who have the requisite skill and experience to keep track of the many details that go into producing a book length work. On this project, Marlene Moulder served in this capacity and with her usual calm manner assisted us in keeping track of everything, both big and small that needed care and attention and for this we are very grateful. Finally, we want to thank the editorial team at Nova Science Publishers, Inc. for bringing this work from idea to printed pages.

In closing, we hope that readers find this work informative and that they will come way from reading the material in this book well equipped to understand the roles and responsibilities of advanced practice nurses both now and in the future. We share the vision statement from the Committee on the Robert Wood Johnson Foundation Initiative on the Future of Nursing at the Institute of Medicine.

> "The committee envisions a future system that makes quality care accessible to the diverse populations of the United States, intentionally promotes wellness and disease prevention, reliably improves health outcomes, and provides compassionate care across the lifespan. In this envisioned future, primary care and prevention are central drivers of the health care system. Interprofessional collaboration and coordination are the norm. Payment for health care rewards value, no volume of services, and quality care is provided at a price that is affordable for both individuals and society. The rate of growth of health care expenditures slows. In all these areas, the health care system consistently demonstrates that it is responsive to individuals' needs and desires through the delivery of truly patient-centered care."

Institute of Medicine (IOM). 2011.
The Future of Nursing: Leading Change, Advancing Health.
Washington, DC: National Academy Press. (pg 22).

Eileen R. Giardino, PhD, RN, ANP-BC, FNP-BC
Robert G. Hanks, PhD, FNP-C, RNC
Angelo P. Giardino, MD, PhD
Houston, TX
May 2014

References

Institute of Medicine (IOM). 2001. *Crossing the Quality Chasm: A New Health System for the 21st Century.* Washington, D.C: National Academy Press.

Landau, E. (2011) Nurse practitioners were 'Lone Rangers,' founder says. CNN.com. http://www.cnn.com/2011/09/30/health

Institute of Medicine (IOM). 2011. *The Future of Nursing: Leading Change, Advancing Health.* Washington, DC: National Academy Press.

About the Editors

Eileen R. Giardino PhD, APRN, FNP, ANP, RN.

Dr. Giardino is an Associate Professor at the School of Nursing at the University of Texas Health Science Center at University of Texas Health Science Center at Houston School of Nursing with a focus is in both clinical practice and nursing education. Dr. Giardino is board certified as an adult nurse practitioner and as a family nurse practitioner. She has served as director of the Family Nurse Practitioner track at UT Health-Houston and teaches in the graduate and doctoral programs for family nurse practitioners and doctor of nursing practice students.

Dr. Giardino supervises clinical preceptorships and advises students in the MSN and DNP programs. Her advanced nursing practice is focused on college health and currently practices at the Student Health Services of University of Houston Downtown. Academic accomplishments include editing text books in the areas of child maltreatment and intimate partner violence. She presents at professional meetings on issues related to physical assessment and interpersonal violence. She is the nursing faculty for the LEND program at UT Health and provide the nursing perspective on caring for children on the spectrum for autistic and neurodevelopmental disabilities.

Dr. Giardino received her bachelor's and doctoral degrees at the University of Pennsylvania, and her master's degree in nursing at Widener University. She was recently awarded the John P. McGovern Outstanding Teacher Award 2012 in recognition of outstanding teaching in the School of Nursing.

Robert Hanks, PhD, FNP-C, RNC

Dr. Hanks has been in the nursing profession his entire adult life, and is currently a nursing faculty member at the University of Texas Health Science Center at Houston School of Nursing in Houston, Texas. Dr. Hanks is currently the Graduate Nurse Education Demonstration Project Manager and has a faculty practice in a college health services position. He has a background in family nursing at the advanced practice level and medical-surgical nursing at the registered nurse level.

Dr. Hanks holds a doctorate, master's, and baccalaureate degree from the University of Texas Medical Branch in Galveston, Texas and is currently recognized as both a registered nurse and family nurse practitioner.

Dr. Hanks has a research interest in nursing advocacy for patients. He has several publications regarding nursing advocacy and has expanded his publication base to include social advocacy as exemplified by his article "Social advocacy: A call for nursing action" published in *Pastoral Psychology*. Dr. Hanks is currently engaged in research examining online content delivery methods and simulation activities in nursing education and has presented at regional and national conferences on these research efforts.

Dr. Hanks' was recently awarded the John P. McGovern Outstanding Teacher Award 2013: Graduate Level in recognition of his teaching expertise.

Angelo P. Giardino, MD, PhD, MPH

Dr. Giardino is a Professor of Pediatrics and Section Chief of Academic General Pediatrics, at Baylor College of Medicine (BCM), Chief Quality Officer for Medicine at Texas Children's Hospital, and Vice-President and Chief Medical Officer at Texas Children's Health Plan in Houston, TX. Dr. Giardino, received his medical degree and doctorate in education from the University of Pennsylvania, completed his residency and fellowship training at The Children's Hospital of Philadelphia, earned a Master's in Public Health from the University of Massachusetts, and completed a Certificate in Medical and Healthcare Management from the Jones School of Business at Rice University. He is Board Certified in Pediatrics, Child Abuse and Medical Quality. A former Robert Wood Johnson Foundation Clinical Scholar, he completed the Patient Safety Certificate Program from the Quality Colloquium and in 2014 was designated a Distinguished Fellow of the American College of Medical Quality. Dr. Giardino has a long standing commitment to nursing education as well having had appointments at the Schools of Nursing at University of Pennsylvania and LaSalle University and currently is Adjunct Professor of Nursing at the University of Texas Health Science Center at Houston School of Nursing. Dr. Giardino has co-edited several books including the Nursing Approach to the Evaluation of Child Maltreatment which is now in its second edition.

PART 1: ROLE, EDUCATION AND PRACTICE PARAMETERS

In: Collaboration with the Advanced Practice Nurse ISBN: 978-1-63321-311-1
Editors: E.R. Giardino, R.G. Hanks and A.P. Giardino

Chapter 1

Advanced Practice Nursing: Role Development and Practice Considerations

Eileen R. Giardino, PhD, RN, APRN
and Robert G. Hanks, PhD, FNP-C, RN
University of Texas Health Science Center at Houston,
School of Nursing, Houston, TX, US

Abstract

Advanced practice registered nurses (APRN) are nurses who practice as certified nurse practitioners (CNP), certified registered nurse anesthetists (CRNA), certified nurse-midwifes (CNM), and clinical nurse specialists (CNS) (APRN Consensus Work Group & National Council of State Boards of Nursing APRN Advisory Committee, 2008). The National Council of State Boards of Nursing APRN Advisory Committee and the APRN Consensus Work Group defined the education process, program accreditation requirements, and national certification and licensure details for APRNs in an effort to standardize and clarify the details of APRN roles, educational backgrounds, and certification issues. Hallmarks of advanced practice nursing are increased clinical skill, knowledge and the delivery of patient care that includes patient assessment, establishment of diagnosis following appropriate diagnostic testing, and development of a management plan (Lowe, Plummer, O'Brien, & Boyd, 2012). This chapter addresses the development of the APRN role, defining factors of APRN roles, relationship of the advanced practice registered nurse to the basic professional nurse who has a BSN degree, and professional issues that the APRN faces regarding certification and practice.

Introduction

The definition of an APRN is a nurse who successfully completed an accredited graduate level educational program that prepared the nurse in one of four recognized APRN roles (APRN Consensus Work Group & National Council of State Boards of Nursing APRN Advisory Committee, 2008). Those four roles are certified registered nurse anesthetist

(CRNA), certified nurse-midwife (CNM), clinical nurse specialist (CNS), or certified nurse practitioner (CNP). The APRN must be licensed as a registered nurse by the state in which the APRN practices, and pass a national certification examination specific for the APRN role. To practice as an advanced practice nurse in a specific role, most states require the APRN to be licensed by a state board of nursing or other oversight regulatory body, and hold certification in the specialty area (APRN Joint Dialogue Group Report, 2008; APRN Consensus Work Group, 2008).

DISTINGUISHING CHARACTERISTICS OF THE APRN

There are distinguishing characteristics of the advanced practice master's or doctorally prepared nurse. The APRN must pass a national certification examination that measures a basic level of competency in the specific role, and then must demonstrate continued clinical competence by recertification by a national certifying body. The educational preparation of the advanced practice nurse allows the APRN to be clinically responsible to provide health promotion, and to assess, diagnose, and manage patient problems by prescribing pharmacologic drugs along with non-pharmacologic interventions (APRN Consensus Work Group & National Council of State Boards of Nursing APRN Advisory Committee, 2008). Given the care responsibilities that go beyond what the registered nurse (RN) is able to do, state boards of nursing regulate advanced practice to ensure that APRNs meet the state board requirements to medically diagnose and treat patients (APRN Consensus Work Group & National Council of State Boards of Nursing APRN Advisory Committee, 2008).

The American Nurses Association (ANA) described essential characteristics of nursing practice that distinguish basic nursing practice from advanced nursing practice. A distinction of advanced nursing practice is the specialization or provision of care for a specific population of patients with complex, unpredictable, and/or intensive health needs. The second is that advanced nursing practice builds on the acquisition or expansion of new knowledge and skills and role autonomy that extend beyond the traditional scopes of nursing practice. The third is advancement, which includes specialization and expansion (American Nurses Association, 2010). See Table 1 for the defining characteristics of an advanced practice nurse. The term advanced nursing practice indicates that the scope of nursing practice in the advanced role extends that of traditional nursing practice to maximize nursing knowledge, increase autonomy in clinical practice, and contribute to professional nursing development (Bryant-Lukosius, DiCenso, Browne, & Pinelli, 2004).

Table 1. Defining Characteristics of an Advanced Practice Registered Nurse (APRN)

	Defining Characteristics
Education	Completes an accredited graduate-level education program preparing for one of the four recognized APRN roles
Certification	Obtains national certification through examination that measures APRN, role & population-focused competencies. Maintains continued competence evidenced by recertification in the role and population through a national certifying body

	Defining Characteristics
Advanced knowledge base	Acquires advanced clinical knowledge and skills to provide direct care and indirect care to patients. A significant component of education and practice focuses on direct care of individuals.
Practice competencies	Practice builds on registered nurses (RN) competencies and demonstrates greater depth and breadth of knowledge, a greater synthesis of data, increased complexity of skills and interventions, and greater role autonomy
Role Expectations	Educationally prepared to assume responsibility and accountability for health promotion and/or maintenance as well as assessment, diagnosis, and management of patient problems (includes use and prescription of pharmacologic and non-pharmacologic interventions)
Licensure considerations	Has clinical experience of sufficient depth and breadth to reflect the intended license
Specific license in the role	Has license to practice as APRN in one of the APRN roles: certified registered nurse anesthetist (CRNA), certified nurse-midwife (CNM), clinical nurse specialist (CNS), or certified nurse practitioner (CNP).
	Adapted from: APRN Joint Dialogue Group Report (2008). Consensus Model for APRN Regulation: Licensure, Accreditation, Certification & Education APRN Joint Dialogue Group Report. pp. 7-8

REGULATION OF ADVANCED PRACTICE NURSING

At this point in time, there is no uniformity of regulation of advanced practice roles among the 50 states, and each of the 50 states determines specific regulatory aspects of each advanced practice role. Although many of the certification requirements are the same from state to state, each state determines its own criteria, and nurses must be certified in each specific state in order to practice. Individual states have similarities in what they require for licensure as a registered nurse and certification and practice at the advanced level for each of the four advanced practice roles. The state board of nursing in each state independently determines specifics for scope of practice, criteria for entry of nurses into advanced practice, and certification examinations required to assess entry-level competence (APRN Consensus Work Group & National Council of State Boards of Nursing APRN Advisory Committee., 2008). While there are nationally recommended components for education, accreditation, and certification, licensing boards of each state regulate who is recognized to practice within their state. Such variations in state regulatory board requirements have created barriers that prevent APRNs to easily move from state to state and then practice in another state before going through an extensive process to validate the credentials of a given APRN (APRN Consensus Work Group & National Council of State Boards of Nursing APRN Advisory Committee, 2008).

A requisite of advanced practice nursing is that the role responsibilities require the nurse to receive additional state or national certification in order to practice at that level. The CNS, CNP, CRNA and CNW roles have to pass a standardized national certification examination and then petition the State Board of Nursing to practice in the advanced practice role (APRN Consensus Work Group, 2008).

Advanced Practice Nursing and Non-Advanced Practice Roles

Every nurse who has a masters or doctoral degree in nursing is not an advanced practice nurse. There are master's level education programs that prepare nurses to work in roles that support the public health, but do not focus on administering direct care to individuals. In those roles, nursing practice does not require regulatory recognition beyond the Registered Nurse license granted by state boards of nursing. Examples of non-APRN masters prepared roles are nursing informatics, public health, nursing education, or nursing administration, to name a few (International Council of Nurses, 2009). For example, a nurse who graduates from a MSN program in Nursing Education and then works as a nurse educator in an inpatient or outpatient setting is not an APRN. Non-APRNs who earn a DNP degree remain as a non-APRN, as in the case of a nurse with an MSN in administration who then completes the DNP degree. The DNP degree does not change the advanced practice status of a nurse who entered the program with a master's degree in a nursing specialty that is not considered an advanced practice role.

Development of the Advanced Practice Role

There is an historical evolution of the educational requirements for each of the four advanced practice nursing roles. The phrase "advanced practice nursing" started to appear in the literature in the 1970s and 1980s (Hanson & Hamric, 2003). The initial educational requirement for a registered nurse to become a nurse practitioner, nurse anesthetist or midwife was to complete a certificate program in the specialty area after the basic nursing program. The nurse graduate of a hospital based diploma program without a bachelor's degree would complete the certification program for the specialty and then practice within the defined guidelines of that role. The shift of APRN education to the master's level curriculum occurred as nursing realized the need to move the baseline education to a higher level to be in compliance with other professions that require a more stringent educational process for practice (Rounds, Zych, & Mallary, 2013; APRN Consensus Work Group & National Council of State Boards of Nursing APRN Advisory Committee 2008). Since the advent of masters education as the required educational baseline for advanced practice in nursing, nurses working in expanded roles who completed certificate programs were usually grandfathered in to continue working in that role. However, even with the grandfathering process, institutions could require their own specific hiring criteria that would or could exclude the clinicians who did not have a master's level education.

Educational Programs for Professional Nursing

There are three levels of educational preparation that comprise professional nursing practice. The entry level is the Bachelor of Science (BSN) in Nursing, followed by the Master of Science in Nursing (MSN), and the clinical doctorate level of the Doctor of Nursing Practice (DNP). The BSN degree is the entry level into professional nursing practice and enables the nurse to seek licensure to practice as a registered nurse. Master's of Science in Nursing degree (MSN) programs prepare advanced practice nurses, nurse administrators, and nurse educators for a variety of roles in education, administration and practice (American Nurses Association, 2014a). For the advanced practice nurse, MSN education provides concepts of nursing theory, role development, and clinical practicum experience to prepare the APRN for the certification examination.

The Doctor of Nursing Practice (DNP) is a clinical practice doctorate that focuses on education related to health care delivery systems, safety, and management. The DNP degree expands the professional knowledge base of the professional nurse. The necessary degree needed for a nurse to apply to a DNP program is either a BSN or an MSN degree, depending on the type of DNP program. The post BSN to DNP program accepts nurses with a BSN degree while the post MSN DNP programs accept masters prepared graduates. A primary goal of the DNP graduate is to translate evidence into practice in ways that improve the quality and safety of patient care and enhance positive patient outcomes (APRN Consensus Work Group & National Council of State Boards of Nursing APRN Advisory Committee, 2008).

There are two program options for the DNP degree, a clinical practice focus and a leadership practice focus. Both DNP programs prepare the graduate to design and implement programs that improve health, health care delivery, improve clinical practice, apply data management and informatics skills to evaluate outcomes, and influence policy decisions (APRN Consensus Work Group & National Council of State Boards of Nursing APRN Advisory Committee, 2008). The post baccalaureate DNP program enables students with a bachelor's degree or higher in nursing to enter directly into a clinical doctorate program. Some post baccalaureate DNP programs offer an MSN degree along the way to the DNP, while other post baccalaureate programs only offer the DNP as the terminal degree. When the DNP is the terminal degree and the graduate does not receive a master's degree during the DNP education, the nurse practitioner graduate is qualified to take the national certification exam for the specific role of focus and apply to the state board of nursing for certification as a nurse practitioner in the way that a master's degree graduate would do.

The Doctor of Philosophy in Nursing is a research focused degree that prepares the nurse to generate evidence that guides safe and effective nursing care. The American Nurses Association states that the PhD degree prepares a nurse to be a nurse scientist and researcher who generates new knowledge. The focus of PhD education is on developing the nurses' ability to perform research rather than the delivery of direct or indirect patient care (American Nurses Association, 2014b). The Nursing doctorate enables nurses to work in roles that require or desire a doctoral degree, such as in higher education, research and administration.

Differences in Basic Nursing Practice and Advanced Nursing Practice

The responsibilities and practice differences of the advanced practice nurse can be understood when one understands the educational background and practice parameters of the basic registered nurse. The three entry pathways to registered nurse practice are: the Associates' Degree, Diploma programs, and the Bachelor of Science in Nursing. Each pathway enables the graduate of the program to take the NCLEX-RN examination and apply for the same licensure as a Registered Nurse (American Association of Colleges of Nursing,

2014). Although diploma, associate's degree and bachelor's degree graduates take the same National Council Licensure Examination for Registered Nurses (NCLEX-RN) examination and share the same licensure requirements, only the baccalaureate degree is considered as the entry degree for professional nursing.

Diploma Nursing Programs

Diploma programs were the major source of registered nurses in the US until the 1970s when a shift in education of nurses from hospital based programs to institutions of higher education continued to arise. There were approximately 1300 diploma schools in operation throughout the United States at the peak of the diploma education trend. During the 1970s, nursing education made a long desired shift from apprentice-type diploma school instruction based in a hospital to education at the college and university level. Diploma program graduates receive a diploma which does not equate to an associate (ADN) or university based baccalaureate degree (BSN). The diploma graduate is qualified to take the NCLEX-RN examination and apply for licensure as a Registered Nurse. Most Diploma schools still in existence are affiliated with colleges or universities that grant college credit for certain courses taken in the Diploma program (Blais, Hayes, Kozier, & Erb, 2006; American Nurses Association, 2014 a; Bureau of Labor Statistics, 2014).

Associate Degree Programs

The Associate Degree in Nursing (ADN) program is typically a two to three year program that prepares nursing graduates for what nursing defines as a technical nurse. The graduate is qualified to take the NCLEX-RN examination and apply for licensure as a Registered Nurse. ADN programs are typically offered in community colleges or higher degree programs that confer the associate's degree (American Nurses Association, 2014a). An associate's degree in nursing (ADN) prepares nurses for an entry level to an intermediate level position in health care sites where a registered nurse is required. An ADN program may require some courses in the arts and sciences, the bachelor of science in nursing (BSN) programs at the university level provides a stronger focus on foundational courses in science and humanities (American Association of Colleges of Nursing, 2014). Sites of practice for ADN graduates include hospitals, clinics, home care, and school health, to name a few. The usual educational route for an ADN who wants to become an advanced practice nurse in any of the four roles is to pursue the BSN degree and then proceed to a masters or DNP program in the advanced practice role of choice.

The Bachelor of Science in Nursing

The graduate of a Bachelor of Science in Nursing (BSN) program completes a four-year academic degree granted by an accredited college or university. The graduate is qualified to take the NCLEX-RN examination and apply for licensure as a Registered Nurse. BSN programs prepare graduates for the professional nursing role with coursework in nursing, science, research, humanities and social sciences. The bachelor's degree affords nursing graduates to practice in positions that include clinical nursing, as well as administrative, research, and consulting positions that might not be available to those with an Associate's Degree in Nursing (Bureau of Labor Statistics, 2014; American Nurses Association, 2014a).

Advanced Practice Registered Nurse Roles

The four APRN roles as defined by the Consensus Model (APRN Consensus Work Group & National Council of State Boards of Nursing APRN Advisory Committee, 2008) are distinct in their clinical focus. The following sections describe each of the advanced practice roles.

Certified Registered Nurse Anesthesia

Nurses have provided anesthesia to patients for more than 100 years. The historical underpinnings of the Certified Registered Nurse Anesthetist (CRNA) to provide anesthesia in all clinical settings is rooted in social, political, and economic forces (MacDonald, Herbert, & Thibeault, 2006). The initial educational requirement for the nurse anesthetist was a certificate or diploma. In 1986, a bachelor's degree in nursing or a related degree was required for admission to nurse anesthesia programs. The Council on Accreditation for Nurse Anesthesia Programs developed educational guidelines that supported the move to a master's degree as the required preparation for practice (AANA, 2014; Horton, 2007). By 1982, the official position of the American Association of Nurse Anesthetists (AANA) board of directors was that nurse anesthetists would first complete a BSN degree and then attend a master's level anesthesia program (Horton, 2007; AANA, 2014). The educational preparation requirement moved to the masters' level by 1998, and in 2007, the AANA adopted the position to move nurse anesthesia education to the doctoral level by 2025 (AANA, 2014).

The CRNA provides a full range of anesthesia care to patients across the lifespan. CRNAs deliver anesthesia to patients across the lifespan in a variety of clinical settings, including inpatient hospital suites, delivery rooms, and outpatient centers such as pain management centers and dental and ophthalmology offices, to name a few. (APRN Consensus Work Group & National Council of State Boards of Nursing APRN Advisory Committee, 2008).

The Nurse Practitioner Role

A certified nurse practitioner (CNP) is an advanced practice registered nurse (APRN) who has completed a masters or doctoral level educational program that provides advanced clinical and theoretical knowledge, beyond what is required for the generalist registered nurse (RN) role. The International Council of Nurses states that an advanced practice nurse practitioner, referred to as a certified nurse practitioner (CNP), has the knowledge base, decision-making skills, and clinical competencies that enable the nurse to expand practice capabilities beyond that of a registered nurse (International Council of Nurses, 2009). CNP education prepares practitioners to competently manage health and illness, including health promotion and disease prevention, regardless of the population served. Graduates gain the knowledge, skills, and abilities that are essential to independent clinical practice (National Organization of Nurse Practitioner Faculty, 2013). The CNP provides direct care through assessment of patient's complaints and identified problems and determines a medical diagnosis and management plan (Lowe et al., 2012).

The need for CNP services has emerged in response to the need to increase the number of clinicians able to provide cost effective and quality care. CNPs are an effective way to maximize resources and expand patient care services in all clinical areas such as emergency departments, primary care, acute and primary pediatric care and specialty practices such as cardiac and endocrine, to name a few.

The role of the nurse practitioner role emerged in the US in the mid-1960s to fill gaps in the delivery of primary health care services to patients across the lifespan, especially in rural areas (McIntosh et al., 2003); (Driscoll, Worrall-Carter, O'Reilly, & Stewart, 2005). At that time, there was a growing demand for primary care medical services, especially in underserved areas, and the realization that nurses could help to meet those needs (Ford, 1982) (McGivern, Sullivan-Marx, & Mezey, 2003). The physician shortage was cited as one reason for the expansion of nurse practitioner programs nationwide (Elder & Bullough, 1990) (McGivern, 1993) (O'Brien, 2003).

In 1965, Dr. Loretta Ford and Dr. Henry Silver, a nurse and a physician, created the first training program for nurse practitioners that focused on child and family health needs, as well as health promotion and disease prevention (Ford, 1986). The short supply of physicians in rural areas identified the need for nurses to provide an advanced level of assessment and clinical management to those in need of medical services (Lowe et al., 2012). The role of the pediatric nurse practitioner started in response to this need.

Nurse practitioner education first started as a post RN level certificate program when the baseline education for the RN was at the diploma level. Nursing leaders initiated a move of the entry level of NP practice from an RN certificate program to a master's degree program. In 2004, a position statement developed by member schools affiliated with the American Association of Colleges of Nursing (AACN) endorse a call to move the current level of preparation necessary for advanced nursing practice from the master's degree to the doctorate-level by the year 2015 (AACN, 2004); (AANP, 2014; APRN Consensus Work Group & National Council of State Boards of Nursing APRN Advisory Committee, 2008). Although CRNA education has formally moved to the doctoral level, as of this time, the AACN position paper recommendation has not been implemented to require the terminal degree for nurse practitioner education to be at the DNP level.

The Clinical Nurse Specialist

The Clinical Nurse Specialist (CNS) role is focused on the improvement of patient care and clinical outcomes through clinical management or case management of patients. The roles of expert practitioner, researcher, educator, consultant and leader are hallmarks of CNS practice internationally (Kring, 2008; Dowling, Beauchesne, Farrelly, & Murphy, 2013). The

CNS integrates clinical care through three interrelated and overlapping spheres of influence: nurse, patient, and system, and each sphere has a distinctive focus. There are many facets to CNS practice. The CNS role includes teaching nurses to show caring behaviors towards patients, implement evidenced based practices to improve patient outcomes, address cultural diversity, and consider ethical decision making principles to guide nursing practice.

The scope of CNS practice is defined and regulated by state boards of nursing. The state boards stipulate the conditions under which a CNS may perform delegated medical acts and prescribe medications (North Carolina Board of Nursing, 2014).The boards of nursing (BON) that regulate advanced practice at the state level generally view the roles of the CNS and CNP as separate and distinct. For example, The Texas Board of Nursing acknowledges that the CNS and CNP scopes of practice may overlap and the amount of overlap varies based on the advanced practice educational preparation of a nurse in each of the roles (Texas Board of Nursing, 2005). CNS scope of practice includes diagnosis and treatment of health/illness states, disease management, and initiation of health promotion and prevention activities for individuals, families, groups, and communities (Lowe et al., 2012); (APRN Consensus Work Group & National Council of State Boards of Nursing APRN Advisory Committee, 2008).

THE CERTIFIED NURSE MIDWIFE

Midwives have been an integral part of society since the beginning of time. There have always been people, mostly women, who have helped in the birthing process. The educational process and requirements for the nurse midwife has evolved over the centuries. At the present time, certified nurse-midwives (CNMs) are educated in a graduate nursing education program, as described by the educational requirements for the APRN, and receive an MSN degree. The Consensus model for APRN regulation states that CNMs provide primary health care services to women across the lifespan, and care to the newborn. CNM services include family planning, gynecologic care, and treating male partners of female clients for sexually transmitted infections. Pregnancy related services include pre and post natal care and childbirth. CNMs provide clinical care in a variety of settings including home, birthing centers, ambulatory care practices, public health clinics, and hospitals (APRN Consensus Work Group & National Council of State Boards of Nursing APRN Advisory Committee, 2008).

ISSUES WITH THE APRN ROLES

The separate and distinct types of clinical practice that each of the four advanced practice roles comprise can cause confusion within nursing and other health care professions. Nurses, patients, consumers, and other health care professionals may find it difficult to understand the differences in the scope of practice of basic registered nurses and advanced practice nurses, as well as the differences of what the scope of practice is in each of the four APRN roles (Lowe et al., 2012). The facets of the APRN roles and oversight that may cause some confusion include: 1) variations in the role responsibilities of APRNs 2) the definition of advanced practice nursing, as opposed to those graduate level roles that are not advanced practice such as administration and education; 3) variations in the scope of practice of the four APRN roles, 4) variations in the credentialing process required to practice as an APRN, and 5) variations in scope of practice from state to state.

Since licensing boards in each state determine the regulations and statutes that oversee the practice of professionals and basic requirements for advanced practice, there are state to state variations in the scope of practice and the oversight of APRN practice as outlined by the nurse practice acts present in each state. The fact that oversight of CNP practice can vary significantly from state to state is a cause of confusion among and between health care professionals. The reality that there is no uniform model of regulation of APRN practice regulations across the states is consistent with other health care related professions. Practice requirement variations occur with other professions that have state board oversight of professional practice, such as with physicians, attorneys, psychologists, dentists, and chiropractors, to name a few. All professions and vocations that require state board oversight face state to state variations in legal scope of practice, specific criteria to enter practice, and certification examinations required to assess an entry-level competence (APRN Consensus Work Group & National Council of State Boards of Nursing APRN Advisory Committee, 2008).

Conclusion

The development of advanced practice nursing has been an evolutionary process, especially since the early 1960s when nurses saw a need for expansion of their practice responsibilities and took opportunities to provide care where needed in both primary and acute care areas of practice. The consensus model for APRN regulation has helped to formalize the educational requirements and professional standards required for advanced practice roles. It is important for nurses and other health care professionals to understand the scope of practice that advanced nursing affords so that they can work collaboratively and effectively with APRNs to improve patient care and health care practices.

References

AACN. (2004). AACN position statement on the practice doctorate in nursing. American Association of Colleges of Nursing [On-line]. Available: http://www.aacn.nche.edu/publications/position/DNPpositionstatement.pdf.

AANA. (2014). History of nurse anesthesia practice. American Association of Nurse Anesthetists [On-line]. Available: http://www.aana.com/aboutus/documents/historynap.pdf.

AANP. (2014). DNP Fact Sheet: The Doctor of Nursing Practice (DNP). American Association of Colleges of Nursing [On-line]. Available: http://www.aacn.nche.edu/media-relations/fact-sheets/dnp.

American Association of Colleges of Nursing. (2014). Fact Sheet: The Impact of Education on Nursing Practice. American Association of Colleges of Nursing [On-line]. Available: http://www.aacn.nche.edu/media-relations/fact-sheets/impact-of-education.

American Nurses Association. (2010). *Nursing's social policy statement: The essence of the profession*. Silver Spring, MD: Nursesbooks. org.

American Nurses Association. (2014a). How to Become a Nurse. American Nurses Association, Inc [On-line]. Available: http://nursingworld.org/EspeciallyForYou/What-is-Nursing/Tools-You-Need/RegisteredNurseLicensing.html.

American Nurses Association. (2014b). Frequently Asked Questions about the Doctor of Nursing Practice. American Nurses Association [On-line]. Available: http://www.nursingworld.org/dnpfaq

APRN Consensus Work Group & National Council of State Boards of Nursing APRN Advisory Committee. (2008). *Consensus model for APRN regulation: Licensure, accreditation, certification & education National Council of State Boards of Nursing.*

Blais, K., Hayes, J., Kozier, B., & Erb, G. (2006). *Professional nursing practice: Concepts and perspectives*, (5 ed.) Upper Saddle River, NJ: Pearson Prentice Hall.

Bryant-Lukosius, D., DiCenso, A., Browne, G., & Pinelli, J. (2004). Advanced practice nursing roles: development, implementation and evaluation. *Journal of Advanced Nursing, 48,* 519-529.

Bureau of Labor Statistics. (2014). Occupational Outlook Handbook, 2014-15 Edition [On-line]. Available: http://www.bls.gov/ooh/healthcare/registered-nurses.htm#tab-4.

Bureau of Labor Statistics. (2014). How to Become a Registered Nurse. Occupational Outlook Handbook, 2014-15 Edition [On-line]. Available: http://www.bls.gov/ooh/healthcare/registered-nurses.htm#tab-4

Dowling, M., Beauchesne, M., Farrelly, F., & Murphy, K. (2013). Advanced practice nursing: A concept analysis. *International Journal of Nursing Practice, 19,* 131-140.

Driscoll A, Worrall-Carter L, O'Reilly J, & Stewart S. (2005). A historical review of the nurse practitioner role inAustralia. *Clinical Excellence for Nurse Practitioners, 9,* 141-152.

Elder, R. G. & Bullough, B. (1990). Nurse practitioners and clinical nurse specialists: are the roles merging? *Clinical Nurse Specialist, 4,* 78-84.

Ford, L. (1982). Nurse practitioner: history of a new idea and predictions for the future. In Aiken L.H & Gortner SR (Eds.), *Nursing in the 1980's: crises, opportunities, challenges.* Philadelphia: Lippincott.

Ford, L. (1986). Nurse, nurse practitioners: the evolution of primary care. *Image Journal of Nursing Scholarship, 18,* 177-178.

Hanson, C. M. & Hamric, A. B. (2003). Reflections on the continuing evolution of advanced practice nursing. *Nursing Outlook, 51,* 203-211.

Horton, B. (2007). Upgrading Nurse Anesthesia Education Requirements (1933-2006) - Part 2: Curriculum, Faculty and Students. *American Association of Nurse Anesthetists Journal, 75,* 247-251.

International Council of Nurses. (2009). Nurse Practitioner/Advanced Practice Nurse: Definition and Characteristics: Nursing Matters Fact Sheets. The International Council of Nurses (ICN) [On-line]. Available: http://www.icn.ch/images/stories/documents/publications/fact_sheets/1b_FS-NP_APN.pdf.

Kring, D. L. (2008). Clinical nurse specialist practice domains and evidence-based practice competencies: a matrix of influence. *Clinical Nurse Specialist: The Journal for Advanced Nursing Practice, 22,* 179-183.

Lowe, G., Plummer, V., O'Brien, A. P., & Boyd, L. (2012). Time to clarify: the value of advanced practice nursing roles in health care. *Journal of Advanced Nursing, 68,* 677-685.

MacDonald, J., Herbert, R., & Thibeault, C. (2006). Advanced practice nursing: Unification through a common identity. *Journal of Professional Nursing, 22,* 172-179.

McGivern, D. O. (1993). The evolution to advanced nursing practice. In (New York: Springer Publishing Company.

McGivern, D. O., Sullivan-Marx, E. M., & Mezey, M. D. (2003). Advanced practice nursing: Preparation and clinical practice. In D.O.McGivern, E. M. ullivan-Marx, & M. D. ezey (Eds.), *Nurse Practitioners: Evolution of Advanced Practice, Fourth Edition* (pp. 3-36).

McIntosh, E, Nagelkerk, J, Vonderheid, S, Poole, M. Dontje, K, & Pohl, J. (2003). Financially viable nurse-managed centres. *The Nurse Practitioner, 28,* 46-51.

National Organization of Nurse Practitioner Faculty. (2013). Independent practice and the certified nurse practitioner: a white paper. National Organization of Nurse Practitioner Faculty [On-line]. Available: http://c.ymcdn.com/sites/www.nonpf.org/resource/resmgr/Docs/IndepenPracPPRFinal2013.pdf.

North Carolina Board of Nursing. (2014). Collaborative Practice Guidelines. North Carolina Board of Nursing [On-line]. Available: http://www.ncbon.com/dcp/i/nursing-practice-nurse-practitioner-collaborative-practice-guidelines.

O'Brien, J. M. (2003). How nurse practitioners obtained provider status: lessons for pharmacists. *American Journal of Health-System Pharmacy, 60,* 2301-2307.

Rounds, L. R., Zych, J. J., & Mallary, L. L. (2013). The consensus model for regulation of APRNs: Implications for nurse practitioners. *Journal of the American Academy of Nurse Practitioners, 25,* 180-185.

Texas Board of Nursing. (2005). Practice - APRN Scope of Practice. Texas Board of Nursing [On-line]. Available: http://bon.state.tx.us/practice_scope_of_practice_aprn.asp.

In: Collaboration with the Advanced Practice Nurse ISBN: 978-1-63321-311-1
Editors: E.R. Giardino, R.G. Hanks and A.P. Giardino © 2014 Nova Science Publishers, Inc.

Chapter 2

THE DOCTOR OF NURSING PRACTICE ADVANCED PRACTICE NURSE: EDUCATION, ROLES AND PRACTICE ISSUES

Joanne V. Hickey, PhD, RN, ACNP-BC, FAAN, FCCM, Sarah L. Livesay, DNP, RN, ACNP-BC, CNS-BC and Laura L. Rooney, DNP, APRN, FNP-BC, DCC, FAANP

The University of Texas Health Science Center at Houston, School of Nursing, Houston, TX, US

ABSTRACT

This chapter reviews the development of advanced practice nursing with a focus on the practice doctorate and the major issues related to the development, the implementation, and the future of the doctor of nursing practice (DNP) degree. Numerous stakeholders both within and outside the profession of nursing have provided input and leadership in the rapid development of the DNP degree and programs. The leadership of the American Association of Colleges of Nursing (AACN) assumed the primary role of conceptualizing the DNP degree based on an urgent national need for radical changes in health care delivery and how health care professionals of educated for practice. Through ongoing vision and political savvy, AACN has led the national movement for DNP education. Other professional organizations such as the National Organization of Nurse Practitioner Faculty (NONPF) and specialty organizations have influenced and contributed to the shaping of the practice doctorate in nursing. Many questions are still unanswered about the DNP degree, curriculum, and roles of graduates, but the evolution of the DNP degree and graduate is sure to continue along a rapid path of development.

INTRODUCTION

The extraordinary development of advanced nursing practice in the United States during the last decade parallels rapid changes in societal needs for health care as well as the maturing of the profession of nursing. An educational pathway for entry level professional nursing practice through the baccalaureate degree is followed by masters and doctoral level options for advanced practice preparation. Compelling societal demands to address unmet health care needs of the nation are reflected in new roles for advanced practice nurses for transitions in care, coordination of care, health policy, and population health. The unprecedented *Future of Nursing: Leading Change, Advancing Health* (2011) report published by the prestigious Institute of Medicine (IOM) was the first IOM report to focus solely on the profession of nursing. The report was in response to an urgent need to assess and transform the nursing profession to meet gaps in access to care and previously identified issues with quality. The IOM report would make recommendations for an action-oriented blueprint for the future of nursing (IOM, 2010). The two-year project was supported by the Robert Wood Johnson Foundation and the IOM. Based on evidence rather than consensus, the multidisciplinary committee crafted four key messages for the future of the nursing profession. They included the following:

- "Nurses should practice to the full extent of their education and training.
- Nurses should achieve higher levels of education and training through an improved education system that promotes seamless academic progression.
- Nurses should be full partners, with physicians and other health care professionals, in redesigning health care in the United States.
- Effective workforce planning and policy making require better data collection and information infrastructure" (IOM, 2011, p. 4).

The report not only sparked a national dialogue about the role of nursing in meeting the current and future health care needs of the nation, but also created an unequaled call to action of all constituents of the nursing profession and others to work collaboratively to create and implement an action plan designed to meet the recommendations of the report through a national and state by state grassroots effort. The magnitude of such an action plan and the national and state cooperation is unmatched in comparison to previous efforts. The call to action has encompassed a critical examination of education of nurses, practice roles, and the many issues that prevent full implementation of nursing to meet societal needs. This chapter will review the development of advanced practice nursing with a focus on the practice doctorate and the major issues related to development, implementation, and future of the doctor on nursing practice (DNP) degree.

Historical Background of Advanced Practice Nursing and the Practice Doctorate

In order to understand the educational evolution of the practice doctorate in nursing, it is important to understand the role of society in the shaping of the profession. Historically, nursing has responded to societal needs by changing educational models and improving educational programs, striving to increase professional competency and the overall numbers of practitioners. More recently, technological advances, personnel shortages, and the greying of America has presented nursing with unique opportunities to demonstrate the capability of the profession to address the complex and changing needs of a society with the development of a clinical doctorate degree for advanced practice nurses. As nursing faces yet another challenge with health care reform and unprecedented numbers of people joining the ranks of the insured, the resounding question is who will fill the gap and provide care for the vast numbers of the newly insured?

At the turn of the century, nurses were found in informal apprentice-type programs directly affiliated with hospitals. Nursing students provided around the clock service to hospitals 24/7 while attending interspersed classroom instruction often on "days off" or after working a night shift. This model provided a source of inexpensive labor for the institutions while giving students an opportunity to learn skills (Grace, 1978). Upon graduation, many of the graduates transitioned into private duty nursing. The Great Depression of 1929 had a profound impact on nursing because many citizens could no longer afford private duty nurses. This change resulted in an excess of nurses without jobs because hospitals were still relying on the nursing student labor pool, leaving no room for the graduated nurse. Concurrently, nursing education experienced very little expansion until the socioeconomic and political challenges brought on by World War II absorbed the nursing labor force leading to the first nursing shortage which had a profound impact on the nursing profession. In response to a severe nursing shortage, Franklin Delano Roosevelt signed the Bolton Act of 1943 enacting the U.S. Cadet Nurse Corps. Referred to as one of the single most important pieces of legislation for nursing education, the Bolton Act awarded $160 million for nursing education (Haase, 1990).

Roots of Graduate Education for Nurses

During these early transitional years, nurse leaders pushed for formalized educational programs to standardize the practice of nursing. Politically, states were developing their individual Nurse Practice Acts which would regulate practice within individual states, protecting the public from harm (Hartigan, 2011). Creating formal educational programs required faculty with advanced degrees. The Doctor of Education (EdD) is considered the first doctoral program for nursing. Established at Teachers College of Columbia University in 1924, the EdD was later followed by the first Philosophy of Science degree in nursing at New York University in 1934 (Apold, 2008). But many years would intercede before doctoral education would become more accessible to nurses. These early programs focused on learning theories, curriculum development, and developing nursing science.

Throughout the years, nursing and political leaders have worked aggressively to advance the standards in nursing education, striving to advance nursing as a profession. Yet attempts to advance education were met with resistance both from within the profession and outside the profession, demonstrating conflicting visions and leading to a lack of uniformity. For example, the American Nurses Association (ANA) recommended that the baccalaureate degree be the entry to professional nursing practice (Committee on Nursing Education, American Nurses Association, 1965). The target date of 1985 for full implementation of this transition is still to be met.

Advanced practice nursing has witnessed similar evolutions in educational requirements. Originally consisting of non-degree certificate programs in 1965 when the role of the nurse practitioner was first developed, today's nurse practitioner must graduate from an accredited institution of higher learning with a graduate or post-graduate degree in order to be eligible for certification and subsequent licensure to practice (American Association for the Colleges of Nursing [AACN], 2011). The National Organization of Nurse Practitioner Faculties (NONPF) endorsed graduate level preparation as foundational for advanced practice nursing (O'Sullivan, Carter, Marion, Pohl & Werner, 2008). Over the years, as health care became more complex and fragmented, and health disparities increased, nursing organizations looked to educational institutions to prepare nurses with advanced skills and competencies to work effectively within health care organizations in order to care for these complex patients. Change was slow to come.

Development of Current DNP Preparation and Title

Nursing education has continued to evolve, often times in response to provider shortages or societal challenges, yet as the health care system grows ever more complex and the patient population more challenging with chronic co-morbidities, nurse leaders strive to meet societal demands. There have been considerable changes in doctoral education during the time period since the emergence of the advanced practice nurse. The EdD was the first doctoral degree developed in 1924 to prepare and produce educators to assist with the current academic challenges. The 1970's and 1980's, however, brought a new era with new challenges. Technology, changing roles of nurses and advanced practice nurses, and emerging interdisciplinary practice models demanded a different type of nursing professional. Advanced practice nurses faced increasingly complex clinical challenges and growing responsibilities in the clinical setting.

The Doctor of Nursing Science (DNSc/DNS/DSN) was created in 1970. Although it was described as the first practice based doctoral degree, the DNSc/DNS/DSN retained curricula that were similar to the PhD (AACN, 2004). The 1970s was an era in which doctoral education, whether it was a practice based program or a PhD program, flourished. Clearly, a renewed interest in advancing the body of nursing science through research had arrived as well as the desire to be on par with other health professions and social scientists.

In 1979, the first nursing doctorate (ND) at Case Western Reserve University was developed with a vision for parity with other disciplines such as medicine, optometry, and dentistry that required an entry level doctorate for practice (Clinton & Sperhac, 2007). This first ND was a doctoral degree open to non-nurses as well as nursing professionals, and prepared providers to enter practice at a doctoral level. However, if a student wanted to *practice* as an advanced practice nurse, that student would still need to earn a master's degree in nursing, which was the requirement of many state regulatory boards (Marion et al., 2003; AACN, 2004). This model was clearly inefficient. Despite the inefficiencies, more clinical doctorate programs developed, all with a goal of producing clinical leaders educated to function in a complex environment. The doctorate of nursing practice (DrNP) was next to follow. This degree was developed for advance practice nurses with a goal of independent practice in *primary care* (Apold, 2008; AACN, 2004). However, the rapid growth in clinically based doctoral programs was not without flaw. There was no standardization amongst program curricula, with no clear educational goals, thus prompting AACN to form a task force to study the problem and present recommendations to the nurse leadership of AACN.

Fundamental Changes in Health Care Delivery and Professional Nursing Education

As the idea of an advanced nursing practice doctorate continued to gain momentum, the first in a series of independent reports identified serious concerns with health care, and the education of health care workers. This report, *Reforming Health Care Workforce Regulation: Policy Considerations for the 21st Century* (Pew Health Professions Commission, 1995), studied the current health care system and made 10 recommendations for the future of health care and its workforce. Ironically, just as nursing was experimenting with a new model in advanced practice nursing education, the Pew Health Professions Commission called upon leaders to completely redesign health care education. Skyrocketing cost and inefficiencies defined the current health care system, and the only way to address these inefficiencies was through a total redesign. Although the report contained a number of recommendations for education of health care providers, two of the more noteworthy recommendations included a call for states to adopt entry into practice standards, and a call to allow competent professionals to practice to the full extent of their scope of practice, recommendations to be echoed in future reports (Pew Health Professions Commission, 1995). The Pew report sparked significant debate about the challenges faced by the current health care educational system. In response, schools of nursing began to examine their current educational models, and the need for a practice doctorate continued to gain momentum.

Shortly after the publication of the Pew Report, the Institute of Medicine (IOM) began to look closely at the health care system, and as a result, produced a series of reports that would serve as catalysts for change. The IOM's assessment revealed a fragmented, broken system fraught with inefficiencies. Resources, including the human resource of the health care professional, were not being utilized to the fullest potential. Recommendations to transition education and health care delivery to a team based approach were made based on the premise that it would create a more efficient system. In *To Err is Human: Building a Safer Health System* (1999), the IOM stunned the public, health care community, and legislators by reporting the number of deaths attributed to medical errors at an estimated 98,000 deaths annually. The report noted that preventable errors cost the nation between $17 billion and $29 billion annually. Fragmentation was identified as a major contributing factor to waste. A follow up report, *Crossing the Quality Chasm: A New Health Care System for the 21st Century* (IOM, 2001) called for health care providers to deliver care that is "safe, effective, patient-centered, timely, efficient, and equitable" (IOM, 2001, p.6). *Health Professions Education: A Bridge to Quality* (IOM, 2003a) noted that all health professionals including nurses are not being adequately prepared to provide the highest quality and safest health care possible, and there is insufficient assessment of their ongoing proficiency. The report went on to say that educators and accreditation, licensing and certification organizations should ensure that students and working professionals develop and maintain proficiency in five core areas including:

- delivering patient-centered care,
- working as part of interdisciplinary teams,
- practicing evidence-based medicine,
- focusing on quality improvement and
- using information technology.

The publication of these ground breaking reports paralleled the growing debate about the role of nursing in a redesigned health care system for the 21st century. This debate began in light of the growing need for providers prepared to care for a complex patient in a dynamically changing healthcare environment. In response, AACN (2002) convened a task force charged with reviewing doctoral education in nursing, identifying trends and needs for faculty and providers, as well as anticipating implications for advanced practice nursing. From the task force came the notable *Position Statement on Doctoral Practice* (2004), which stated that due to increasingly complex social, economic, and political forces, entry to advanced nursing practice required a more complex and clinically based curriculum. AACN, therefore, recommended the practice doctorate become the standard degree required for entry to practice (AACN, 2004). This report highlighted the difference between research based programs (PhD), and practice based programs. This position statement was approved by the AANC membership in 2004.

Comparison of MSN and DNP Curriculum and Educational Pathways in Nursing

For years, master's programs have educated advanced practice nurses and supplied the public with licensed professionals skilled to provide care and achieve outstanding patient outcomes (Mundinger, 2000). However, as the health care system grew in complexity and people were living longer, experts began to express concern that perhaps the advanced practice registered nurse (APRN) was not qualified to care for these complex patients, which in turn, questioned APRN educational preparation. Meanwhile, other health care professionals such as physical therapists, pharmacists, and audiologists were struggling with similar concerns as they strived to be recognized as equal members of the health care team. Advanced education for entry into these professions migrated from master's degrees to doctoral degrees (Clinton & Sperhac, 2008). In accordance with this trend, nursing looked to the clinical doctorate as a way to strengthen depth and breadth of practice, while supporting parity with health care colleagues.

Schools of nursing initially responded to the IOM reports by expanding content to address identified gaps in educational preparation within existing master's programs. Educational trends revealed the addition of both clinical and didactic coursework to address knowledge gaps (Stanley, 2012). This additional content created master's programs already heavily loaded with content and credit, with new content and additional credit hours. The hours required to earn a master's degree in nursing now significantly exceeded the number of hours required to earn a master's degree in other graduate programs of other professions (O'Sullivan et al., 2005). Despite the additional content, AACN still found content to be lacking. Most often these areas were in health policy, practice management, information technology, risk management, evidence-based practice, and advanced diagnosis and management of complex conditions (Marion et al., 2005). With the development of new and complex technology, rapidly expanding amounts of evidence being generated to guide practice, programs overloaded with content, and professionals seeking to specialize, experts believed that the information needed to practice in this complex and dynamically changing environment would require clinical leaders with enhanced skills. The time had come for the doctor of nursing practice degree program.

There were eight (8) doctoral programs in existence when AACN put forth a proposal that the practice doctorate become the entry for advanced nursing practice (AACN, 2004). Each existing program had developed a curriculum according to the unique needs of their student population, so uniformity was lacking. Yet AACN proposed that by 2015 the practice doctorate should become the entry into practice. This recommendation paralleled the publication of the IOMs landmark reports described earlier which highlighted a broken health care system fraught with costly medical errors and inefficiencies (IOM 1999; IOM 2001). To respond to these reports, a dramatic shift in how health care professionals were educated would be needed. New content such as patient-centered care, interdisciplinary teams, quality improvement, and evidence-based care became common findings in nursing syllabi objectives.

In 2004 when AACN proposed the clinical doctorate as entry to practice, a national spotlight focused on the poor quality of health care. The clinical doctorate was viewed as a way to improve quality by creating clinical leaders educated to practice at the highest level. However dramatic changes in the socioeconomic climate in the United States ensued in the following years. Projected provider shortages and the passage of the Affordable Health Care Act (2013) changed the landscape for APRNs. With unprecedented numbers of people now seeking healthcare and shrinking numbers of providers to deliver this care, APRNs find themselves in a position to fill yet another gap in healthcare, much like that of 1965 when the first nurse practitioner program was founded. Although some believe we must rely upon our historically successful master's programs to deliver providers quickly and expeditiously, others believe nursing should heed the rationale to better meet societal needs and adopt the recommendations of the AACN for the clinical doctorate.

Examination of the AACN MSN *Essentials* for the master's degree and the AACN DNP *Essentials* for the practice doctorate, reveal that these documents are quite similar (AACN, 2006; AACN, 2011). This is not without deliberate design because the DNP program was originally envisioned to build on the MSN Essentials. The DNP Essentials take the current MSN Essentials and expand them to include a focus on population health. The practice doctorate also addresses the gaps previously identified in master's programs such as practice management, health policy, information technology, risk management, utilization and translation of evidence based practice, and advanced diagnosis and management (Apold, 2008). [see Chapter X: Administration] Both the MSN and DNP Essentials provide a roadmap for nursing curricula, and although individual Essential titles are similar, there is significant progression in content from the master to the doctoral level. For example, master's students are expected to have a basic foundation and background from science and humanities, while doctoral students must have an understanding of the laws of science which govern all life forces. Theory is a component of both programs of study. The topics may be similar, such as chaos or complexity theory, but the DNP student is expected to not only learn theories, but also to utilize theories from other disciplines, to serve as a framework for practice and development of new models of care (AACN, 2006).

Comparison of the two programs of study demonstrate similarities, yet the practice doctorate takes topics introduced in the master's program and expands upon them. For example leadership is a central competency for both MSN and DNP programs of study. This refers not only to leadership in patient care, but in equitable use of resources and maintaining cost-effective use of resources. The practice doctorate, however, includes content on the use of interprofessional teams to address inefficiencies and waste within settings. Both programs address practice scholarship. But while the master's prepared nurse is educated in translating scholarship into practice, the DNP creates a scholarly practice through the use of quality improvement methodologies, thus identifying unsafe practices and improving the products of health care delivered to an individual, group, or population (AACN, 2006). Technology and its equitable use has become a major factor in health care. This is evident in the use of electronic health records, and the encouragement of health care settings to make efficient use of resources through electronic communication. Therefore, each program contains components of information technology education although at different levels of objectives and expected outcomes. Each program expects its graduates to participate in health policy and advocacy for social justice.

In review of the inefficiencies of U.S. health care, the IOM has called for the use of interprofessional teams to deliver the complex care required in today's health care delivery environment. Both programs of study contain essential elements to meet these demands. As clinical leaders, the DNP graduate receives education in defining and developing an interdisciplinary team. Finally, each of the Essentials address the fact that our nation is becoming burdened with chronic disease and co-morbidity, and therefore knowledge of population health is foundational. While the master's prepared APRN is expected to be familiar with disease specific content, the DNP is prepared to be the leader in population health. The DNP is the innovative visionary for new population health programs, relying on knowledge of advanced practice nursing, population health, and economics of health policy in order to create sustainable and effective programs.

As evident by this discussion, the two levels of study may be viewed as complimentary and a progression of one to the next, facilitated by similar course content. This is not without significant thought devoted to the development and refinement of the two programs of study. The master's degree may or may not culminate with some form of a written product such as a thesis while the doctoral degree culminates with a substantive scholarly product called a capstone project as evidence of clinical competencies. Quality improvement projects, pilot studies, or other demonstrations of clinical excellence are examples of clinical expertise. Graduates of each program contribute to meeting patient needs through complimentary and unique contributions, but it is becoming increasingly evident that in today's health care setting, a higher level of practice is needed to maneuver the system. The level of clinical expertise expected from each program is also noteworthy. If one thinks of clinical expertise along a continuum from beginning skills for practice to practice at the highest level of professional practice, the master's prepared nurse makes an important and valuable contribution, but is not expected to practice at the highest level of professional practice as a clinical scholar.

National certification and licensure to practice as an APRN depend upon successful completion and subsequent graduation from an accredited master's degree program. For this reason, there is much more consistency in master's programs in order to ensure entry level competency. Since there are no licensing requirements tied to the practice doctorate, and therefore no legal obligations for minimum practice hours, many doctoral programs have interpreted the doctoral Essential which speaks to APRN practice differently (AACN, 2006). While some doctoral programs choose a rigorous course for their graduates, requiring up to an additional 720 clinical hours, some programs have no additional clinical hours at all. This lack of uniformity reignites an age-old debate surrounding the problem of standardization and lack of consistency in the training for nursing professionals.

Essentials of Doctoral Nursing Practice Education

AACN played a pivotal role in DNP role and competency definition, and educational preparedness through the development of the *DNP Essentials of Doctoral Education for Advanced Practice Nursing* published in 2006 (Algase, 2010; AACN, 2006). The document details the background and context for the DNP degree, and outlines the elements and competencies expected from a program conferring the DNP degree. Additional elements of the DNP degree such as planning, program length, DNP capstone project, and DNP program quality are also addressed.

The competencies and program elements that serve as the foundation for the role must be addressed by a DNP program and operationalized in the DNP role are organized into eight (8) Essentials. The first DNP Essential addresses the scientific underpinnings for practice. The scientific underpinnings for practice are rooted in nursing concepts, and address the laws and patterns of human behavior guiding well-being and illness. With this foundational knowledge, the DNP graduate is prepared to implement actions that result in positive health changes. The DNP is an expert in nursing science, as well as the utilization of science from other disciplines including biology, medicine, psychology and other social sciences. The DNP integrates current and emerging theories as frameworks to improve health. (AACN, 2006).

The second DNP Essential is organizational and system leadership for quality improvement and systems thinking. The DNP graduate is prepared to conceptualize new care delivery models to improve health, eliminate health disparities, and promote high quality and safe care. The DNP graduate is prepared to conduct such activities within the national, organizational, political, cultural, and economic cultures of healthcare organizations. High quality communication skills and sensitivity to organizational culture are key to the DNP graduate's success in meeting this competency.

The third DNP Essential addresses clinical scholarship and analytical methods for evidence-based practice. DNP graduates are prepared to demonstrate clinical scholarship through evaluation of evidence, translation of evidence into practice, leadership in high level quality improvement projects, generating internal evidence (Melnyk, 2013), informing ongoing research, and generating clinical questions to initiate research. DNP graduates are posed as experts at delivering care, and also evaluating outcomes of practice and improving practice at a system and population level. The fourth DNP Essential is information systems and patient care technology for improvement and transformation of health care. As technology continues to revolutionize healthcare, DNP leaders are equipped to manage individual and aggregate patient information to evaluate programs of care, outcomes of care, and care systems. DNP graduates are also competent and contribute to the evaluation and resolution of legal and ethical issues surrounding technology in health care.

Health care policy for advocacy in health care is the fifth DNP Essential. DNP graduates are educated in policy issues and competent to design, influence, and implement healthcare policies to improve patient care, access to care, and health care systems. Participation in the policy process and advocacy are core competencies for the DNP graduates. Participation in the process of policy development and advocacy may translate into advocacy for ethical principles in all healthcare settings and discussions. The sixth DNP Essential is interprofessional collaboration for improving patient and population health outcomes. DNP education should support and model team-based care and DNP graduates have foundational knowledge in the team science of high performance teams and the relationship between team work and outcomes in healthcare. DNP graduates display competency in leading and participating in interprofessional teams.

The seventh DNP Essential is clinical prevention and population health for improving the nation's health. DNP graduates are educated to understand complex health and population issues impacting populations. DNP graduates are prepared to evaluate the health of populations, and intervene by developing and implementing population level solutions. DNPs also have competency in evaluating community, environmental, and occupational care models including keeping communities healthy though a focus on prevention and health promotion. The final DNP Essential is the clinical care provided by the DNP as an advanced practice nurse. The DNP APRN provides clinical care including the comprehensive assessment of health and illness, planning and implementing therapeutic interventions, and evaluating the outcomes of those interventions for underserved populations at the highest level of advanced practice.

Table 1. Key Dates in the Development of DNP Programs

1979	Nurse Doctorate (ND) offered at Case Western Reserve
1999	Institute of Medicine's *To Err is Human: Building a Safer Health System* published
2001	Institute of Medicine's *Crossing the Quality Chasm* published
2001	Doctor of Nursing Practice (DNP) program opened at the University of Kentucky
2003	Institute of Medicine's *Health Professions Education: A Bridge to Quality* published
2004	Member schools affiliated with the American Association of Colleges of Nursing (AACN) voted to endorse the ***Position Statement on the Practice Doctorate in Nursing*** on October 25, 2004.
2005	Columbia University begins the Doctor of Nursing Practice Program and awards DrNP initial (changed in the future in respond to AACN's plan to only accredit programs leading to a DNP degree).
2006	AACN member institutions voted to endorse the *Essentials of Doctoral Education for Advanced Nursing Practice* on October 30, 2006 after a two-year consensus-building process.
2008	Commission on Collegiate Nursing Education (CCNE) launches an accreditation program for DNP programs in the Fall of 2008.
2010	Institute of Medicine's *The Future of Nursing: Leading Change, Advancing Health* published
2014	AACN commissions the ANCC Task Force on Implementation of the DNP Program

The Essentials of doctoral education for advanced nursing practice define curricula development for DNP programs, and define the DNP roles embodied by DNP graduates. As the DNP degree is relatively new and experienced DNP practitioners practicing in healthcare are gaining momentum, research demonstrating the outcomes of DNP practice is necessary to demonstrate impact on outcomes.

The Impact of Professional Organizations on DNP Role Definition

Multiple nursing organizations have published position statements regarding the DNP degree, and several have published opinion papers guiding educational preparedness and role definition. The National Organization of Nurse Practitioner Faculties (NONPF) published several relevant reports. NONPF published several position statements in 2008. One addressed the use of the term *doctor* by DNP graduates and supported its use by doctorally prepared nurses pointing out that the term "doctor" is a generic academic title bestowed on to those who earn a doctoral degree. DNP graduates are entitled to use the title. The position statement emphasized that the use of the term doctor demonstrates parity between professional with doctoral degrees. The statement further emphasized that while the terms 'medical doctor' and 'doctor of osteopathy' may be protected by state law, the term 'doctor' is not a protected title (NONPF, 2008). NONPF also emphasized the difference between academic degrees and certification for licensure. In addressing certification, NONPF continues to support the examinations currently in place for various nurse practitioner specialties offered to graduates of the master's program, and does not advocate an additional certification with the addition of a doctorate degree (NONPF, 2008).

In 2013, NONPF recognized the inconsistency between programs in curriculum and titling of the scholarly project (dissertation equivalent) required for DNP graduation. NONPF published a paper describing the variability in DNP curricula, and faculty constraints which have occurred as DNP programs developed over the past decade. The statement recognized that until sufficient time has elapsed during which DNP graduates readily fill faculty positions in DNP programs, programs will continue to be facilitated by non-DNP prepared faculty and by faculty without recent clinical practice experience. The paper highlights the over-reaching goal of the DNP project which is to create practice knowledge and demonstrate the Essentials of DNP education and competency. A NONPF conducted survey identified 33 different names for the final DNP capstone project or other body of work to demonstrate doctoral scholarly work. NONPF recommended the generic title of DNP project for the final demonstration of doctoral scholarly work. They also recommended a number of modalities for dissemination of the project, including written papers, public presentation, and published manuscripts (NONPF, 2013).

Finally, NONPF has published an opinion statement on DNP residency hours in an effort to standardize the minimum number of patient contact hours necessary for DNP programs (NONPF, 2013). NONPF endorsed previous AACN publications mandating a minimum of 1000 graduate level clinical practice hours. Most advanced practice masters programs require 500 patient contact hours for graduation and to be eligible for board certification. However, not all graduate nursing programs are clinically focused or offer patient contact hours. The

DNP graduate must have completed at least 1000 clinical practicum hours by the completion of the program (NONPF, 2013)

As the DNP degree has expanded to include other advanced practice roles such as clinical nurse specialists (CNS)s, nurse midwives, nurse anesthetists (NAs) as well as other nursing roles such as nurse executives, other professional nursing organizations and societies will likely define the role and educational expectations, and doctoral level competencies. The chapter has already addressed the position of NONPF which is the major organization representing nurse practitioners. The following provides a brief description of the positions taken by the organizations representing the other three APRN roles.

The National Association of Clinical Nurse Specialists (NACNS) supports CNS education at both the master's level and the doctoral level although it does not support the elimination of MSN programs to move to the DNP as entry into CNS practice. The NACNS Board of Directors commissioned the development of doctoral level CNS competencies, which have been endorsed by NACNS and several other organizations. In addition, the Society from Clinical Nurse Specialists Education has endorsed the DNP and developed curriculum guidelines for CNS options within DNP programs.

The American Association of Nurse Anesthetists (AANA) has mandated that all certified registered nurse anesthetist (CRNA)s program transition to a practice doctorate by 2022. By 2025, all new CRNA graduates must have a practice doctorate to be eligible to take the national certification examination (AANA, 2007). In addition, the AANA Council on Accreditation has said that they will no long accredit new master's degree programs for CRNAs after 2015 (Raines, 2010).

The American College of Nurse-Midwives supports the master's degree as the basic educational preparation for midwifery practice although they support doctoral degree options for midwifery programs. Currently, they do not require a DNP for certification or require midwifery programs to offer a DNP for entry into practice or for program accreditation. As noted with other professional organization, they plan to develop competencies for midwifery education at the doctoral level (American College of Nurse –Midwifery, 2011).

It is clear form this brief discussion that there is variability among the requirement for advanced practice nursing, acceptance of the DNP degree for entry into advanced practice, DNP competency development, and requirements for accreditation of programs.

CONTROVERSIES RELATED TO THE DNP PRACTITIONER

Any change in professional titles and roles is accompanied by controversy. The controversies associated with the DNP degree generally apply to role definition and educational preparedness.

An ongoing discussion regarding DNP education is debated over the need for another nursing doctorate degree option and conflict with existing doctorates. Doctoral preparation of nurses has evolved over several generations as discussed above, with various doctoral degrees offered to nurses including the Doctor of Education and Doctor of Philosophy. The advent of a nursing focused doctorate began as a minor focus of study in the late 1960s, and evolved over time into a PhD in nursing or a Doctor of Nursing Science Degree (Zaccagnini & White, 2014). In recent years, a flurry of doctoral degree options and titles were developed, including the Nursing Doctor (ND) and Doctor of Nursing Science (DNS) (Brown-Benedict, 2008). Initial opponents of the DNP doctorate argued the addition of another doctoral degree pathway only confused the already muddled doctoral degree pathways and had the potential to further fracture the nursing role. However, proponents of the DNP doctorate option argue the DNP offers uniformity in role preparation and role identity for nurses seeking a practice focused doctorate rather than a research focused doctorate (Brown-Benedict, 2008).

Another controversy surrounding the DNP degree is opposition from current practicing APRNs. The opposition may be marred by the association of the degree with AACN's pursuit of establishing the DNP degree as the entry level degree for advanced practice. The proposal of the degree, as mandatory for entry level into practice, ignited significant debate within the advanced practice community with some APRN groups voicing dissent and concern. A significant argument against the DNP degree as the entry level to advanced practice is the lack of evidence that the APRN prepared with a DNP produces superior outcomes compared to the APRN prepared at the MSN level (Brown-Benedict, 2008). Others in the nursing community argue against the need to establish such evidence because the DNP degree does not change scope of practice.

Financial and human resource consumption is a concern voiced in opposition to the DNP degree and the AACN position statement mandating the DNP degree as entry to advanced practice (Brown-Benedict, 2008). Doctoral education places an additional cost burden on the student who wishes to function as a DNP advanced practice nurse. This constraint comes at a time when current healthcare reform initiatives are contributing to a shortage of physicians, and APRNs are increasingly predicted to fill the gap as primary care providers over the next decade. The addition of the DNP degree and mandate for the degree as entry level to practice places additional burdens on already constrained university resources (Brown-Benedict, 2008). Nursing faculty shortages are a significant concern throughout universities, and the rapid increasing need for faculty resources necessary to fully implement DNP programs may burden an already overburdened system (Brown-Benedict, 2008).

The doctoral nursing pathways are consolidated into two major degree pathways, the PhD as a research doctorate, and the DNP as a practice doctorate. While the differentiation between research and practice seems clear, the roles and education preparedness is a significant concern and controversy continues to evolve regarding the relationship between the PhD prepared nurse and the DNP prepared nurse. Concern regarding the DNP graduate being viewed as inferior and less rigorous than the PhD is a theme often voiced in opposition to the DNP doctorate (Brown-Benedict, 2008). Further concern exists regarding the lack of uniformity and varied program rigor in current accredited programs.

Initial opposition to the DNP degree pathway included concern around role and title confusion, as multiple nursing doctoral degrees are available with multiple titles conferred to graduates. However, the AACN took steps to reduce the role and title confusion in 2004 when they recommended standardized practice doctorate language. The nursing educational system has generally followed suit on the recommendations, with the emergence of DNP degree and title as the primary practice doctorate alternative to the PhD. As the various APRN roles such as gerontological nurse practitioner (GNP), acute care nurse practitioner (ACNP), and other roles have gained acceptance and recognition, the health care in the general public, some argue that the DNP title and role will add to the general APRN role and title confusion.

A final controversy in DNP education relates to the variation in DNP program curricula and program rigor. While program accreditation is available, great variability in coursework, clinical hours, doctoral project scope and implementation, and fellowship experiences exists between currently accredited programs.

Current Issues and Future Trends with DNP Education, Roles and Practice

The DNP programs focus on preparing clinical scholars who are leaders in translation of science into practice, systems-level changes, clinical scholarship, and practice at the highest level of advanced nursing practice (Sebastian & Delaney, 2013). The DNP degree prepares a new level of practitioner to serve current and emerging interests and needs of the public (Cronenwett et al., 2011). With the seismic changes in health care and the consequential realities surrounding nursing education and practice, numerous trends are shaping the future of advanced practice nursing. Grey (2013) points out that there is consensus within the profession about the intent to expand the role of the advanced practice nurse to include population health, health policy, and leadership are well outlined in the DNP Essentials. However, many areas of controversy urgently await resolution and include: expected outcomes and competencies of the DNP graduate; curricular models; purpose and nature of the capstone project; and the impact of DNP programs on schools of nursing (Cronenwett et al., 2011; Dennison & Payne, 2012; Frantz, 2013; Grey, 2013; Kirkpatrick & Weaver, 2013; Melnyk, 2012; Slyer & Levin, 2012). The following discussion briefly addresses some of the major areas of concern in education, roles, and practice issues.

Rapid Development of DNP Programs

On October 25, 2004, the member schools affiliated with the American Association of Colleges of Nursing (AACN) voted to endorse the *Position Statement on the Practice Doctorate in Nursing* which supported a transformational change in the education required for professional nurses who will practice at the most advanced level of nursing from the master's degree to the practice doctorate (AACN, 2006, pp. 4-5). Multiple factors influenced this recommendation including the expansion of scientific knowledge required for safe nursing practice, the growing concerns about quality, safety, and patient outcomes, and the enhanced complexity of health care delivery. The position statement also broadly defined advanced nursing practice as:

> "any form of nursing intervention that influences health care outcomes for individual or populations, including the direct care of individual patients, management of care for individuals and populations, administration in nursing and health care organization, and the development and implementation of health policy" (AACN, 2004 p. 2).

Once the *Position Statement on the Practice Doctorate in Nursing* was approved in 2004, AACN assembled a taskforce to outline the curricular elements and competencies required for conferring of the DNP degree. The taskforce produced the *Essentials of Doctoral Education for Advanced Nursing Practice* which includes eight Essentials described as foundational outcome competencies deemed essential for all graduated of a DNP program regardless of specialty or functional focus (AACN, 2006). Some recommendations about the curriculum were also made such as the minimum number of practice hours required. The Essentials were approved by the AACN membership in 2006 and serve as the framework for DNP programs throughout the United States.

If year 2004 is used as the benchmark for the inception of DNP education in the United States, the new practice doctorate in nursing is 10 years old. From a handful of DNP programs in 2004, to 241 currently enrolling students and 59 programs in the planning stage, there has been extraordinary growth and interest in DNP program (AACN, 2014). From 2012 to 2013, the number of students enrolled in DNP programs increased from 11,575 to 14,699. During that same period, the number of DNP graduates increased from 1,858 to 2,443 (AACN, 2014). To address standards for DNP educational programs, the Commission on Collegiate Nursing Education (CCNE) began accrediting DNP programs in the fall of 2008. As of January of 2014, 125 DNP programs have been accredited by CCNE (AACN, 2014). At what point will there be a leveling off of new DNP programs remains to be seen.

Competencies and Expected Outcomes

The expected outcome competencies of the DNP product are well described in the DNP Essentials and are related to practice. The DNP is a practice degree, not a role. However, there is great variation in the translation and interpretation of the Essentials into a curriculum and program of study. The intent of the DNP educational pathway is to produce graduates for advanced practice nursing who will provide care to individuals and populations at the highest level of advanced practice nursing. In reality, many DNP graduates are assuming roles as faculty members and administrative roles in health care facilities (Frantz, 2014). It remains unclear what roles DNP graduates are expected to fill. Faculty members also struggle with identifying the terminal competencies of the graduates within a dynamic ever changing health care system of escalating costs, increased chronic illness, a growing aging population, and the unclear rollout the Affordable Care Act. Lack of clarity around societal needs as a driving force adds confusion in shaping the role of providers. These factors contribute to the variability in translating the DNP Essentials into the education and practice arenas.

When nurse leaders at a summit meeting in 2013 were asked to respond to the question, "do the DNP Essentials need revision", there was overwhelming agreement that the current DNP Essentials should be maintained with the caveat that some clarifications such as broadening of Essential IV to include self-care management were needed (Frantz, 2014). This recommendation, along with others, is now being addressed by the *AACN Task Force on Implementation of the DNP Program* which will report back to the AACN Board of Directors in June 2015.

Curriculum

The great variation in the curriculum and program of studies for DNP programs across the country is stunning. As one nurse leader noted, if you see one DNP program, you have seen one DNP program. There is no generalizability from one DNP program to another. In the development and design of any curriculum, the starting point is a clear understanding of the intended audience (student) and the expected terminal competencies and educational outcomes of the program. With two entry points to DNP education for students (BSN to DNP and post MSN to DNP), students come with variations in previous nursing practice experience and knowledge at either the baccalaureate level or the post MSN level which impacts on curriculum design and course content. DNP curricula build on traditional master's programs by providing education in evidence-based practice, quality improvement, and systems leadership, among other key areas (AACN, 2014). However, how to build such a curriculum is challenging as evidenced by the wide variation in curricula. There is urgency for the profession to address these concerns and to set standards.

The complexity and multi-layers of today's health care environment requires the collective contributions of health professionals with competency in interprofessional collaborative practice models. Team care provided by interdisciplinary teams is well recognized as best practice in delivering high quality care that leads to optimal patient outcomes (IOM, 2001; IOM, 2003; O'Neil, 1998; AACN, 2004). DNP Essential VI, Interprofessional Collaboration for Improving Patient and Population Health Outcomes, recognizes the need for DNP graduates to be competent in working effectively in interprofessional teams both as leaders and followers, depending on changing patients' needs, and the work to be done. This means that the DNP curriculum must prepare students not only with didactic content in interprofessional teams, but also clinical experiences in which students work in interprofessional teams in real world health care environments. Recent surveys of DNP programs found that classes are generally not interprofessional and clinical experiences are intraprofessional rather than interprofessional experiences. The mismatch between the need for competency in interprofessional practice and the current methods of preparing DNP students must be eliminated and substituted what new models to meet societal needs for quality and safe health care.

For example, TeamSTEPPS, developed by the Agency for Healthcare Research and Quality (AHRQ) and the Department of Defense, is an evidence-based teamwork system aimed at optimizing patient outcomes by improving communication and teamwork skills among health care professionals. It includes a comprehensive set of ready-to-use materials and a training curriculum to successfully integrate teamwork principles into any health care system (TeamSTEPPS, 2014). The program is free and provides excellent materials as well as training for those who wish to become master trainers in TeamSTEPPS. These and other excellent resources are available for integration into DNP curricula.

An examination of required credits for completion of a DNP program varies widely from 52 to 103 credits (average 80.2) for BSN to DNP program, and from 24 to 75 credits (average 38.8) for post MSN programs (Udelis & Mancuso, 2012). Course titles and content have great variability. The clinical experiences in the program vary considerably from the counting of a student's job related practice hours to one that requires a separate site from the student's normal work environment with a designated preceptor overseeing a planned experience based on written objectives. The wide variation in programs is a challenge to the rigor of a program in meeting the number of required practice hours and the appropriate focus of the clinical experiences for the development of DNP competencies.

The rapid development of instructional technology and computer based learning is revolutionizing all levels of education providing a broad spectrum of teaching and learning strategies for integration into the curriculum. Simulation, social networks, and computer supported learning are all examples of the current educational landscape. More and more students are interested in on-line learning. Working professionals, including nurses, like the idea of on-line programs for convenience purposes or because of a belief that on-line programs are easier. Many programs that advertise themselves as an on-line program do require some on campus meetings. However, the trend to on-line education in nursing and other educational programs is reflective of a general trend in education.

Because the DNP is a new degree, it is not surprising that there is great variation in DNP curricula. However, it is critical that standards and uniformity occur so that the expected outcomes of graduates are clear and attainable.

Capstone Projects

All doctoral programs require some substantive high level scholarly product from the student as an indicator of scholarship. The PhD program requires a dissertation describing original research conducted by the student. The DNP program focuses on a capstone project which is a scholarly product that is a high level practice focused project. The "capstone" project is called by many different names such as practice inquiry project and practice improvement project. However, the purpose of the capstone project is the demonstration of completed scholarly work through evidence synthesis, leadership projects, and evidence-based change projects (Melnyk, 2013). Requirements vary widely among programs from the writing of a proposal without implementation while others require implementation of the project. What constitutes a capstone project has no clear definition across DNP programs and has wide variations including a case study, systematic review of the literature, integrated review of the literature, quality improvement project, and qualitative or quantitative research.

There is broad variation across DNP programs in providing a written report of the capstone project. Some programs require only an executive summary while others programs require a 5-chapter report similar to a dissertation format. Of interest is that some programs have adopted the SQUIRE format which stands for **S**tandards for *QU*ality Improvement *R*eporting *E*xcellence, a format designed for reporting of quality improvement projects (Ogrinc et al,. 2008), as more appropriate for the quality improvement work completed by many DNP students. It is clear that there continues to be confusion between the differences of a PhD dissertation and a DNP capstone project and the scope and expected deliverables of scholarship from DNP students (Kirkpatrick & Weaver, 2013). Clarification of the purpose, title and the scope of the capstone project are urgently needed to support national standards and the credibility of scholarly achievement by DNP graduates.

Roles

These are tumultuous time in the health care delivery system and nursing education as the leaders in the profession work to align societal needs for health care and realign professional nursing roles to meet those needs. The IOM *Future of Nursing* report is also a driving force for both the redesign of health care and roles of nursing. The original intent of creating a practice doctorate in nursing was to prepare advance practice nurses to practice at the highest level of advanced practice to provide primary care to individuals and populations. However, many DNP graduates are assuming faculty roles or administrative roles in health care organizations rather the intended direct practice roles. There is a call in the profession to clarify what roles DNP graduates are expected to fulfill, and AACN has established a taskforce of experts to address this and other urgent issues.

Practice Issues

The emergence of DNP graduates has created questions about their role and unique contributions to health care delivery. Many questions regarding the differences between a master's prepared advanced practice nurse and the DNP prepared advanced practice nurse have been raised as discussed above. There is also consideration of certification. Currently there is no certification for DNP graduates nor are there any regulatory differences in licensure or approval to practice. Keeping in mind that the DNP is a degree and not a role, adds to the confusion of role clarification and optimal utilization of DNP graduates. With any new degree or new addition to the cadre of health care professionals, it takes time for clarification of the competencies brought by the graduates which is the foundation for utilization and integration of these graduates into the health care system. This is not a new scenario in the history of nursing. However, with the wide variability in the DNP educational programs and the lack of clarity about expected roles and contributions to health care, integration of graduates will be stymied. Therefore, it falls to the leaders and professional organizations in nursing, to address these issues immediately and provide clarity. If nursing does not do this critical and time sensitive work, someone else will.

In response to the needs for clarification and direction, AACN has established the *AACN Task Force on Implementation on the DNP*. The charge to the task force is to produce a white paper on the evolution and current development of DNP programs and report back to the AACN Board of Directors by June 2015. The task force will address clarification of the clinical practice requirements, purpose of the DNP final project, exemplars of scholarly projects, and other critical issues important to DNP programs. The complete list of the items to be address by the task force can be found on the AACN website.

CONCLUSION

There has been a tumultuous road traveled by nurses and the nursing profession to create and develop advanced practice nursing and especially the DNP degree program. However, the impetus for the vision and purpose for making change rests on the sacred trust placed on profession to provide service to society. For the profession of nursing, that trust is directed at meeting the needs of a multidimensional society for high quality and safe nursing care delivered by an individual advanced practice nurse or as a member of an interprofessional team. For the highest level of advanced practice in nursing, the practice doctorate, known as the doctor of nursing practice, is projected to be the educational route to prepare this high level practitioner. The degree and educational program are only a decade old. Many areas related to education, roles, and integration into practice still await resolution, but that is not unexpected with a new degree for practice. It will be interesting to see how the process unfolds, and how the goals for the DNP degree and DNP graduates are realized especially in light of the IOM recommendations found in *The Future of Nursing: Leading Change, Advancing Health (2010) report.*

REFERENCES

Algase, D. L. (2010). Essentials of scholarship for the DNP: Are we clear yet? *Research and Theory in Nursing Practice, 24*(2), 91-93.

American Association of Nurse Anesthetists. (2007). *AANA position on doctoral preparation of nurse anesthetists.* Available at: http://www.aana.com/ceandeducation/educationalresources/Documents/AANA_Position_DTF_June_2007.pdf. Accessed February 11, 2014.

American Association of Colleges of Nursing (AACN). *DNP fact sheet, January 2014.* Available at: http://www.aacn.nche.edu/media-relations/fact-sheets/dnp. Accessed January 26, 2014.

American Association of Colleges of Nursing. (2006). *The essentials of doctoral education for advanced nursing practice.* Retrieved January 4, 2014, from http://www.aacn.nche.edu/DNP/pdf/Essentials.pdf.

American Association of Colleges of Nursing. *The essentials of master's education in nursing.* (2010). Available at: www.aacn.nche.edu/

Apold, S. (2008). The doctor of nursing practice: Looking back, moving forward. *The Journal of Nurse Practitioners.* Available at: www.npjournal.org.

Brar, K., Boschma, G., & McCuaig, F. (2010). The development of nurse practitioner preparation beyond the master's level: what is the debate about? *Internaitonal Journal of Nursing Education Scholarsiph, 7*, Article9. doi: 10.2202/1548-923X.1928.

Brown-Benedict, D. J. (2008). The Doctor of Nursing Practice degree: lessons from the history of the professional doctorate in other health disciplines. *Journal of Nursing Education, 47*(10), 448-457.

Chase, S. K., & Pruitt, R. H. (2006). The practice doctorate: innovation or disruption? *Journal of Nursing Education, 45*(5), 155-161.

Clinton, P. & Sperhac, A.M. (2006). National agenda for advanced practice nursing: The practice doctorate. *Journal of Professional Nursing, 22*(1), 7-14.

Committee on Nursing Education, American Nurses Association. (1965). American Nurses Association citation's first position on education for nursing. *American Journal of Nursing, 65*(12), 106-107.

Cronenwett, L., Dracup, K., Grey, M., McCauley, L., Meleis, A. & Salmon, M. (2011). The doctor of nursing practice: A national workforce perspective. *Nursing Outlook, 59*, 9-17. DOI: 10.1016/j.outlook.2010.11.003.

Dennison, R. D., & Payne, C. (2012). The doctorate in nursing practice: Moving advanced practice nursing even closer to excellence. *Nursing Clinics of North American, 47*, 225-240. doi: 10.1016/j.cnur.2012.04.001.

Draye, M.A., Acher, M. & Zimmer, P.A. (2006). The practice doctorate in nursing: Approaches To transform nurse practitioner education and practice. *Nursing Outlook, 54*, 123-129. DOI: 10.1016/j.outlook.2006.01.001

Edwardson, S.R. (2010). Doctor of philosophy and doctor of nursing practice as complementary degrees. *Journal of Professional Nursing, 26*(3), 137-140.

Frantz, R.A. (2014). Reflections on the future of doctoral programs in nursing: DNP. Presented at American Association of Colleges of Nursing 2014 Doctoral Education Conference, Naples, FL, January 30, 2014.

Frantz, R. A. (2013). Resource requirements for a quality doctor of nursing practice program. *Journal of Nursing Education, 52*(8), 449-452. doi: 10.3928/014834-20130713-01.

Grace, H.K.(1978). The development of doctoral education in nursing: In historical perspective. *Journal of Nursing Education, 17*(4), 17-27.

Grey, M. (2013). The doctor of nursing practice: Defining the next steps. *Journal of Nursing Education, 52*(8), 462-465. doi 10.3928/014834-20130719-02.

Hartigan, C. (2011). APRN regulation: The licensure-certification interface. *AACN Advanced Critical Care, 22*(1), 50-65.

Institute of Medicine (1999). *To Err is Human: Building a safer health system.* Washington, DC: National Academies Press.

Institute of Medicine (2001). *Crossing the quality chasm.* Washington, DC: National Academies Press.

Institute of Medicine (2003a). *Health professions education: A bridge to quality.* Washington, DC: National Academies Press.

Institute of Medicine (2010). *The future of nursing: Leading change, advancing health.* Washington, DC: National Academies Press..

Kirkpatrick, J. M., & Weaver, T. (2013). The doctor of nursing practice capstone project: Consensus or confusion? *Journal of Nursing Education,52*(8), 435-441. doi 10.3928/014834-20130722-01.

Marion, L., Viens, D., O'Sullivan, A., Crabtree, K., Fontana, S. & Mizell, M. (2003). The Practice Doctorate in nursing: Future or fringe? Available at: http://www.medscape.com/viewarticle/453247_print.

Melnyk, B. M. (2013). Distinguishing the preparation and roles of the Doctor of Philosophy and Doctor of Nursing Practice graduates: National implications for academic curricula and health care systems. *Journal of Nursing Education, 52,*__442-448. doi: 10.3928/014834-20130719-01.

Midwifery education and the doctor of nursing practice (DNP) position statement. American College of Nurse-Midwives;2011. Available at: http://www.midwife.org/ACNM/files/ACNMLibraryData/IPLAODFILENAME/000000000079/Midwifery%20Ed%20and%20DNP%207.09.pdf. Accessed February 11, 2014.

Mundinger, M.O., Kane, R.L., Lenz, E.R., Totten, A. M. & Tsai, W. (2000). Primary care outcomes in patients treated by nurse practitioners or physicians: A randomized trial. *Journal of the American Medical Association, 283*, 59-68.

National Association of Clinical Nurse Specialists. White paper on the nursing practice doctorate (2009). Available at: http://www.nacns.org/docs/PositionOnNursing Practice Doctorate.pdf. Accessed February 11, 2014.

National League for Nursing, (2010). *Master's Education in Nursing..* Available at: http://www.nln.org/aboutnln/reflectikon_dialogue/refl_dial_6.htm. Accessed January 3, 2014.

National Organization of Nurse Practitioner Faculties, (2008). *Nurse practitioner DNP education, certification, and titling: A unifying statement.* Retrieved January 14, 2014, from http://c.ymcdn.com/sites/www.nonpf.org/resource/resmgr/imported/DNP Unified Statement0608.pdf.

National Organization of Nurse Practitioner Faculties. (2013). *Titling of the doctor of nursing practice project.* Retrieved January 14, 2014, from http://c.ymcdn.com/sites/ www.nonpf.org/resource/resmgr/dnp/dnpprojectstitlingpaperjune2.pdf.

Ogrinc, G., Mooney, S. E., Estrada, C., Foster, T., Goldmann, D., Hall, L. W., Huizinga, M. M., Liu, S. K., Mills, P., Neily, J., Nelson, W., Pronovost, P. J., Provost, L., Rubenstein, L.,V., Speroff, T., Splaine, M., Thomson, R., Tomolo, A.,M.,& Watts, B. (2008). The SQUIRE (Standards for QUality Improvement Reporting Excellence) guidelines for quality improvement reporting: Explanation and elaboration. *Quality and Safety Health Care, 17* (Suppl 1), 13-32. doi 10.1136/qshc.2008.029058.

O'Neil, E. H., & Pew Health Professions Commissions. (1998). *Recreating health professional practice for a new century: The fourth report of the Pew Health Professions Commission.* San Francisco, CA: Pew Health Professions Commissions.

O'Sullivan, A.L., Carter, M., Marion, L., Pohl, J.M. & Werner, K.E. (2005). Moving forward together: The practice doctorate in nursing. *The Online Journal of Issues in Nursing: A Scholarly Journal of the American Nurses Association, 1*0(3). Available at: www.nursingworld.org/MainMenuCategories/ANAMarketplace/ANAPeriodicals?OJIN/TableofContents/Volume102005/No3Sept05/tpc28_416028.aspx.

Udlis, K. A., & Mancuso, J. M. (2012). Doctor of nursing practice programs across the United States: A benchmark of information. Part I: Program Characteristics. *Journal of Professional Nursing 28*(5), 265-273.

Pew Health Professions Commission. (1995). *Reforming health care workforce regulation: Policy Considerations for the 21st century.* San Francisco, CA: Pew Health Professions.

Raines, C. F. (2010), The doctor of nursing practice: a report on progress. Paper presented at the American Association of Colleges of Nursing Spring Annual Meeting. Washington, DC, March 21, 2010.

Robert Woods Johnson Foundation (2013). *Charting nursing's future: Reports on policies that can transform patient care.* Available at: http://www.rwjf.org/content/dam/farm/reports/issue_briefs/2013/rwjf407597 Accessed on January 3, 2014

Rosseter, R. J. (2014). *The impact of education on nursing practice.* Retrieved January 14, 2014 from http://www.aacn.nche.edu/media-relations/fact-sheets/impact-of-education

Sabastian, J. G., & Delaney, C. W. (2013). Doctor of nursing practice programs: Opportunities for faculty development. *Journal of Nursing Education, 52*(8), 453-46i. doi 10.3928/014834-20130722-02

Stanley, J.M. (2012). Impact of new regulatory standards on advanced practice registered Nursing: The APRN consensus model and LACE. *Nursing Clinics of North America 47,* 241-250. DOI: 10.1016/j.cnur.2012.02.001

Slyer, J., & Levin, R. F. (2012). On the doctor of nursing practice (DNP*). Research and Theory in Nursing Practice: An International Journal, 26*(1), 6-9.

TeamSTEPPS. Retrieved February 2, 2014 from http://teamstepps.ahrq.gov/aboutnationalIP.htm.

In: Collaboration with the Advanced Practice Nurse ISBN: 978-1-63321-311-1
Editors: E.R. Giardino, R.G. Hanks and A.P. Giardino

Chapter 3

ADVANCED PRACTICE NURSING: CERTIFICATION, LICENSURE, OVERSIGHT AND REIMBURSEMENT

Deborah Guida, ARNP, PhD
School of Nursing The University of Texas School Health Science Center at Houston, US

ABSTRACT

Advanced Practice Registered Nurses (APRN or APN) are licensed independent practitioners who practice in a variety of clinical settings under specific rules and laws that govern their practice. This chapter discusses the types of laws that underlie advanced nursing practice, the association of the nurse practice act on scope of practice of the APN, and the effect of the practice environments of a state on the nursing practice that can take place in a state. There is discussion of the Consensus Model for APRN practice is relation to the ARN education, and practice.

INTRODUCTION

The legally protected title Advanced Practice Registered Nurse (APRN or APN) is a collective term that encompasses the clinical roles of certified nurse practitioners (CNP), certified nurse midwives (CNM), certified registered nurse anesthetists (CRNA) and clinical nurse specialists (CNS) (National Council of State Boards of Nursing & National Council of State Boards of Nursing, 2008). Each of the four advanced practice roles is a licensed independent practitioner who is governed by the nurse practice act in the state in which they practice.

The Nurse Practice Act and Types of Laws

Each state board of nursing (BON) is a government agency charged to protect the public through regulation of nursing practice within that state only. The BON ensures that nurses are competent to practice and that nurses and organizations meet their standards of nursing practice. The state BON ensures that nurses comply with the state nurse practice act (American Nurses Association, 2012; Texas Board of Nursing, 2005). The rules governing advanced nursing practice are derived from three types of law: statutory law, administrative law and judicial law. Each type of law is enacted by a different legislative body or administrative body for the purpose of to body is defined below.

Statutory Law

Statutory law is the basis of the Nurse Practice Act (NPA) in each state. Statutory law is written and passed by a legislative body at the state or federal level and is referred to as a statute or, more commonly, as an "act." A statute is a written law passed by a legislature on the state or federal level. Statutes apply to specific situations and may act to direct or forbid certain acts, make a declaration, or put mechanisms in place that aid society. The Nurse Practice Act is an example of state statutory law. A statute may direct or forbid a certain act, define a role, or set forth governmental mechanisms of enforcement. In some states, a "regulation" serves a similar function by giving a regulatory board authority to define a role and its expectations.

Each state has a Nurse Practice Act with the intent to protect the public health and safety by broadly defining the legal scope of nursing, and by extension advanced practice nursing (American Nurses Association, 2012). The NPA includes laws that define nursing scope of practice, nursing responsibilities, services and range of activities, and what is required to qualify a person to practice nursing (American Nurses Association, 2012). The intent of a NPA is to protect patients from harm resulting from unsafe or incompetent practice, or unqualified nurses. An NPA states what constitutes unprofessional conduct or misconduct, and what nurse behaviors may warrant disciplinary actions that could be taken against a nurse. Although there are similarities among and between the NPA of each state, the NPA of most state defines the term Advanced Practice Register Nurse (APRN) and then defines each of the four roles of the APRN Table 1 is an example of terminology and specific criteria that a state board of nursing includes in a nurse practice act.

At the State level, a Nurse Practice Act is usually stated in broad generalities, which in turn makes it open to interpretation. The Nurse Practice Act varies from state to state and may include attention to a variety of issues that pertain to nursing practice. Table 2 shows major components of a nurse practice act.

At the federal level, statues often pertain to reimbursement issues relating to Medicare and Medicaid. A final rule titled CY 2014 Physician Fee Schedule Final Rule established a requirement for a face-to-face encounter for written orders prior to delivery for certain items of durable medical equipment (DME) (77 Federal Register 68892) (Centers for Medicare & Medicaid Services, 2014). It is necessary for the clinician to evaluate a patient in a face-to-face encounter where an assessment shows the need for each covered item of DME. A face-to-face encounter may be accomplished via a telehealth encounter if all Medicare telehealth requirements are met (McDermott, Will & Emery, 2014)

Table 1. South Carolina Nurse Practice Act: Definitions of APRN & the Four Roles

Role	Role Characteristics
Advanced Practice Registered Nurse" or " APRN"	Prepared for an AP role through an advanced formal education program of nursing in a specialty area approved by the board. APRN categories are nurse practitioner, certified nurse-midwife, clinical nurse specialist, and certified registered nurse anesthetist. An APRN shall hold a doctorate, a post-nursing master's certificate, or a minimum of a master's degree that includes advanced education composed of didactic and supervised clinical practice in a specific area of advanced practice registered nursing. Those activities considered the practice of registered nursing, an APRN may perform delegated medical acts.
Certified Nurse-Midwife" or "CNM	APRN who holds MSN in specialty area and provides nurse-midwifery management of women's health care, focusing particularly on pregnancy, childbirth, postpartum, care of the newborn, family planning, and gynecological needs of women.
Certified Registered Nurse Anesthetist" or " CRNA"	APRN who: (a) successfully completed an advanced, organized formal CRNA education program at master's level accredited by the specialty area's national accrediting organization and that is recognized by the board; (b) is certified by a board-approved national certifying organization (c) demonstrates advanced knowledge and skill in delivery of anesthesia services
Clinical Nurse Specialist" or "CNS"	APRN is a clinician with a high degree of knowledge, skill, and competence in a practice discipline of nursing. Holds an MSN with an emphasis in clinical nursing. CNS is directly available to the public through the provision of nursing care to clients and indirectly available through guidance and planning of care with other nursing personnel. A CNS who performs delegated medical acts is required to have physician support and practice within approved written protocols. A CNS who does not perform delegated medical acts is not required to have physician support or to practice within approved written protocols as provided in Section 40-33-34.
Nurse Practitioner" or "NP"	Has completed an advanced formal education program at the master's level acceptable to the board, and who demonstrates advanced knowledge and skill in assessment and management of physical and psychosocial health, illness status of persons, families, and groups. NPs who perform delegated medical acts must have a supervising physician or dentist who is readily available for consultation and shall operate within the approved written protocols.

Adapted from South Carolina Nurse Practice Act (Legislative Council, 2013).

Table 2. Components of a Nurse Practice Act

Components
• Requirements for licensure
• Scope of practice
• Prescribing authority
• Collaborative or supervisory oversight
• Circumstances for license suspension, revocation or nonrenewal
• Standards of practice
• Requirements of educational programs
• Authority, power and composition of a board of nursing
• Types of titles for advanced practice nurses
• Grounds for disciplinary action, other violations and possible remedies

Adapted from: (Trilla & Patterson, 1998; American Nurses Association, 2014; American Nurses Association, 2012; Russell, 2012) (Trilla & Patterson, 1998; National Council of State Boards of Nursing, 2014) [nurse practice act].

Although statutory law may be passed at the federal or state level, state level statutory law may not grant privileges or authority specifically prohibited at the federal level. Since there are significant variations between APRNs and related state statutes, rules and regulations, it is necessary for the APRN and those who employ them to understand the state definition of scope of practice and the laws and regulations that pertain to the state regulatory agency (American Nurse Association, 2014; Klein, 2007).

Administrative Law

Administrative law is legislated by Congress or state legislatures and specifically gives agencies authority to carry out intentions of statutes. In the case of the Nurse Practice act, authority for administration may be given to a Board of Nursing or a Board of Nursing in conjunction with a Board of Medicine.

Judicial Law

Judicial law is made by courts and may be referred to as *case law*. It is the interpretation and application of the law to a particular set of facts contested by litigants in a court of law. It involves an exercise of discretion in interpretation based upon an evaluation of the evidence presented at a hearing. While statutes are the primary source of law, judicial decisions also have the force of law. As state statutes such as the Nurse Practice Act do not cover every conceivable situation, the courts may need to interpret specific situations in terms of the broad nature of its language. A judicial decision determines the outcome of the particular case, and also may regulate future conduct of all persons within the jurisdiction of the court.

The Sermchief v. Gonzalez was a landmark case in Missouri that exemplifies a judicial law decision (Blumenreich, 1998). Sermchief v. Gonzalez addressed the question of whether advanced practice nursing constituted the practicing of medicine. Two nurse practitioners providing family planning and women's health services were accused by physicians of practicing medicine without a medical license. The Missouri Nurse Practice Act described advanced practice professional nursing in general terms that indicated dependence upon degree of specialized training and education, judgment and skills, and did not mandate physician oversight of nurse practitioner practice. Nurse practitioners acts such as diagnosing and managing patient care were found to be within the nursing scope of practice as the nurse practitioners had the necessary education and training to perform the tasks. *Sermchief v Gonzales* is still widely quoted as an interpretation of where the dividing line between advanced practice nursing and medical practice stands. The answer, as so clearly stated by the Missouri Supreme Court, is that there is no clear defining line between the professions (Blumenreich, 1998). There are numerous overlapping areas and activities which constitute the practice of nursing when performed by nurses and the practice of medicine when performed by physicians.

Scope of Practice and State Boards of Nursing

The term scope of practice refers to professional activities that advanced practice nurses are permitted to perform under their professional license and certification as determined by law in a particular state or jurisdiction. A scope of practice defines the permissible activities for APRNs as determined by the nursing profession, professional and specialty organizations, the state in which the practitioner practices, and possibly the institution of practice (American Nurses Association, 2014).

Categories that make up the scope of practice may include but are not limited to:

- Education and training
    - The APRN must meet the academic requirements that are set by the professional organizations and the state qualifications as stated in the nurse practice act
- Governing body
    - The state, district, province or federal government that oversees the skill or profession must allow (or not explicitly disallow) the practice activities
- Institution
    - The institution's policies and procedures that define acceptable advanced nursing practice activities and skills

Scope of practice for APNs addresses the issues of diagnosis, treatment, prescribing and managing care of patients. It also addresses the subject of oversight or supervision of APNs. In some states, the board of nursing maintains control over administration of the Nurse Practice Act, whereas in other states, the board of nursing maintains oversight of advanced practice issues in conjunction with the medical board. For example, the South Carolina nurse practice act stipulates that a licensed NP who performs "delegated medical acts must do so under the general supervision of a licensed physician or dentist who must be readily available for consultation" (Legislative Council, 2013).

In most states, the government agency called the State board of nursing oversees the regulation of nursing practice, and protects the public by ensuring that standards of nursing practice are met and nurses are competent in their practice. In general, State boards of nursing ensure that nurses and nurse related organizations are in compliance with state nurse practice acts (American Nurses Association, 2012)[FAQ Boards of nursing re]. The following are typical powers and duties of a board of nursing (American Nurses Association, 2012):

- Interprets and enforces the state nurse practice act
- Administers nurse licensure by overseeing exams to grant licenses
- Takes action against licenses of nurses who have exhibited unsafe nursing practice
- Accredits or approves nurse education programs
- Develops nursing practice standards as per regulations
- Develops policies, administrative rules and regulations
- Investigates complaints regarding nurse compliance with the nurse practice law holds hearings for license holders,
- Determines and administers disciplinary actions based on evidence of law violations

(Adapted from: (American Nurses Association, 2012)

In all four of the APRN roles, the nursing board in each of the 50 states, the District of Columbia, and a number of US territories regulate what each of the roles can do related to professional nursing practice. In all of the states, except Nebraska, APRN's are regulated by the same board that oversees the practice of RN's. The National Council of State Boards of Nursing (NCSBN) is a collective voice of all of the independent boards of nursing, and was instrumental in developing the Consensus model for APRN practice (National Council of State Boards of Nursing & National Council of State Boards of Nursing, 2008).

State specific APRN Scope of Practice is often affected by forces outside of the nursing profession. The medical boards in many states may have a strong physician lobby against allowing APRNs to take on practice responsibilities that the board of medicine does not want the APRN to do. For example, the states that have restricted APRN practice usually face obstacles to standards for prescriptive authority which vary according to the state in which the APRN practices (American Nurses Association, 2014) [scope & standards of practice]. The physician oversight of advanced practice nurses is also described in terms of day to day practice. APNs may have supervised collaborative or independent practice. All models require the APN to be accountable for their own scope of practice (Fairman, Rowe, Hassmiller, & Shalala, 2010). The APRN who practices in states that require collaborative or supervisory practice models is still individually responsible to stay within the scope of legally granted authority. Collaborative practice does not imply that the APN is not responsible for any malpractice or problems that the APN may incur.

The terms independent, collaborative, and supervisory practice may vary widely in interpretation and regulatory definition. The Joint Commission on Accreditation of Healthcare Organizations (JCAHO) defines a Licensed Independent Provider (LIP), as a person who is permitted by law and by the organization to provide patient care and services, without direction or supervision, that is within the individual's scope of practice and consistent with clinical privileges that are granted by an institution or organization (Joint Commission on Accreditation of Healthcare Organizations, 2013) The Department of Health and Human Services, Health Resources and Services Administration support the LIP in their credentialing document for ambulatory health centers (HRSA, 2012); (Hittle, 2010).

Some state laws that require NPs to practice under physician supervision do not specify the requisite extent or form of physician oversight (AANP, 2013; American Nurses Association, 2012) [FAQ – roles of state boards of nursing]. The required physician supervision as defined by type of supervision and extent of supervision ranges from requiring that a physician have a physical presence at the practice site to allowing phone accessibility only. Some states may require regular meetings with the supervisory physician and periodic chart reviews. Supervisory requirements may also depend on practice settings. In most cases, a collaborative model dictates the use of written agreements between supervisor and ANP delineating practice guidelines, methods of communication and a template for review of work product and patient outcomes.

While the term "supervisory" is open to some interpretation, the term collaboration is even more loosely defined in Practice Acts as well as by interested agencies. The Code of Federal Regulations (Title 42) states that collaboration process occurs when a nurse practitioner works with one or more physicians to provide client care that are within the practitioners' scope of expertise, with medical direction and supervision that is determined through guidelines or other mechanisms as determined by the State law (Centers for Medicare & Medicaid Services, 2011) #401).

There are specific practices, procedures, or skills that the CNP may perform that are not evident conclusively in the Nurse Practice Act. Examples include the circumstances under which a CNP perform micro-dermabrasion, or administer IV anesthetics for intractable pain. In those situations, the state regulatory body may address the circumstances under which a CNPs may perform such procedures in the form of an opinion (American Nurse Association, 2014).

State Practice Environments

The American Academy of Nurse Practitioners outlines each state practice category and illustrates those states that allow full independent practice and those requiring some level of oversight (AANP, 2013; American Association of Nurse Practitioners, 2013; Sekscenski, Sansom, Bazell, Salmon, & Mullan, 1994; American Association of Nurse Practitioners, 2013). Table 3 states the level of supervision required in a state and practice implications of the state requirement.

In states that have reduced or restricted practice for APRNs, most require the ANP and the delegated physician to file a document with the administrating agency, usually the Board of Nursing or in some states, the Board of Medicine). The document, usually referred to as a collaborative agreement (CPA), is different than an employment contract. The employment contract spells out terms of compensation, hours of work, interoffice duties and conditions for continued employment or termination. The collaborative agreement fulfills a legal requirement within a state Practice Act. The document must include the names and credentials of the APN and the collaborating or supervising physician and the location at which the agreement will be utilized (Trilla & Patterson, 1998; Clavelle & Bramwell, 2013). At a minimum, the collaborative practice agreement (CPA) describes the functions of the APN and how the physician and APN will cooperate, collaborate and manage the care of the practice population. Details of how the APN practice will be reviewed and what mechanisms are in place for contact with the physician for support are included.

Table 3. State Practice Category Definitions (Required Level of Supervision)

Level of Supervision	Criteria for Practice
Full Practice States	• Licensure authority exclusively by the state board of nursing. • NP can practice without the need for collaborative agreement with an outside health discipline (usually a physician)
Reduced Practice States	• State practice & licensure law reduce ability of NPs to engage in at least one element of NP practice. • State requires regulated collaborative agreement with outside health discipline for NP to provide patient care
Restricted Practice States	• State practice & licensure law restricts ability of NP to engage in at least one element of NP practice. • State requires supervision, delegation or team-management by outside health discipline for NP to provide patient care

Adapted from: (AANP, 2013) & (American Association of Nurse Practitioners, 2013).

The completed and signed collaborative practice agreement document must be filed with the regulatory board(s) and a copy maintained at the place of practice. Samples of collaborative agreements may be found on most state Board of Nursing websites. Understanding APN scope of practice is critical for safe practice for APNs as well as all other health care providers and entities that work with them. APNs, collaborators, supervisors and employers are well advised to review the applicable state Nurse Practice Act and Scope of Practice. An APN who relocates to a new state needs to confirm compliance with the Practice Act under which they will be working. The state's board of nursing website usually defines specific information regarding state requirements for APRN oversight.

Additional oversight of APN practice may be directed by individual facility policy. Health care facilities may institute procedure or policies that limit scope of APN practice. While facilities may limit scope of practice, they may not expand practice scope beyond that allowed by state statute or regulation.

Titling for the APRN and CNP

There are a variety of titles used in the literature and in practice that refer to or signify an advance practice nurse who is a nurse practitioner. For example, a number of nursing organizations refer to the advanced practice nurse practitioner as a certified nurse practitioner (CNP) (National Council of State Boards of Nursing & National Council of State Boards of Nursing, 2008; National Organization of Nurse Practitioner Faculty, 2013; National Organization of Nurse Practitioner Faculty, 2013; National Organization of Nurse Practitioner Faculty, 2013). The term advance practice nurse practitioner (APNP) refers to an advanced practice registered nurse who is certified to practice as a nurse practitioner and has at least a master's level of education Other references to the advanced practice nurse practitioner are simply 'nurse practitioner' (NP). The nurse practitioner who graduates from a DNP program is a CNP with a doctoral degree and can still be referred to as a CNP, an NP, an APNP or a DNP nurse practitioner.

Professional Organizations

Professional organizations that advocate for professional practice, may issue opinions, statements or formal "white papers". Many of the issues professional organizations address are imprecisely or vaguely defined by law. These documents serve to offer definitions or guidance on issues of scope of practice, reimbursement, competencies, educational preparation and issues of independent practice. Professional organizations hold no lawful authority over practice but may be a powerful political change agent. For example, in 1994, the American Association of Colleges of Nursing took the position that all APNs should have a master's degree in order to be nationally certified. Other agencies, including those responsible for reimbursement legislation, soon followed and the majority of certifying organizations now require a master's degree in order for APNs to sit for national certification (National Council of State Boards of Nursing & National Council of State Boards of Nursing, 2008).

One of the important functions of professional nursing organizations is the review and reporting of critical legislative updates that may affect practice. Such reporting intends to inform as well to rally professional support for or against potential changes in practice law. Organizations can represent general nursing issues (American Nurses Association), APN specific issues (American Association of Nurse Practitioners, National Association of Clinical Nurse Specialists) and issues specific to groups of people affecting ANP practice (National Organization of Nurse Practitioner Faculties). Additionally, most states and many municipalities have nursing and advanced practice nursing organization charters.

Licensing and Certification

Licensing requirements and scope of practice for APNs vary from state to state according to the individual state Nurse Practice Act but all require a license as a registered nurse as a prerequisite. All states include language stipulating some level of education beyond the basic requirements for RN licensing. Due to changes in reimbursement law, many states now require national certification for ANP licensing. Certification ascertains that APNs have attained minimum, entry level knowledge for practice.

Each state defines the general scope of practice for the APN but the educational program from which the APN graduates and certification further defines the role within which the APN functions. For example, in Texas, a license may read "Advanced Practice Registered Nurse". Without further information, it is difficult to determine the exact scope of practice of the APN without additionally knowing the educational and certification area. The APN may be educated and hold certification as a family nurse practitioner, pediatric nurse practitioner, a nurse midwife, a nurse anesthetist or any of the other recognized roles. Each of those practice areas entails different skills and knowledge base and the ANP scope of practice is further defined by knowing the certification area of the APN.

National Certification

Board certification is a national process and once attained moves across all state lines with the APN. The purpose of requiring a national certification examination for professional advanced nursing practice is to demonstrate through a written examination that a CNP has entry level knowledge for practice as a nurse practitioner. In order to sit for a certification exam, the candidate must meet the prerequisites of the certifying body. All APN certifying bodies currently require a candidate to complete a Master's degree in a program which is nationally accredited. Successful certification stays in effect for a varying period of time, most commonly five years, after which the APN may renew the certification. Renewal entails demonstrating continued competency through a combination of practice hours and continuing education, or re-testing.

Individual state boards of nursing did not always require APRNs to pass a national certification examination in order to practice as a nurse practitioner in their state. Lack of state uniformity requiring national certification created problems because there was not a standard level of knowledge acquisition required to practice in the advanced practice role (APRN Consensus Work Group, 2008). Any definitions of advanced practice nursing that included language indicating a demonstration of advanced knowledge and skill in patient assessment, and health and illness management, of persons, families, and groups did not pertain to those APRNs working in states that did not have a requirement to pass a national certification exam (Buppert, 2011); (Legislative Council, 2013) #41).

The Consensus Model for APRN Practice

In 2008, over 40 nursing organizations endorsed the "Consensus Model for APRN Regulation: Licensure, Accreditation, Certification, & Education" developed by the APRN Consensus Work Group and the National Council of State Boards of Nursing (APRN Consensus Work Group & National Council of State Boards of Nursing APRN Advisory Committee, 2008). The purpose of the Consensus model was to define and standardize licensure, accreditation, certification and education of advanced practice nurses in order to create a more uniform practice for advanced nursing across the states. Although it is described as a regulatory model, there is no legal means of enforcing the implementation of the Consensus Model.

Through the 1980s and 1990s, the vagaries of such definitions and the increasing utilization of APNs in the health care system gradually led to the employment of APNs in roles for which they were not educationally prepared. A proliferation of specialty and subspecialty practice areas grew without sufficient academic or certification support. Additionally, the lack of a uniform model of APN license across the states is problematic as is lack of clear definition of role. The consensus model for APN regulation states that the individual state independently determines the APRN legal scope of practice, the roles that are recognized, the criteria for entry-into advanced practice and the certification examinations accepted for entry-level competence assessment (APRN Consensus Work Group & National Council of State Boards of Nursing APRN Advisory Committee, 2008). Lack of uniformity of standards for APRN education, practice and licensure has created barriers for APRNs to easily move from state to state and has decreased access to care for patients (National Council of State Boards of Nursing & National Council of State Boards of Nursing, 2008). In order for the recommendations within the model to be fully implemented, all states would need to legislatively adopt the licensure, accreditation, certification and education (LACE) requirements for ANP practice set forth in the document. Aspects of the model have already been adopted by some educational institutions in anticipation of a move toward the Consensus Model in the future and for clearer definition of the APN roles (National Council of State Boards of Nursing & National Council of State Boards of Nursing, 2008).

The Consensus Model provides a clearer definition of APN role (Figure x.2 Consensus Model). According to parameters of the model, an advanced practice nurse is educated and then certified to practice in one of the four APN roles: certified registered nurse anesthetist, certified nurse practitioner, certified nurse midwife or clinical nurse specialist. Within their chosen role, the student is then educated and (after graduation) licensed and certified in a population focus; Family/Individual across the life span, Adult/Gerontology. Neonatal, Pediatrics, Women's Health/Gender related or Psychiatric/Mental health. The Adult/Gerontology and Pediatric foci can be further broken down to educate students in either acute or primary care. After licensing and certification, APNs may choose to specialize in more focused areas within their original role choice but always within their original population focus. For example, a Family Nurse Practitioner may specialize in palliative care across the life span of the individual. A Pediatric Nurse Practitioner may specialize in palliative care but only within the pediatric population (National Council of State Boards of Nursing & National Council of State Boards of Nursing, 2008).

Reimbursement for Nurse Practitioner Services

Reimbursement for the services of advanced practice nurses is accomplished in a variety of ways and may vary from state to state dependent on the rules and regulations of third party payers and state regulations. This section addresses the different types of reimbursement models that enable either the advanced practice nurse or the employer of the APN to receive payment for APN services.

Types of Reimbursement for APN Services

Just as practice parameters can change state to state, APN reimbursement can vary by state, or by type of reimbursement organization or structure. Reimbursement structures can take many forms. Two examples are fee-for-service and capitation.

In the fee-for-service model, each service or procedure is reimbursed at a predetermined amount contained in a negotiated rate schedule. The rate schedule varies geographically as well as by certain provider circumstances. Under this system, the more billable services provided or procedures performed, the more revenue is generated.

Capitation is a system in which a Managed Care Organization pays a provider a monthly amount based on the gender and age of the patient. The set fee is paid for all services agreed on within a negotiated contract. The provider receives no additional payment no matter how many services the patient receives. Conversely, even if a patient receives no services, the monthly amount is still paid to the provider. Under the capitation system, the more patients enrolled under the provider name, the higher the monthly reimbursement.

The traditional fee-for-service and capitation models have minimal mechanisms in affect to take quality of care into account, instead focusing on numbers of patients or services. In 2013, the Centers for Medicare & Medicaid Services launched the Bundled Payments for Care Improvement initiative which has 4 payment models. In the Bundled Payments for Care Improvement initiative, an organization has a payment arrangement that includes financial and performance accountability for episodes of care. The desire is that such arrangements will lead to a more coordinated and higher quality care but a cost that is lower to Medicare (CMS.Gov, 2014).

Under a Health Care Innovation Award, multiple agencies across the US began implementation in 2013. The project will be administrative over 3 years with full evaluation for feasibility of more widespread application

Reimbursement Organizations

There are five main types of reimbursement organizations available. Each has different rules for payment. They are:

- Medicare (federally funded and managed)
- Medicaid (federally funded, state managed)
- Commercial indemnity agencies
- Commercial managed care organizations
- Private pay (may be individuals or businesses)

Medicare Reimbursement

For primary care providers, the outpatient prospective payment system (OPPS) reimburses Medicare providers a pre-set amount by service provided. Medicare reimbursement may be fee-for-service or capitated. In order to obtain permission to bill Medicare for APN service, the APN must meet all Medicare requirements including holding a master's degree, an APN state license and national board certification in a population focus. The APN must be legally permitted to perform the action for which they are billing in the state where they are providing the service. For reimbursement, all APNs must have a collaborative agreement with a physician, even in states where APNs enjoy independent practice. APNs must apply for and receive a Medicare billing number.

The APNs may bill for services considered to be physician services under their own Medicare number. Such services are not nursing services. Reimbursement for APN services billed to Medicare is at 85% of the physician reimbursement rate. However, APNs may receive 100% of physician reimbursement rate by the process of *incident-to* billing in which the charge is submitted under the physician's Medicare number. Medicare mandates that incident-to billing be performed under physician supervision.

Incident-to billing requires but is not limited to the following rules:

- The APN must be employed by or contracted with the physician or the legal entity that employs or contracts with the physician
- Direct supervision in an office setting stipulates the physician to be present in the office suite and available immediately to provide direction and assistance throughout the service visit [physician present in the same office suite and available immediately]. (Buppert, 2012)
- The physician must perform the first visit for the problem and initiate the plan of care. (CMS does not clearly define what constitutes a 'first visit'. It could, in theory, be the first visit to the practice or a first visit for a new problem that will require continuing care)
- The physician must perform subsequent visits at a frequency that indicates active participation in the care of the patient, but the frequency is not specified. This can be as frequently as every other visit or once a year depending on the setting and the complexity of the case.

For example, a patient sees the physician for diabetes. The physician develops and institutes the plan of care. For subsequent visits to manage the diabetes, the APN may see the patient provided the physician is present in the office suite. In this case, each visit may be billed under the physician's Medicare number and will receive reimbursement at 100% of the physician reimbursement amount. Should the patient visit be for a new problem, such as a respiratory infection, the APN may see the patient, but must bill under his or her own Medicare number. Reimbursement for that visit would be at 85% of the physician reimbursement amount for the visit.

Medicaid

Medicaid is a federally funded program for mothers and children who meet poverty guidelines and adults with short term disabilities who meet poverty guidelines. Reimbursement is fee-for-service. APNs must obtain a provider number from their state Medicaid office.

Federal law now requires fee-for-service Medicaid to cover health care services provided by pediatric nurse practitioners, family nurse practitioners and certified nurse midwives. States may individually elect to also cover the services of certified registered nurse anesthetists and clinical nurse specialists. This is particularly important in states where physician coverage may be low, such as in rural communities. Although federal law provides for reimbursement for APN practice, the program is state managed. Individual states are permitted to set reimbursement amounts and typically they are 70-100% of physician fee-for-service rates.

States are permitted to apply for Medicaid waivers, permitting patients to be enrolled in a Managed Care Organization (capitated structure) instead of a fee-for-service model. In addition to being an enrolled Medicaid provider, APNs must then also apply to the appropriate managed care panel.

Commercial Indemnity Organizations

Commercial Indemnity Organizations provide financial coverage for health care services but do not actually provide health care services. Reimbursement is provided in a fee-for-service manner under fee schedules negotiated between the provider and the organization (payer). Cost for coverage is paid by the patient or, under employment contracts, by the employer. Patients often share the cost of medical services via co-pays, deductibles and co-insurance payments. APNs must apply to the organization for authorization to bill for services.

Commercial Managed Care Organizations

Commercial Managed Care Organizations (CMO) are prepaid health care systems offering services to which the member is entitled, as opposed to a set dollar amount guaranteed by an Insurance policy. They combine the functions of health insurance, delivery of care and administration. CMOs may fall into one of several types:

- Health Maintenance Organizations (HMO): usually only pay for care within the network. The patient chooses a primary care provider who manages or coordinates all care.
- Preferred Provider Organizations (PPO): allow patients more selectivity in choosing providers. Patients may choose from in-network or may choose an out-of-network provider and pay a larger portion of the service fee.
- Point of Service (POS) plan: lets the patient choose between an HMO or a PPO each time care is needed.

In each case, APNs must apply to be added to a commercial managed care organizations provider panel before they are able to bill for services. In some states, an MCO cannot discriminate against a provider based on class of license, whether a medical or nursing license. However, the organization can accept or reject any provider in some states.

Private Pay

APNs may choose to work in a cash based practice or for a business that contracts them to perform certain services for a flat fee. Often, the services performed are not billable to a 3rd party payer or are billable in a very limited or restricted manner. Examples are college or university health care offices, clinics run by philanthropic or religious based institutions, and offices that perform cosmetic or esthetic services. In situations where third party billing is performed it is necessary to undergo the process of credentialing. Credentialing serves the purpose of ensuring the safety of the recipients of health care as well as to ensure that the provider has met all the legal requirement of practice. Credentialing can be a lengthy process. In addition to demographics, applicants will be asked to provide:

- Information on educational preparation
- License, certification and specialty information
- Place of practice information
- Complete employment history
- Military service
- DEA, prescribing and NPI numbers
- Professional liability coverage
- Professional references
- Professional sanctions
- History of any malpractice suits

Billing and reimbursement for APN practice is complicated and fraught with many opportunities for reduced, delayed or denied payments. It is critical that both APNs and their MD colleagues be current on federal and state policies regulating APN reimbursement.

CONCLUSION

The practice parameters of advanced practice registered nurses (APRN or APN) are regulated by state and federal laws as well as the individual state boards of nursing in which an advanced practice nurse works. State boards of nursing provide general guidelines for how the individual clinician in a specific advanced role may practice in the state. The purpose of the board of nursing as well as the nurse practice act in each state is to protect consumers and assure that advanced practice is delivered in a lawful and safe manner. Although states define nursing scope of practice, individual institutions may further delineate what the advanced practice nurse can do in the institution. Reimbursement for advanced practice nursing services is complicated and requires knowledge of the rules and regulations that govern advanced practice There is definitive progress towards refining and defining advanced practice roles through education, licensure and certification. The Consensus Model for APRN practice helps advanced practice nurses and those who collaborate with them understand issues of licensure and certification in advanced practice nursing.

Appendix A: Texas Board of Nursing - Decision Tree to Determine If Task or Procedure Is within Scope of Practice

Step One: Is the act consistent with the Texas Nursing Practice Act (NPA)? Do the Board's rules or positions statements address this specific act? (This may be all the information you need to make your decision. If not, continue to the next step).

The following Information available on the BON's web page may be of assistance:

a. NPA, Ch. 301.002(2), Definition of Professional Nursing & Ch. 301.002(5), Definition of Vocational Nursing.

b. Standards of Professional Nursing Practice (BON Rule 217.11)

c. Unprofessional Conduct Rule (BON Rule 217.12)

d. Delegation Rules for RN Delegation to Unlicensed Assistive Personnel (224 & 225)

e. Documents listed under "Scope of Practice" in the Nursing Practice Section on the BON web site.

f. BON Position Statements, Guidelines, & Frequently Asked Questions (FAQ's)

If NO, the act is NOT within your scope of practice;
If YES, continue to the next step.

Step Two: Is the activity appropriately authorized by a valid order when necessary, and in accordance with current policies and procedures? Clarification of the orders(s) should be sought as needed [Rule 217.11(1) (N)].

If NO, the act is NOT within your scope of practice;
If YES, continue to the next step.

Step Three: Is the act supported by positive and conclusive data from nursing literature, nursing research, and/or research from a health related field (such as evidence based practice standards)? Has a national nursing organization issued a position statement, guideline, or standard supporting LVNs, RNs, or both engaging in this practice?

If NO - the act is NOT within your scope of practice;
if YES, continue to the next step.

Step Four:

Do you personally possess current clinical competence to perform the task safely from knowledge acquired in a basic nursing education program, post -basic program, or continuing education program? Documentation to validate competency should be maintained in accordance with agency/facility policy and procedure. Each nurse is also encouraged to maintain his/her own copies of competency forms.

If NO, the act is NOT within your scope of practice;
if YES, continue to the next step.

Step Five: Is the performance of the act within the accepted "standard of care" which would be provided in similar circumstances by reasonable and prudent nurses who have similar training and experience? An additional related question to ask is: If an untoward event/reaction occurs as a result of your nursing actions, can the untoward consequences/reaction be resolved through nursing intervention alone? Rule 217.11(1)(A) states that the nurse (LVN, RN or RN with advanced practice authorization) shall "Know and conform to the Texas Nursing Practice Act and the board's rules and regulations as well as all federal, state, or local laws, rules or regulations affecting the nurse's current area of nursing practice."

Review of the applicable rules in their entirety is recommended for the nurse in this step of the six - step model. In addition, human, material, and equipment resources can vary greatly across the spectrum of possible practice settings, and may contribute to the nurse's decision in a given circumstance.

If NO, the act is NOT within your scope of practice;
if YES, continue to the next step

Step Six: Are you prepared to accept the consequences of your actions?
If NO, the act is NOT within your scope of practice;
if YES, then: Perform the act –based upon valid order when necessary, and in accordance with appropriately established and current policies and procedures; and Assume accountability for provision of safe care.

Insert TBON Six step Decision Tree

From: Texas Board of Nursing Decision Tree – A six step process for determining if a task or procedure is in one's scope of practice. (with permission from the Texas Board of Nursing)

REFERENCES

AANP. (2013). State Practice Environment. American Association of Nurse Practitioners [On-line]. Available: https://www.aanp.org/legislation-regulation/state-legislation-regulation/state-practice-environment

American Association of Nurse Practitioners. (2013). 2013 Nurse Practitioner State Practice Environment. State Nurse State Practice Acts and Administration Rules, 2012 [On-line]. Available: http://www.aanp.org/ images/documents/state-leg-reg/stateregulatorymap.pdf

American Nurse Association. (2014). State law and regulation. American Nurse Association [On-line]. Available: www.nursingworld.org/statelawandregulation

American Nurses Association (2012). Frequently Asked Questions: Roles of State Boards of Nursing: Licensure, Regulation and Complaint Investigation. American Nurses Association, Inc [On-line].

American Nurses Association. (2014). Model of Professional Nursing Practice Regulation. American Nurses Association Nursing world [On-line]. Available: http://www. nursingworld.org/EspeciallyForYou/ AdvancedPracticeNurses/Scope-of-Practice-2/Scope-of-Practice/Model-of-Practice-Regulation.html

American Nurses Association (2014a). Scope and Standards of Practice. Nursing World ANA [On-line]. Available: http://www.nursingworld.org/scopeandstandardsofpractice

ANA Factsheet on Medicaid Reimbursement. (2013). Retrieved January 30 2014, from http://www.nursingworld.org/MainMenuCategories/Policy-Advocacy/ExpiredContent-GOVA/HCFA/HCFAFCT211690.html

APRN Consensus Work Group & National Council of State Boards of Nursing APRN Advisory Committee (2008). Consensus model for APRN regulation: Licensure, accreditation, certification & education National Council of State Boards of Nursing.

Blumenreich, G. (1998). The overlap between the practice of medicine and the practice of nursing. Journal of the American Association of Nurse Anesthetists, 66, 11-15.

Buppert, C. (2011). *Nurse practitioner's business practice and legal guide*. Sudbury MA: Jones & Bartlett Publishers.

Buppert, C. (2012). Nurse practitioners business practice and legal guide. *Federal regulations of the nurse practitioner program.* (p 151). Sudbury, Md: Jones, Bartlett Learning.

Buppert, C. (2002). Billing For Nurse Practitioner Services: Guidelines for NPs, Physicians, Employers, and Insurers. *Medscape*. Jan 24, 2002. Retrieved from http://www.medscape.com/viewarticle/422935_3

Centers for Medicare & Medicaid Services (2014). Physician Fee Schedule: CY 2014 Physician Fee Schedule Final Rule with Comment Period. CMS.gov [On-line]. Available: http://www.cms.gov/Medicare/Medicare-Fee-for-Service-Payment/Physician FeeSched/index.html?redirect=/physicianfeesched

Centers for Medicare & Medicaid Services, D. o. H. a. H. S. (10-1-2011). 42 CFR 410.75 - Nurse practitioners' services. 4-21-2014.

Clavelle, J. & Bramwell, K. (2013). Nurse Practitioner/Physician Collaborative Practice: An Integrative Model for Professional Peer Review. *Journal of Nursing Administration*, 43, 318-320.

CMS.Gov: Bundled Payments for Care Improvement Initiative Fact Sheet (2014). retrieved January 30, 2014 from http://www.cms.gov/Newsroom/MediaReleaseDatabase/Fact-Sheets/2014-Fact-sheets-items/2014-01-30-2.html

Department of Health and Human Services Centers for Medicare & Medicaid Services. (2011). *Medicare Information for Advanced Practice Registered Nurses, Anesthesiologist Assistants, and Physician Assistant.* Medicare Learning Network. Washington DC.

Fairman, J. A., Rowe, J. W., Hassmiller, S., & Shalala, D. E. (2010). Broadening the Scope of Nursing Practice. *New England Journal of Medicine*, 364, 193-196.

Frequently Asked Questions: Roles of State Boards of Nursing: Licensure, Regulation and Complaint Investigation. American Nurses Association [On-line]. Available: http://www.nursingworld.org/mainmenucategories/tools/state-boards-of-nursing-faq.pdf

Hittle, K. (2010). Understanding certification, licensure, and credentialing: A guide for the new nurse practitioner. *Journal of Pediatric Health Care,* 24, 203-206.

HRSA (2012). Clarification of Bureau of Primary Health Care Credentialing and Privileging Policy outlined in Policy Information Notice 2001-16. Health Resources and Services Administration [On-line]. Available: http://bphc.hrsa.gov/policiesregulations/policies/pin200222.html

Joint Commission on Accreditation of Healthcare Organizations (2013). Comprehensive Accreditation Manual for Hospitals: The Official Handbook. Joint Commission Resources.

Klein, T. (2007). Scope of Practice and the Nurse Practitioner: Regulation, Competency, Expansion, and Evolution. Topics in Advanced Practice Nursing eJournal [On-line]. Available: http://www.medscape.org/viewarticle/506277

Legislative Council (2013). Title 40 - Professions and Occupations, CHAPTER 33. NURSES ARTICLE 1. NURSE PRACTICE ACT. South Carolina Code of Laws [On-line]. Available: http://www.scstatehouse.gov/code/t40c033.php

McDermott Will & Emery (2014). Overview of 2013 Final Rule on DME Written Order and Face-to-Face Encounter Requirements. McDermott Will & Emery [On-line]. Available: http://www.mwe.com/Overview-of-2013-Final-Rule-on-DME-Written-Order-and-Face-to-Face-Encounter-Requirements-11-13-2013/?PublicationTypes=d9093adb-e95d-4f19-819a-f0bb5170ab6d

National Council of State Boards of Nursing & National Council of State Boards of Nursing (2008). Consensus model for APRN regulation: Licensure, accreditation, certification & education National Council of State Boards of Nursing.

National Council of State Boards of Nursing (2014). Nurse Practice Act, Rules & Regulations. National Council of State Boards of Nursing (NCSBN) [On-line]. Available: https://www.ncsbn.org/1455.htm

National Organization of Nurse Practitioner Faculty (2013). Independent practice and the certified nurse practitioner: a white paper. National Organization of Nurse Practitioner Faculty [On-line]. Available: http://c.ymcdn.com/sites/www.nonpf.org/resource/resmgr/Docs/IndepenPracPPRFinal2013.pdf

Russell, K. A. (2012). Nurse Practice Acts Guide and Govern Nursing Practice. *Journal of Nursing Regulation,* 3, 36-42.

Sekscenski, E., Sansom, S., Bazell, C., Salmon, M. E., & Mullan, F. (1994). State practice environments and the supply of physician assistants, nurse practitioners, and certified nurse-midwives. *New England Journal of Medicine*, 331, 1266-1271.

Stantz, R. (2013). Demystifying Medicare's 'incident to' billing by nurse practitioners, physician assistants. Retrieved January 30, 2014 from http://medicaleconomics.modernmedicine.com/medical-economics/news/demystifying-medicares-incident-billing-nurse-practitioners-physician-assista?page=full

Texas Board of Nursing. (2005). Practice - APRN Scope of Practice. Texas Board of Nursing [On-line]. Available: http://bon.state.tx.us/practice_scope_of_practice_aprn.asp

Trilla, F., & Patterson, A. (1998). Physicians and nurse practitioners in collaborative practice. In *Harvard Risk Management Foundation. Forum. Winter.*

U.S. National Library of Medicine from the National Institutes of Health. (2013). Retrieved January 30, 2014, from http://www.nlm.nih.gov/medlineplus/managedcare.html

In: Collaboration with the Advanced Practice Nurse ISBN: 978-1-63321-311-1
Editors: E.R. Giardino, R.G. Hanks and A.P. Giardino

Chapter 4

NURSE PRACTITIONERS AND PHYSICIAN ASSISTANTS: EDUCATION, PRACTICE AND REGULATION

Vicki A. Keough*[1]*, PhD, APRN-BC, ACNP FAAN,
Susan Bednar*[1,2]*, RN-C, ANP and Alison Ruiz*[1,2]*, PA-C, MS
[1]Marcella Niehoff School of Nursing, Loyola University, Chicago, US
[2]NorthShore University Health System

ABSTRACT

Nurse practitioners (NPs) and physician assistants (PAs) have been providing care to residents of the US for almost 50 years. Often the public does not know the difference between the two professions and even more surprising, even NPs and PAs have a difficult time describing the differences. This chapter provides an overview of the similarities and differences in NP and PA education, practice and regulatory issues. The most evident difference is that NPs practice and are educated within a nursing education framework and PAs practice are educated within a medical model framework. Most NP students enter NP school having an initial Bachelor of Science in Nursing (BSN) degree, an RN license, experience as an RN and then go to NP school part-time to obtain a Master's Degree, accumulating approximately 700 additional post-baccalaureate clinical hours in their NP program (Bednar, Atwater and Keough, 2007). NP education typically takes between 2-3 years after the BSN degree. Most PA students enter the program with some health-care related experience, about 1-2 years of pre-requisite courses and attend PA school full-time for 27 months accumulating approximately 2,000 hours of clinical throughout their programs. Practice foci and populations are often the same for NPs and PAs. There is no difference with regard to expected patient outcomes and standards of care applied to their practices.

With regard to regulatory issues, PAs must have supervisory oversight by a physician while NPs have varying requirements for physician collaboration depending on the state in which they practice. Some states require no physician collaboration for NPs and allow NPs to practice independently, some states require the NP to have collaborative practice agreements with physicians in order to practice and very few states require direct physician supervision for NPs.

Keywords: Nurse Practitioner Education, Nurse Practitioner Practice, Nurse Practitioner Regulation, Physician Assistant Education, Physician Assistant Practice, Physician Assistant Regulation

INTRODUCTION

Nurse Practitioners (NP) and Physician Assistants (PA) are an important component of the healthcare workforce and may be the best kept secret in healthcare. These healthcare professionals provide excellent care, are well-educated and often underutilized throughout the US.

In our nation, there is a perfect storm in health care arising that will help to increase the visibility and the utilization of NPs and PAs. There is an aging population of consumers who because of longevity have a host of co-morbid conditions that require frequent monitoring such as heart disease, diabetes, arthritis, etc. and not enough physicians to handle this increase (Clabo et al., 2013); due to the increase in access to care as a result of the affordable care act, there are millions of individuals who now have access to health care who previously could not afford care (Dower and O'Neil, 2011); and finally, due to media support there is increased public knowledge about the value of NP and PA care. Due to this increased public awareness of the values NPs and PAs bring to healthcare, legislation is being proposed that will allow for these practitioners to practice to the full scope of their education (Clabo et al, 2013; Institute of Medicine [IOM], 2011).

Currently there are approximately 106,000 NPs and 77,000 PAs providing care throughout the nation (BLS, 2012). Very often NPs and PAs are serving in the same roles, providing care to similar populations and demonstrating excellent outcomes and patient satisfaction scores (Laurant et al., 2010; Moote, Krsek, Kleinpell and Todd, 2011). In a study by Peterson, Phillips, Puffer, Bazemore and Peterson (2013) between 1999 and 2009 the utilization of NPs, PAs and Certified Midwives in physician offices teams increased from 25% to 50%.

According to the Bureau of Labor Statistics (BLS, 2012) the NP and PA definitions are similar. "Nurse practitioners (NPs) are registered nurses with specialized graduate education. They may diagnose and treat acute, episodic, or chronic illness, either independently or as part of a healthcare team. NPs may focus on health promotion and disease prevention, perform or interpret diagnostic tests, and prescribe medications". "Physician assistants (PAs) graduate from an accredited educational program for physician assistants. They provide healthcare services under the supervision of a physician that are typically performed by a physician. PAs conduct complete physical examinations, provide medical treatment, prescribe medication, and counsel patients" (BLS, 2012).

NPs and PAs provide care in a variety of settings including primary care offices, tertiary care centers (typically medical surgical hospitals), surgical centers, outpatient centers and home care (BLS, 2012; Peterson et al., 2013; Bednar, Atwater, and Keough, 2007). According to the BLS (2012), the majority of NPs and PAs provide care in primary care offices, while general medical/surgical hospitals are the second largest employer of NPs and PAs followed by outpatient care centers.

A logical question for both health care consumers and health care providers would be, so what is the difference between NPs and PA's? This chapter will provide a discussion as to the differences between the two groups of highly qualified health care professionals. Perhaps after understanding the rigorous educational and practice standards for both professions the reader might ask, "So why are we wasting our time trying to find/define the differences?"

HISTORY

It is interesting that both NPs and PAs came into existence in the US around the same time. NPs and PAs entered the health care arena in 1965 and have been providing care throughout the US ever since. NP programs first began when nurse Loretta Ford and pediatrician Henry Silver developed a pediatric NP program at the University of Colorado as a 4 month post-baccalaureate certificate program (Pulcine and Wagner, 2002; Tumolo, 2004). Similarly, in 1965, a physician by the name of Stead began the first PA program at Duke University. His intent was to help alleviate the severe physician shortage and provide access to health care. Stead's initial program consisted of a group of Navy corpsmen with health training from the military which was not recognized in the civilian health care arena (Stead, 1966).

EDUCATION FOR PAS AND NPS

Physician Assistant Education

In general, PA education consists of at least 2 years of prerequisite college courses with a focus in the sciences, an average of 3 years of healthcare experience, and completion of a 27 month full time PA program. The prerequisite college courses are modeled after the pre-medical school prerequisites including chemistry, physiology, anatomy, microbiology and biology.

The healthcare experience required for admission would typically include patient contact experiences such as paramedic, EMT, nurse, nursing assistant (Physician Assistant Education Association [PAEA], 2013).

Currently the terminal degree for PAs is a master's degree. However, one can still enter the profession with a certificate, bachelors, or master's degree. There are 181 accredited PA programs across the country and 165 award master's degree, 10 award baccalaureate degree, 2 award an associate degree, and 4 award a certificate (Accreditation Review Commission of Education for the Physician Assistant (ARC-PA) (ARC-PA 2014). PA students are educated based on a set of standards set by the accrediting body, the ARC-PA. Therefore, regardless of whether the student is receiving a bachelor's degree or master's degree, the basic didactic and clinical content has to meet the same standard set by the accrediting body (Bednar et al., 2007).

PA school is on average 27 months in length and requires full time commitment of 40 hours per week, there is no option to be part-time. PAs are trained from a generalist or primary care approach (Hooker and Everett, 2011). PA school consists of full time immersion in core curriculum and clinical training that mimics the medical model of education (AAPA, March 2011) (Figure 1).

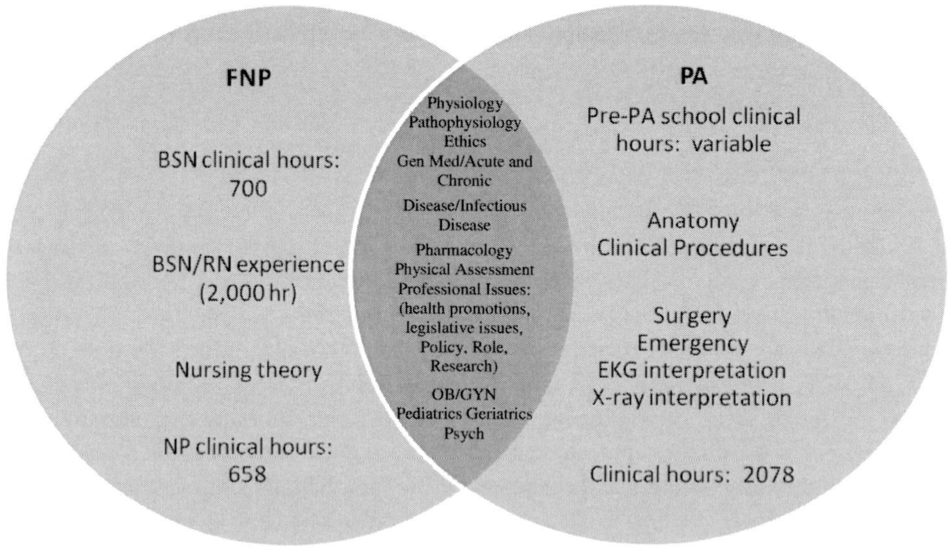

*The FNP program was chosen in order to compare the generalist NP program that would most closely resemble the PA p generalist program. Master's degree programs were used as comparisons between both the NP and PA educational models.

**The American Association of Colleges of nursing endorses the Doctor of Nursing Practice as the terminal degree for the Nurse Practitioner by 2015. This degree required a minimum of 1,000 clinical hours and additional doctoral theory not reflected in the diagram above.

Figure 1. FNP and PA educational similarities and differences.

Nurse Practitioner Education

Typically, NP education requires a Bachelor of Science in Nursing degree, an RN license, varying nursing experience post baccalaureate degree completion and completion of a master's degree NP program (Figure 1) (American Association of Colleges of Nursing (AACN) (AACN, 2014). Entry level preparation for NP practice is at the master's, post-master or doctoral level (ANP, 2013). The American Association of Colleges of Nursing (AACN) endorsed the position that all NPs will be prepared at the doctorate level by 2015 (AACN, 2006). However, that endorsement has not been implemented at the state or national level as a requirement for nurse practitioner practice.

An NP typically enters school with a BSN degree prior to pursuing one of the six advanced NP roles (US Bureau of Labor Statistics, 2012). Some schools offer a bridge program which allows for those candidates who do not have a bachelor's degree in nursing but have an associate's degree or a diploma in nursing to go on and obtain a master's degree and incorporate the bachelor's degree content within the master's degree program. In addition, there are post baccalaureate programs in nursing which allow individuals with a bachelor's degree in a field other than nursing to complete coursework required to take the

RN licensure exam and then continue right on to complete course and clinical NP requirements to obtain a master's or doctorate degree and take the NP certification exam (BLS, 2014).

All nursing schools in the US are expected to meet accrediting body standards and become accredited in order to confer the Master's (NP) degree. There are two major accrediting bodies for schools of nursing: the National League for Nursing (NLN) and the American Association of Colleges of Nursing (AACN).

NP education is population specific and not a generalist education. Therefore, all NP students first determine the specialty focus on which they want to concentrate before they are accepted into an NP program and begin their course work and clinical education (Figure 2) (Bednar et al., 2007). NP education focuses on the completion of NP core requirements. In 2011, the National Organization of Nurse Practitioner Faculties (NONPF) developed nine core competencies that must be demonstrated by all NP students upon graduation regardless of specialty focus (Table 1).

Since NPs enter the profession as specialists, they are certified to provide care within the boundaries of their certification and education (Keough, Stevenson, Martinovich, Young and Tanabe, 2011). For example, NPs interested in primary care could choose to specialize in primary care of the adult (Adult/Gerontology NP), family (Family NP), pediatrics (Pediatric NP) or women's health (Women's Health NP), etc. (Figure 2). In a similar fashion, NPs who chose acute care typically focused on an adult population (Adult/Gerontology Acute Care NP) or pediatrics (Pediatric NP). Since individual states do not recognize the same NP certification criteria, there is confusion regarding the current NP specialty population-focused model. In order to address this confusion, in 2008 the National Council of State Boards of Nursing (NCSBN) convened a specialty workgroup to develop an "Advanced Practice Registered Nurse Consensus Model" (Advanced Practice RN Consensus Workgroup and National Council of State Boards of Nursing (APRN/NCSBN) to explain NP certification and practice options (Figure 2) (APRN/NCSBN, 2008; Keough et al., 2011). This APRN Consensus Model consists of 4 "advanced practice" roles: certified registered nurse anesthetist (CRNA), certified nurse midwife (CNM), clinical nurse specialist (CNS), and certified nurse practitioner (CNP). APRNs are trained in one of these 4 roles and if the CNP role is chosen, then the CNP will choose at least one of six identified population foci specified in the paragraph above.

SUMMARY OF NP/PA EDUCATION

There are a great deal of similarities between NP and PA education (Table 1). In 2008, NONPF defined nine core competencies where graduating NPs must demonstrate successful achievement in order to graduate and continued competency. Achievement of these core competencies are described as a more accurate tool to measure goals than the total number of didactic and clinical hours completed.

Similarly, the Physician Assistant organization's (American Academy of Physician Assistants [AAPA], ARC-PA, PAEA and National Commission on Certification of Physician Assistants [NCCPA]) describe core competencies that graduated and licensed PAs must demonstrate through continuing education in order to maintain licensure and certification

(Table 1). Though NP core competencies are tied to an academic degree and PA core competencies are aligned with life long learning goals, the bottom line is that the core competencies for these professions are quite similar. One of the biggest differences in NP/PA education/profession is that PAs enter their profession and are educated as generalist while NPs enter the profession and are educated in a specialty area (Figure 2).

Table 1. NP and PA Core Competencies

6 PA Core Competencies *(AAPA, ARC-PA, PAEA, NCCPA)	9 NP Competencies **(NONPF)
Medical Knowledge Demonstrate core medical knowledge, surgical principles, disease prevention, health promotion; expected to demonstrate investigative and analytic thinking approach to clinical situations, analyze and understand evidence-based medicine. Understand a variety of clinical scenarios.	Scientific Foundation Critically analyzes data and integrates knowledge within the context of nursing science; develops new practice approaches based on research, theory and practice
Interpersonal and Communication Skills Encompasses verbal, nonverbal, written and electronic exchange of information. Includes the ability to effectively communicate information to patients, patients' families and physicians or other professional associates. Demonstrate emotional resilience and stability, adaptability, flexibility and tolerance to ambiguity and anxiety	Technology and Information Literacy Demonstrates information literacy skills and integrates technologies to improve healthcare
Patient Care Assessment, evaluation and management of patients. Delivers care that is effective, safe, high quality and equitable. Demonstrate compassionate and respectful behaviors when interacting with patients. Develop and implement patient care plans. Counsel and educate patients. Use information technology to support patient care decisions.	Practice Inquiry Leads practice inquiry, analyzes clinical guidelines, applies clinical investigative skills to improve health outcomes
Professionalism Expressing positive values and ideals as care is delivered. Must acknowledge their own limitations. Must maintain high level of responsibility, ethical practice, sensitivity to diversity in patient population. Adherence to legal and regulatory requirements.	Leadership Policy Ethics Assumes complex and advanced leadership roles to initiate and guide change. Advocates for ethical policies that promote access, equity, quality and cost.

6 PA Core Competencies *(AAPA, ARC-PA, PAEA, NCCPA)	9 NP Competencies **(NONPF)
Demonstrate professional relationships with physicians and other healthcare team members. Commitment to excellence and on-going professional development. Commitment to education of students and other healthcare professionals.	Demonstrates and understanding of the interdependence of policy and practice. Applies ethically sound solutions to complex issues related to individuals, populations and systems of care.
Practice-Based Learning & Improvement This is the process in which PAs critically analyze their own practice, the medical literature and resources for the purpose of self and practice improvement. Utilize information technology to manage information. Recognize and address personal biases, gaps in medical knowledge and physical limitations.	
Systems-Based Practice This includes the societal, organizational and economic environments in healthcare delivery. PAs must be aware and respond to the healthcare system. Effectively interact with different types of medical practice and delivery systems. Understanding funding sources and payment systems that provide coverage for patient care and use the systems effectively. Continue to focus on the patient with awareness of balancing quality and cost. Promote a safe environment for patients. Apply concepts of population health to patient care.	Health Delivery System Competencies Quality Facilitates the development of healthcare systems that address the needs of culturally diverse populations, providers and other stakeholders. Evaluates how organizational structure, care processes, financing, marketing and policy decisions impact the quality of healthcare. Applies skills and peer review to promote a culture of excellence.
	Independent Practice Functions as a licensed independent practitioner; Provides patient-centered care recognizing cultural diversity and the patient or designee as a full partner in decision making. Demonstrates the highest level of accountability for professional practice.

* AAPA (American Academy of Physician Assistants), ARC-PA (Accreditation Review Commission on Education for the Physician Assistant), PAEA (Physician Assistant Education Association), NCCPA (National Commission on Certification of Physician Assistants) (2012).

** NONPF (National Organization of Nurse Practitioner Faculty) (2012).

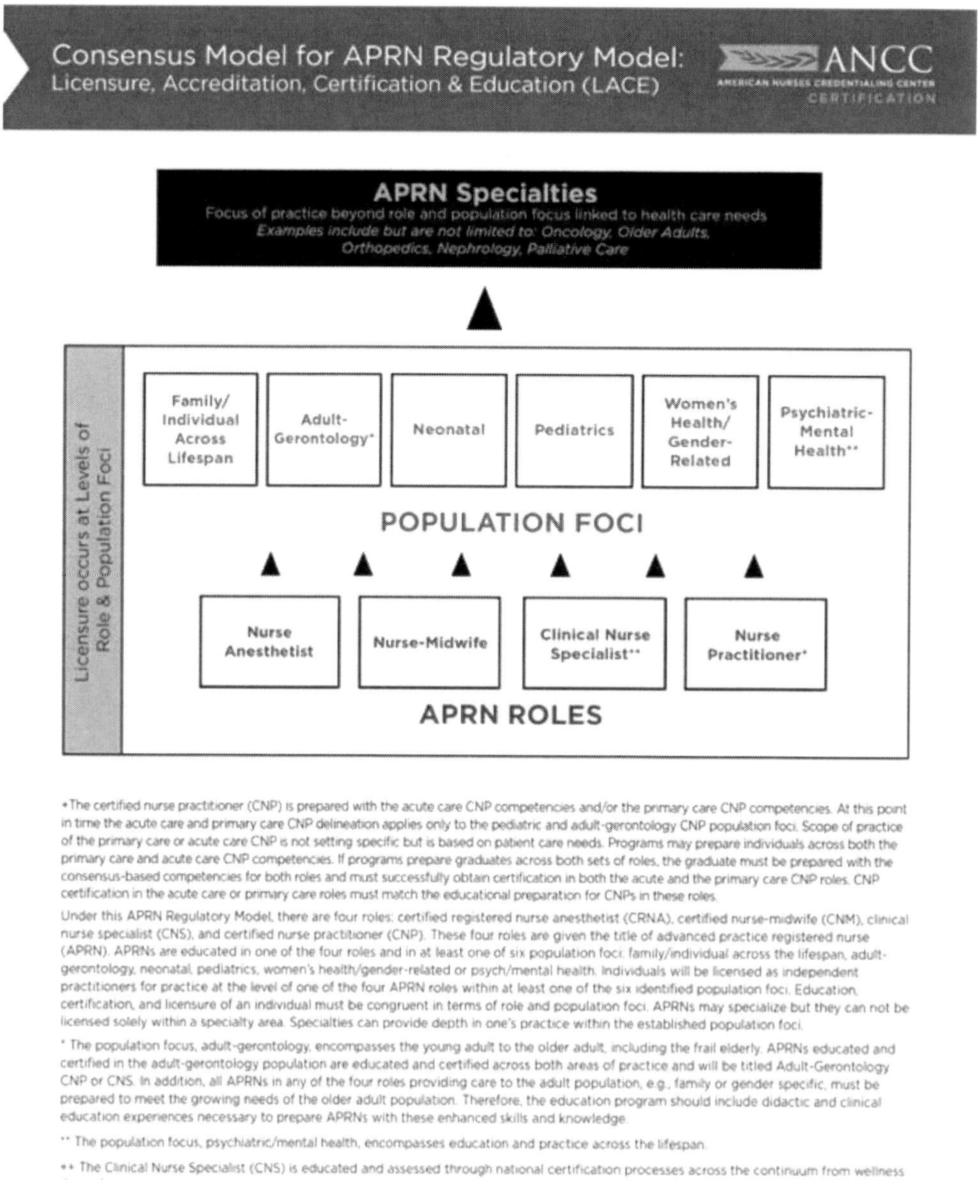

Figure 2.The Consensus Model for APRN Regulatory Model.

Certification and Licensure (Lifelong Learning)

Physician Assistants Certification and Licensure

Upon completion of the PA program, PAs must take a national certifying exam. In addition, PAs must re-certify every 6 years (and starting in 2014, every 10 years) and must complete 100 hours of continuing medical education (CME) every two years. PA certification requirements mandate that PAs must earn CME credits of performance improvement (PI)

CME and/or self-assessment CME every two years (NCCPA, 2013). This recertification model aligns with the recertification medical board model and encompasses 6 core PA competencies developed by NCCPA, AAPA, PAEA, and ARC-PA (AAPA, 2012). These competencies were initiated in order to promote the concept of team-based practice and improve patient outcomes. In addition, the core competencies will provide a template for the documentation of competences and accountability (see Table 1) (AAPA, 2012).

PA Expansion of Specialized Skills

Once certified, PAs are licensed by the state and once licensed, they have an option to expand their level of training and certification. There are several options for PAs to develop more specialized skills and experiences in one particular area of medicine. One way to achieve this is to attend a specialty residency program. There are a total of 43 residency programs registered with the Association of Postgraduate PA Programs (APPAP) throughout the country (APPAP, 2014). For example, Duke University has a PA residence program in surgery, Johns Hopkins has a post-graduate critical care residency for PAs, and Mayo Clinic in Arizona has a PA fellowship in hospital internal medicine. Northshore University Health Systems in Evanston, Ill has just begun a new PA fellowship program in emergency medicine (The Jane R. Perlman NP/PA Fellowship in Emergency Medicine).

PAs also have an opportunity to obtain a "certificate of added qualification" (CAQ). The NCCPA developed CAQs in order to acknowledge the unique set of specialized knowledge and skills required to work in specialty practices. In order for the PA to obtain certification in a specialty or subspecialty area, the PA must acquire addition continuing medical education (Category I CME), one to two (1-2) years of experience, procedures and medical cases specific to the specialty, and pass specialty exam (Table 2). Currently, CAQ is available in the following specialty areas: Emergency medicine, CV and Cardiothoracic surgery, Hospital medicine, Nephrology, Orthopedic surgery, Pediatrics, and Psychiatry. CAQ certification maintenance is on a 10 year cycle (NCCPA, 2013).

Table 2. Eligibility Requirements for Specialty CAQs

Eligibility Requirements for Specialty CAQs
1. Must hold "PA-C" designation
2. Must have a "valid/unrestricted" state PA license to practice as a PA or "unrestricted privileges" to practice as a PA for a governmental agency (All licenses held if there are more than one, must be "valid and unrestricted")
3. Minimum of 150 credits of specialty CME
4. Procedures and patient case logging appropriate for the specialty
5. 2,000-4,000 hours of experience working as a PA in the specialty
6. Take the specialty exam

Nurse Practitioner Certification and Licensure

NPs are certified in their specialty areas. Certification for NPs occurs through the American Nursing Credentialing Center (ANCC), the American Academy of Nurse Practitioners (AANP), or specialty organizations. The ANCC is a subsidiary of the American Nurses Association, the organization that represents all nurses in the US. Other professional organizations that credential NPs include the American Association of Critical Care Nurses (AACC), the National Organization of Obstetrics and Gynecology, National Association of Pediatric Nurse Practitioners, to name a few.

Certification for NP practice is required in most states and once certified, NPs are licensed by the specific state in which they practice. Individual states then regulate NP Practice.

Recertification is dictated by each certification body but in general requires a specified number of continuing education hours (CEUs) and documented practice hours every 3-5 years. As discussed earlier, the APRN Consensus Model provides some level of standardization for NP certification among states.

Currently there is no seamless path for NPs to switch specialty certification without returning to a formal NP program and obtaining additional certification and licensure. This process is in contrast to the PA generalist model. For example if an Adult NP wishes to add pediatric patients to her/his scope of practice, that NP would be required to enter an FNP or Pediatric NP post master's program in order to obtain certification and licensure to treat pediatric patients.

At this point in time, graduates of nurse practitioner programs are not required to complete a residency program, similar to PA graduates. There are several post-graduate residency programs for NPs that have developed throughout the nation. However, these programs are few and currently in the infancy stage of development. Residency programs provide NPs with additional didactic and clinical experience opportunities to advance their knowledge and skills in a specialty area (Flinter, 2012).

Credentialing and Privileging

Over the years, NP and PA roles have expanded to provide more of the functions historically provided by physicians (IOM, 2011). In 2011, Centers for Medicare and Medicaid Services (CMS) amended the definition of medical staff to include NPs and PAs (CMS, 2011). In response to the changes at CMS and as the number of NPs and PAs increase, the Joint Commission medical staff credentialing and privileging process for PAs and NPs has changed over the years to more closely resemble that of the physician provider (Joint Commission on the Accreditation of Hospitals Organization [JCAHO], 2011). In a growing number of institutions, PAs and NPs who provide "medical level of care" must now be credentialed and privileged by medical staff departments (as opposed to human resources). This decision was made in order to align the standards of the JCAHO with that of the CMS. According to the JCAHO, all PAs and NPs who provide "medical level of care" must use the medical staff processes for Ongoing Professional Performance Evaluation (OPPE) and Focused Professional Performance Evaluation (FPPE) for credentialing and privileging NPs and PAs (this requirement excludes non-CMS hospitals).

OPPE/FPPE are evaluation tools required by the joint commission and are intended to assure ongoing evaluation of a practitioner's privileges. Focused performance evaluation (FPPE) is a process used to evaluate competency in a specific "requested" privilege. In addition, if a specific patient care issue arises with a particular healthcare provider, FPPE could be the process used to monitor that particular provider's performance regarding a specific privilege. Institutions may choose to restrict state defined and legislated scope of practice of the NP/PA, however, they may never exceed it.

Scope of Practice

The PA profession emphasizes the value of the physician-PA team. The AAPA, AAFP and the AMA endorse a physician-led team with a strong physician-PA relationship to deliver high quality care (AAPA, March 2011a). The PA's license to practice is directly tied to the license of the physician. PAs work as a team member under the supervision of a physician with "delegated-autonomy". This means that the PA must be able to reach the physician if necessary, but the physician does not have to be physically present and directly supervising the PA while he or she is providing care to patients. The physician must be available by telecommunication or other means at all times. The level of autonomy and scope of practice of the PA is typically determined by the physician who ultimately is the most familiar with the PA's capabilities. The scope of practice for PAs emphasize patient centered care, with a focus on primary care and advanced specialized knowledge within their specialty area of practice (AAPA, Oct. 2011).

NP practice varies from state to state and is dependent on state nursing regulation (American Association of Nurse Practitioners [AANP], 2013). This regulation varies from total independence where NPs can practice independently without physician collaboration to NPs required to practice under the supervision of the physician (Figure 3).

Depending on specialty certification of the NP, the scope of practice for NPs emphasizes health promotion, disease prevention, chronic and acute care and patient advocacy. NPs combine the roles of mentor, provider, educator, administrator and researcher. NPs are accountable for promoting the best possible health care outcomes. In order to achieve this, NPs require national certification, measurement of clinical outcomes, a code for ethical practice, continuing professional development and maintenance of clinical skills. In addition, the AANP supports the concept of team based care as described in the IOM report (IOM, 2011) where interprofessional collaboration and coordination are the norm.

One major difference between NP and PA practice centers on licensure and supervision. Some states allow NPs to practice independently, without a physician collaborator. However, in all states PA practice must be linked with a physician license.

Inter-professional collaboration is a consistent theme among NP and PA education and practice initiatives. There are incentives among NP and PA programs to enhance and highlight opportunities for team collaboration among all health care professionals (Interprofessional Education Collaborative Expert Panel, 2011).

Practice Settings

NPs and PAs often practice in the same settings (BLS, 2009). The primary practice setting for both NPs and PAs is within a primary care physician practice.

State Variation in Scope-of-Practice Laws Governing Nurse Practitioners

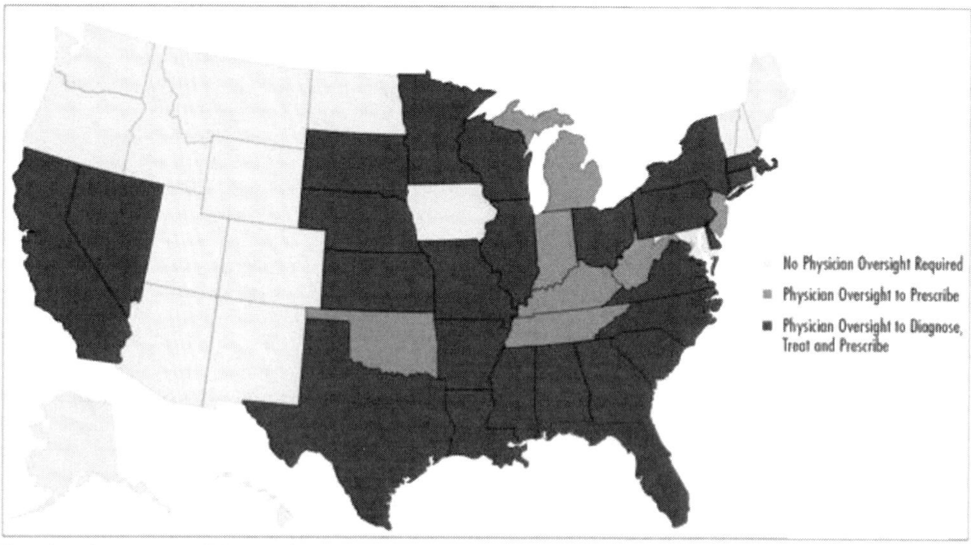

Note: Arkansas has two categories of NPs: registered nurse practitioners (RNPs) and advanced nurse practitioners (ANPs). RNPs are subject to physician oversight for diagnosing and treating and may transmit physicians' medication orders for noncontrolled substances. ANPs are subject to physician oversight for prescribing only.

Source: Pearson, Linda. The 2012 Pearson Report: A National Overview of Nurse Practitioner Legislation and Health Care Issues, *NP Communications, LLC, Monroe Township, N.J.*

Figure 3. NP practice variations by state.

The second most common practice areas are in general medicine and surgery. NPs and PAs also work in other practice setting such as government agencies, public health, retail clinics, and medical and surgical sub-specialties. NP managed clinics also exist (Robinson, 2000).

Utilization of both NPs and PAs has grown in academic medical centers across the country. Reasons cited for this increased utilization include accreditation, Accreditation Council for Graduate Medical Education (ACGME) resident duty hour restrictions and increase in patient throughput (Moote, 2011). A study involving the enhanced utilization of NPs and PAs at a level 1 trauma center in Pennsylvania revealed a significant reduction in ICU length of stay with no increase in rate of complications (Gillard, 2011). A published productivity assessment of NPs and PAs in an oncology setting by Moote (2011) revealed that though NPs and PAs reported similar activities, there was a high rate of variability in productivity. Productivity measurement for NPs and PAs can be challenging for a variety of reasons.

Many NPs and PAs working in tertiary care centers often do not bill for their services leaving no direct financial relationship between provider and patient. In addition, though academic centers have made a significant investment in NPs and PAs, measuring the financial impact has not yet become a priority. Though utilization of these providers has grown, only

69% of academic medical centers have measured the financial impact of NPs and PAs (Moote, 2011).

Although the NP and PA describe slightly different educational frameworks, clinical practice for both professions is nearly identical in many settings. According to an article in JONA investigating the debate of hiring an NP or PA by assessing the use of NPs and PAs in a specific oncology setting, it was found that the clinical role of both professions was quite similar (Reid Ponte, 2013). Both NPs and PAs manage patients, made assessments and diagnoses, and developed treatment plans. The level of involvement and communication with the attending oncologist was the same for both the NP and PA. In summary the similarities among the roles far outweighed the differences and a recommendation was made that hiring be based on whatever candidate best met the role requirements.

Legal Considerations for NPs and PAs

All healthcare professionals are held to a legal standard which hold them accountable to practice within the bounds of their education and certification (AAPA, March a, 2011; APRN/NCSBN, 2008). Whether their profession requires physician supervision or independent practice, PAs and NPs are accountable for the care they provide. All professionals are required to practice only within the scope of their education and certification.

NPs practicing in a collaborative relationship with a physician and PAs practicing under a supervisory relationship with a physician share legal accountability (Moses and Feld, 2007). When NPs practice in states that allow for independent practice, there is no shared legal accountability with a physician.

It is typical that malpractice insurance coverage is provided for NPs and PAs by their employers. NPs and PAs have the option to purchase medical malpractice insurance independent of their practice setting.

There are three major types of liability: Vicarious liability; negligent supervision; negligent hiring (Moses and Feld, 2007). Vicarious liability is a major area of concern. When a NP or PA is employed under a supervisory relationship with a physician and engages in an erroneous act, the physician can also be held liable for the actions of the NP or PA. Negligent supervision means that a physician is responsible for the PA or NP negligent acts if there was insufficient supervision. This issue is tied directly to lack of adequate supervision. Negligent hiring occurs when the physician provider knows that a NP or PA applicant is not competent to perform the duties required but hires the NP or PA anyway.

CONCLUSION

Although NPs and PAs are often educated in separate academic programs, in the practice setting, they often practice side-by-side, using the same standards of practice, seeing the same patients, performing similar assessment, diagnosis and treatment plans. In fact, the number of universities training NPs and PAs at the same institution has more than tripled, increasing from 21 to 66 across the country since 2006 (PAEA, 2014; AANP, 2014; Bednar et al., 2007).

This chapter demonstrates the similarities of the competencies for NPs and PAs which is becoming the standard for the measurement of educational outcomes. Competency based assessment focuses on outcomes and is moving away from more traditional measurements of NP and PA preparedness.

Both roles are filling gaps in the provision of healthcare in primary and acute care settings. The NP and PA professions began in the 1960's because there was a severe shortage of physician providers. Access to care and lack of adequate physician providers continues to be a challenge in today's healthcare environment. According to Association of American Medical Colleges (AAMC), there will be a shortage of 91,000 physicians by 2020 (AAMC, 2010).

The delivery of healthcare is moving toward a "Team-Based Approach" where teams of healthcare providers value, appreciate and depend on the success of the team to obtain the best outcomes for their patients. Moving the patient to the center of the care model challenges the team to breakdown the silos of conventional models of care toward a collaborative model of care with the best outcomes for the patient driving the model. The key to moving healthcare delivery toward a team based model is to fully utilize the growing NP/PA workforce, the sleeping giants. NPs and PAs have the education, the skills and the capacity to expand the healthcare teams and access to care for the nation. They remain the best kept secret in healthcare.

REFERENCES

Accreditation Review Commission of Education for the Physician Assistant. (2014). Accredited Programs. http://www.arc-pa.org/acc_programs/, Retrieved January, 2014.

Advanced Practice RN Consensus Workgroup and National Council of State Board of Nurses. (2008). Consensus Model for APRN Regulation: Licensure, Accreditation, Certification and Education. http://www.aacn.nche.edu/education APRNReport.pdf

American Academy of Physician Assistants. (2012). Competencies for the Physician Assistant Profession (Originally adopted 20c05; revised 2012). http://www.aapa.org/uploadedFiles/content/Your_PA_Practice/Practice_Regulation/Resource_Items/Competencies%20for%20the%20PA%20Profession%20-%20Approved%202012.pdf Retrieved January, 2014.

American Academy of Physician Assistants. (March, 2011). Professional issues. Issue Brief. Physician Assistant Education-Preparation for Excellence. http://www.aapa.org/uploadedFiles/content/The_PA_Profession/Federal_and_State_Affairs/Resource_Items/PI_PAEducation_v3.pdf Retrieved January, 2014.

American Academy of Physician Assistants. (March 2011a). Professional Issues. Issue Brief. The Physician-PA Team. https://www.aapa.org/uploadedFiles/content/The_PA_Profession/Federal_and_State_Affairs/Resource_Items/PI_PhysicianPATeam_v3.pdf. Retrieved January 2014.

American Academy of Physician Assistants. (March 2011b). State Law Issues. Issue Brief. The 6 Key Elements of a Modern Physician Assistant Practice Act. https://www.aapa.org/uploadedFiles/content/Common/Files/SL_KeyElements_v3.pdf Retrieved, Jan. 18, 2014.

American Academy of Physician Assistants. (Oct, 2011). Professional Issues. Issue Brief. Physician Assistant Scope of Practice. https://www.aapa.org/uploadedFiles/content/The_PA_Profession/Federal_and_State_Affairs/Resource_Items/PI_PAScopePractice_110811_Final.pdf. Retrieved Jan. 18, 2014.

American Association of Colleges of Nursing. (2006). The Essentials of Doctoral Education for Advance Nursing Practice. American Association of Colleges of Nursing, Washington DC.

American Association of Colleges of Nursing. (2014). Your Guide to Graduate Nursing Programs. http://www.aacn.nche.edu/publications/brochures/GradStudentsBrochure.pdf. Retrieved February 26, 2014.

American Association of Nurse Practitioners. (2014). NP Program Search. http://npprogramsearch.aanp.org/search. Retrieved 2/17/2014.

American Association of Nurse Practitioners (2013). Scope of Practice for Nurse Practitioners. https://www.aanp.org/images Retrieved Jan. 18, 2013.

American Association of Nurse Practitioners. (2010). Nurse Practitioner Curriculum. http://www.aanp.org/images Accessed 2/17/2014.

American Nurses Association. (2014). Masters Nursing Programs. http://www.aacn.nche.edu/publications/brochures/GradStudentsBrochure.pdf Retrieved February 26, 2014.

Association of American Medical Colleges. (2010). Physician Shortages to Worsen without Increasing Residency Training. AAMC Center for Workforce Studies, June 2010 Analysis. https://www.aamc.org/download/286592/data/ retrieved Jan. 18, 2013.

Association of Post-Graduate PA Programs. (January 2014). APPAP Programs by Specialty. http://www.appap.org/LinkClick.aspx?fileticket=z%2bAXVB1RUOE%3dandtabid=58 Retrieved January, 2014.

Bednar, S., Atwater, A., Keough, V. (2007). Educational Preparation of Nurse Practitioners and Physician Assistants. An Exploratory Review. *Advance for Emergency Nursing Journal.* 29, (2), 158-171.

Bureau of Labor Statistics (BLS). (2012). Occupation, Employment and Wages, May 2012. www.bls.gov/oes/current/oes291171.htm Accessed on Dec. 29, 2013.

Bureau of Labor Statistics (BLS). (2014). How to Become a Nurse Anesthetist, Nurse midwife, or Nurse Practitioner, January 2014. http://www.bls.gov/ooh/healthcare/nurse-anesthetists-nurse-midwives-and-nurse-practitioners.htm#tab-4. Retrieved February 26, 2014.

Clabo, L. L, Giddens, J., Jeffries, P., McQuade-Jones, B., Morton, P., Ryan, S. (2013). A Perfect Storm: A Window of Opportunity for Revolution in Nurse Practitioner Education. *Journal of Nursing Education*, 51(10), 539-541.

Department of Health and Human Services Center for Medicare and Medicaid. (2011). CMS Manual System, Pub. 100-07, State Operation Provider Certification. http://www.cms.gov/Regulations-and-Guidance/Guidance/Transmittals/downloads/R78SOMA.pdf Retrieved February, 26, 2014.

Dower, C., and O'Neil, E. (2011). Primary care health workforce in the United States. *Research Synthesis Report No. 22*. Princeton, N. J.: Rood Wood Johnson Foundation.

Flinter, M. (2012). From New Nurse Practitioner to Primary Care Provider: Bridging the Transition through FQHC-Based Residency Training. *Online Journal of Issues in Nursing,* 2012, Jan. 17 (1).

Gillard, J. N., Szoke, A., Hoff, W., Wainwright, G. A., Stehly, C., Toedter, L. J. (2011). Utilization of PAs and NPs at a Level 1 Trauma Center: Effects on Outcomes. *Journal of Am Acad of Physician Assistants,* 24:7, 34-43.

Hooker, R. S. and Everett, C. M. (2011). The Contributions of Physician Assistants in primary care systems. *Health and social care in the Community*, 20(1), 20-31.

Institute of Medicine. (2011). The future of nursing: leading change, advancing health. Washington, DC: National Academies Press.

Interprofessional Education Collaborative Expert Panel. (2011). Core competencies for interprofessional collaborative practice: Report of an expert panel. Washington, D.C.: Interprofessional Education Collaborative.

Joint Commission for the Accreditation of Hospitals (2011). Standards BoosterPak for Focused Professional Practice Evaluation and Ongoing Professional Practice Evaluation. http://www.mc.vanderbilt.edu/documents/CAPNAH/files/Forms/Competency%20Evaluation%20Forms/TJC%20Booster%20Pack%20FPPE-OPPE.pdf Retrieved February, 2014.

Keough, V., Stevenson, A., Martinovich, Z., Young, R., Tanabe, P. (2011). Nurse Practitioner Certification and Practice Settings: Implications for Education and Practice. *Journal of Nursing Scholarship,* 43 (2), 195-202.

Laurant, L. M., Reeves, D. Hermens, R., Braspenning, J., Gorl, R. and Sibbald, B. (2006). Substitution of Doctors by Nurses in Primary Care. The Cochrane Database of Systematic Reviews, Issue 1.

Moote, M., Krsek, C., Kleinpell, R., Todd, B. (2011). Physician Assistant and Nurse Practitioner Utilization in Academic Medical Centers. *American Journal of Medical Quality,* 26 (6), 452-460.

Moses, R, and Feld, A. (2007). Physician Liability for Medical Errors of Non-Physician Clinician: Nurse Practitioners and Physician Assistants. *American Journal of Gastroenterology,* 102, 6-9.

National Commission on Certification of Physician Assistants. (2013). Certification Maintenance. http://www.nccpa.net/CertMain. Retrieved January, 2014.

National Commission on Certification of Physician Assistants. (2013). Specialty Certification of Added Qualification (CAQ). http://www.nccpa.net/SpecialtyCAQs. Retrieved January, 2014.

National Organization of Nurse Practitioner Faculties. (2012). Nurse Practitioner Core Competencies.http://c.ymedn.com/sites/www.nonpf.org/resource/resmgr/competenciies/npcorecompetenciesfinal2012.pdf Retrieved 2/17/2014.

Physician Assistant Education Association. (2014). PAEA program directory. http://directory.paeaonline.org/. Retrieved January, 2014.

Physician Assistant Education Association. (2013). Twenty-seventh Annual Report (2010-2011): Physician Assistant Educational Programs in the United States. Alexandria, VA. http://www.paeaonline.org/index.php?ht=a/GetDocumentAction/i/149930 Retrieved January,2014.

Peterson, L. E., Phillips, R. L., Puffer. C., Bazemore, A. and Peterson, S. (2013). Most family physicians work routinely with nurse practitioners, physician assistants or certified nurse midwives. *J. Am. Board Fam. Med.,* 26 (3), 244-245).

Pulcine, J. and Wagner, M. (2002). Nurse practitioner education in the United States: A success story. *Clinical Excellence for Nurse Practitioners*, 6(2), 51-56.

Reid Ponte, P, O'Neill, K. (2013). Hiring into Advanced Practice Positions; The Nurse Practitioner versus Physician Assistants Debate. *The Journal of Nursing Administration*, 43(6) 329-335.

Robinson, K. R. (2000). Nurse-managed primary care delivery clinics. *Nursing Clinics of North America,* 35 (2), 471-9.

Stead, E. (1966). Conserving costly talents: Providing physician's new assistants. *The Journal to the American Medical Association,* 198(10), 182-183.

Tumolo, J. (2004). Captains of their ships. Four NPs who took the plunge and started their own practices. *Advance for Nurse Practitioners*, 12(6), 47-50.

US Bureau of Labor Statistics (2012). http://www.bls.gov/ooh/healthcare/nurse-anesthetists-nurse-midwives-and-nurse-practitioners.htm#tab4. Retrieved 2/17/2014.

PART 2: CLINICAL SETTINGS FOR PRACTICE

In: Collaboration with the Advanced Practice Nurse ISBN: 978-1-63321-311-1
Editors: E.R. Giardino, R.G. Hanks and A.P. Giardino

Chapter 5

PRIMARY CARE NURSE PRACTITIONER

Rebecca Tsusaki, PhD, RN, WHNP-BC, Daisy Mullassery, MSN, RNC-OB, WHNP-BC, Rebecca Helmreich, PhD, RN, WHNP-BC and Diane Wind Wardell, PhD, RN, WHNP-BC
School of Nursing, The University of Texas School Health Science Center at Houston, Houston, Texas, US

ABSTRACT

The role of the advanced practice registered nurse (APRN) in providing primary care to patients across the lifespan has developed since the 1960s. Over the past 40 years, APRNs have evolved to meet strict educational requirements, training, skill sets, accreditation, and certification requirements. The services provided by APRNs have become an integral part of today's healthcare system. This chapter addresses the educational background of primary care nurse practitioners, the types of primary care nurse practitioners, and regulations of practice. There is discussion of the consensus-based entry-level primary care objectives that represent the nurse practitioner population foci of adult, gerontology, pediatric and women's health and their use in conjunction with the APRN core competencies that determine graduate nursing education curriculum in four population concentrations.

INTRODUCTION

Primary care in the United States (U.S.) has been historically under-addressed and the ill effects related to lack of primary care understudied. Even though the U.S. spends substantially higher amounts of money than other developed countries for healthcare, the results are not commendable. In reality, the morbidity and mortality of the U.S. population is far worse than other industrialized countries (U.S. Department of Health and Human Services, 2014). Besides, the upward trajectory of healthcare expenses is not displaying any signs of recession. About 75% of our healthcare dollars are spent to manage chronic conditions which points to the acute need for improved primary care (Centers for Disease Control [CDC], 2009). When death rate of individuals belonging to the age group of less than 75 years was compared among 19 industrialized countries, all the countries except the U.S. showed an adjusted decrease in death rate of 16% whereas the U.S. had a decline of only 4% (Nolte & McKee, 2008). While the etiology for such a disparity is multifaceted, lack of systematized primary care efforts is cited as one of the major reasons. Countries with well-structured primary care programs seem to improve quality of life, prevent diseases, and decrease mortality rate (Starfield & Shi, 2002).

Approximately 75% of Advanced Practice Registered Nurses (APRN) work in primary care in the adult-gerontology, family, pediatric, women's health and midwifery specialties in the United States (Naylor & Kurtzman, 2010). APRNs or nurse practitioners (NPs) have worked as primary care providers since the 1960's and their number continues to grow to meet the changing needs of health care delivery. The pioneering NPs blended the art and science of nursing with the provision of illness management traditionally administered by physicians. Seeking to establish new roles and collegial relationships with physicians and administrators, pioneering nurse practitioners worked hard to define their role as quality primary care providers while facing obstacles to the autonomous provision of this care (Brown & Draye, 2003). NPs face many of the same obstacles today in providing primary patient care. Resistance from physician groups, insurers, and regulatory bodies often inhibit the ability of the NP to practice at the full potential of their education and training (Reagan & Salsberry, 2013). There also lacks a consensus on the nurse practitioner scope of practice among the individual state regulatory agencies, which further confounds definition of the nurse practitioner role in providing primary care.

The American Association of Medical Colleges (AAMC) reports a projected primary care physician shortage of 65,800 by year 2025 (AAMC, 2010). This projected shortage comes at a time of increasing primary health care need since health reform in the United States will continue to increase the demand for primary care providers. The predicted future shortfall of the primary care workforce increases the need for certified nurse practitioners (NP). In response, graduate nursing programs have increased by 61% to try and meet these increasing needs (Naylor & Kurtzman, 2010).

The Patient Protection and Affordable Health Care Act (ACA) allocates funds for the development and function of community-based and nurse managed primary health care clinics (Liu, Finkelstein, & Poghosyan, 2014). Nurse practitioners are in a unique position to mediate the shortages of primary care providers and contribute significantly to the provision of quality comprehensive, cost-effective and holistic care to those in the community, whether they choose to work as part of an inter-professional team or as an independent provider (Poghosyan, Lucero, Rauch, & Berkowitz, 2012). This chapter will examine how primary care is defined, the effect of the Consensus Model on primary care roles, the current APRN primary care roles and the future trends in the provision of primary care.

Initiation of Regulations

Training and certification curriculum guidelines were loosely defined in the early days and were originally created by the AAP and later jointly with the American Nurses Association. These early guidelines were informal and most university or hospital-based programs varied in length from four to 18 months (AANP, 2013b). The Association of Faculties of Pediatric Nurse Practitioners (AFPNP) was established in 1972 and began to create curriculum standards. In 1978, the AFPNP established the first national pediatric nurse practitioner certification examination that was administered by the National Certification Board of Pediatric Nurse Practitioners and Associates (NCBPNP/A), currently known as the Pediatric Nursing Certification Board (PNCB) (AANP, 2013b; Berg, Hawkins-Walsh, Gaylord, Lindeke, & Docherty, 2011). In 1973 the National Association of Pediatric Nurse Associates and Practitioners (NAPNAP) was established after a group of pediatric nurse practitioners from six states met informally in Ohio to determine if they should affiliate with other professional nursing and medical associations. The group eventually decided to remain an independent organization and currently serves over 7,500 members (NAPNAP, 2013).

In 1970, the ANA proposed modification of the role definition of nursing to include APN scopes; Idaho became the first state to redefine nursing to include APNs and many states followed suit (Fontenot & Hawkins, 2011). The American College of Nurse-Midwives began offering certification programs so that nurse midwives could be credentialed as Certified Nurse Midwives (CNMs) in 1971 (ACNM, 2009). Similarly ANA began credentialing services including certification for nurse practitioners and in 1978 APNs predominantly caring for women were offered certification as maternal-gynecologic practitioners (ANA, 1978). Later on, in mutual agreement with ANA, the Nurses Association of the American College of Obstetricians and Gynecologists (NAACOG) started credentialing OB/GYN nurse practitioners and the designation of OB/GYN nurse practitioner was changed to women's health nurse practitioner (WHNP) in 1995 reflecting care provided by them for women across the life span. The NAACOG later assumed its current name, the Association of Women's Health, Obstetric, and Neonatal Nurses (AWHONN) (Fontenot & Hawkins, 2011). The credentialing body was named National Certification Corporation (NCC) in 1993, overseeing credentialing of WHNPs and Neonatal Nurse Practitioners (NNPs) exclusively (NCC, 1999).

As noted by Fontenot and Hawkins (2011), pioneer NPs had to face many hurdles to practice and most of it stemmed from lack of regulations, statutes, and even lack of understanding among healthcare personnel including nurses about the scope of practice of a NP. In the beginning there was a great deal of discrepancy in roles and functions of NPs between states that continues today. Early on NPs may have been under both the board of nursing and board of medicine, with medical tasks being delegated to them by the physicians whom they worked, and almost all NPs had to depend on physicians to write prescriptions or order tests. Lack of protocols and guidelines was another issue and NPs had to depend solely on their collaborating physicians for practice support. Another challenge was third party reimbursement; there was no way a nurse practitioner would be reimbursed directly by insurance companies, they lacked legal provider status and identification numbers (Fontenot and Hawkins, 2011).

In the early years there were a variety of specialties (i.e. oncology nurse practitioner, perinatal nurse practitioner, emergency nurse practitioner) but in order to create more consistency in education, training, and certification these specialties were either merged or eliminated. By doing so, programs were also able to broaden the student base by offering more general fields like family and adult health. This also increased the flexibility of the NP in employment.

The American Association of Colleges of Nursing (AACN) in 2002 prepared the report *Nurse Practitioner Primary Care Competencies in Specialty Areas: Adult, Family, Gerontological, Pediatric, and Women's Health* for the Department of Health and Human Services, Health Resources and Services Administration, Bureau of Health Professions, Division of Nursing (NONPF & AACN, 2002). The consensus-based entry-level primary care objectives were developed by nine professional nursing organizations that represented the nurse practitioner population foci of adult, gerontology, pediatric and women's health to use in conjunction with the APRN core competencies to determine graduate nursing education curriculum in these four population concentrations.

Effect of Consensus Model

To further define competencies NONPF again worked with multiple other professional nursing organizations to develop a statement on primary and acute care certified NPs based on the 2008 Consensus Model of APRN Regulation. The 2008 Consensus Model recognizes that the CNP is prepared for the nurse practitioner role and that any description of the acute and/or primary care role with delineation occurs at the level of the population foci. Currently the delineation between acute and primary care is only applied to the Adult Gerontology and Pediatric NP population foci (NONPF, 2013).

Traditionally, the acute care setting was determined to be the hospital setting and the primary care setting in the community. The scope of practice of primary and acute care CNPs is actually non-specific to the practice setting, but based on educational preparation of the CNP and the needs of the patient. The acute and primary care settings occur along a continuum of care venues that may overlap and graduate or doctoral programs may prepare nurse practitioners for both roles (APRN Consensus Work Group & the National Council of State Boards APRN Advisory Committee, 2008; NONPF, 2012). The Consensus Model does not specifically define primary care, but the description of the CNP includes the concepts commonly included in most definitions of primary care and includes the provision of comprehensive care, health screening, health promotion and education, and diagnosing and treating patients with both acute and chronic illnesses (NONPF, 2013). Nurse practitioners are prepared at the graduate or doctoral level to provide primary care across settings both at first patient contact and the continued provision of health care (AANP, 2013a). Patient-centered health promotion and education, fundamental concepts of the nursing profession, are integrated into the primary care practices of diagnosing and treatment of acute and chronic illnesses. Models of health care delivery in the United States are rapidly changing with the Affordable Care Act, growth in aging population, and chronic illnesses. Focus on the future of primary health care needs in all sectors of American population with the rapid transformation of health care gives rise to opportunities for the CPN to expand their practice and fulfill these needs.

PRIMARY CARE ROLES

There are certified nurse practitioners (CNP), midwives (CNM), clinical nurse specialists (CNS) and nurse anesthetist (CRNA) outlined in the Consensus Model for APRN Regulation in which an APRN has prepared for through an accredited graduate-level or post-graduate advanced nursing education program that builds on the competencies of registered nurses (APRN Consensus Work Group & the National Council of State Boards APRN Advisory Committee, 2008). In the CNP role there are four primary care focused roles that include pediatrics, women's health, adult-gerontology and family; and additional primary care role is also held by CNMs. The Consensus Model recommendation to combine the adult and gerontology roles was done in recognition of the population and roles that NPs working with adults will encounter.

Passing a national certification examination that measures the APRN role and focused competencies is required for licensure. Irrespective of the specialty branch, all NPs are trained to evaluate an individual's health, diagnose health and medical conditions, manage health problems by developing a viable individualized plan of care, and promote health by providing screening, preventive services, patient teaching, and counseling.

PEDIATRIC NURSE PRACTITIONER

The certified pediatric nurse practitioner (PNP) provides primary and/or acute care services to the pediatric population from birth to age 21. The PNP is educationally prepared to provide primary care to the pediatric population by assessment, diagnoses, and management of patient problems across health-wellness-illness continuum using both pharmacologic and non-pharmacologic measures. Holistic provision of care also includes health promotion and education. The PNP can further specialize beyond the role of PNP, but official state board licensure occurs in one of the four defined Consensus Model APRN roles and within the pediatric population foci (APRN Consensus Work Group & National Council State Boards of Nursing, 2008).

The specific competencies of the PNP are identified to provide care of children from birth through young adult with an in-depth knowledge and experience in pediatric primary health care including well child care and prevention/management of common pediatric acute illnesses and chronic conditions. This care is provided to support optimal health of children within the context of their family, community and environmental setting.

They assess all aspects of the patient's health status, including health promotion needs, health protection, and disease prevention. Obtaining a relevant and thorough health history of children, allows for age-appropriate screening for developmental and behavioral concerns such as speech/ language development, learning disabilities and behavioral and mental health concerns. Assessing the child's developmental status allows for the recognition of individual differences, in temperament, reactions to selected developmental tasks, situational crises and coping styles and strategies. Further, the impact of such factors as genetic background, prenatal factors, parenting style and significant life events are assessed and analyzed. Family systems are evaluated to identify factors that influence the health of the child and adolescent including, but not limited to family dynamics, communication style, values, beliefs, risk factors and health indicators such as physical activity and eating disorders.

They are engaged in the diagnosis of health status using the diagnostic process of critical thinking, differential diagnosis, and the integration and interpretation of various forms of data. They differentiate between normal and abnormal development in relation to anatomical, physiological, motor, cognitive, psychological findings, and social behavior of children. Identification of developmental considerations, pathogenesis, and clinical manifestations of common disease process are often aided by ordering and interpreting age and situation appropriate screening, labs and other diagnostic tests. These labs and tests may include but not limited to, hematocrit, lead level, tuberculosis testing, ova and parasites. The PNP collaborates with the health care team in the diagnosis of children with special health needs and disabilities.

Another competency of the role for the practitioner is in stabilizing the patient, minimizing physical and psychological complications, and maximizing the patient's health potential. Among the behaviors of this competency is to promote healthy nutritional practices and intake considering food preferences and avoidance of food sensitivities. The PNP is also acutely aware of and focused on providing interventions to modify behavior associated with health risks such as tobacco and substance abuse, lack of physical activity, nutritional patterns, sexual activity and violence. Making referrals for children in need to appropriate community agencies and for family support and specialty care as needed, and incorporating health objectives into individual educational plans for children with special needs are also within their scope of practice.

The PNP is also cognizant of the practitioner-patient relationship as it relates to therapeutic patient outcomes. Communication is the key to impart knowledge and associated psycho-motor skills to patients. Acting in the role as a coach involves skills of interpreting and providing individualized therapies through the activities of advocacy, modeling, and tutoring to assist the child in assuming responsibilities for self-care and healthy behaviors in accordance with age and developmental readiness. The PNP demonstrates a commitment to the implementation, preservation, and evolution of their role. The PNP also maintains current knowledge regarding state and federal programs for child and family health care. Monitoring public issues that impact the delivery of health services for children and their families, and recognizing the influence of cultural variations on child health practices, including child rearing are also competencies esteemed by the PNP.

WOMEN'S HEALTH AND MIDWIVES

Women's Health Nurse Practitioners (WHNP) are trained to care for women across the life span whereas Certified Nurse Midwives (CNM) concentrate on care for childbearing age women including pregnancy and delivery. The focus in this section will be on the WHNP.

It is the expectation that a WHNP once graduated and certified will be able to take care of women's health issues across the life span and also care for men with infertility issues, sexual dysfunction and sexually transmitted Infections (STIs). This is a very different picture when compared to the programs designed in the 1970s. The OB/GYN or FPNPs of those days were only expected to care strictly for issues related to OB, GYN, and Family Planning (Marecki, 2006).

During the teen and adolescent years, the WHNP concentrates on providing services including but not limited to immunizations, sexual health and safe sex practices, birth control, and gynecological issues. During childbearing years the WHNP manages birth control, prenatal care, infertility issues and post-partum care. Some WHNPs provide care for special needs such as high risk antepartum patients and follow them throughout their pregnancy and post-partum period. Also, they take care of various gynecologic issues that child bearing age women experience. During transitional years in a women's life the WHNP manages menopause and associated hormonal imbalances and other special needs related to the process of aging. In addition, WHNPs identify, treat, and refer primary care problems common to this age group. For the older women, the WHNPs role differs slightly as they pay more attention to general health issues of women that are gender related such as osteoporosis, breast health issues and cardiovascular problems to name a few.

During any of the life phases mentioned above, women benefit from a holistic approach to healthcare leading to optimum outcomes. When healthcare delivery systems get fixated on associating women with child bearing, overall health promotion and management of chronic problems get overlooked (Walker & Tinkle, 1996). This becomes even more important since we know now that different disease occurrences, manifestations and management is greatly different between men and women. Closing this gap can only be achieved by incorporating primary care in to practice. One of the major roles for WHNPs practicing in primary care settings is to screen women for general health problems such as heart disease, hypertension, diabetes, and manage or refer these patients appropriately.

WHNPs approach gender specific events as normative transition and help women to overcome physical and mental issues related to those normal developmental changes. They are specially trained to recognize unique health care needs of the marginalized and non-traditional patients. Special attention is paid to disease manifestations specific to women thus addressing them more effectively. It is safe to say the role of WHNPs that began as very focused and narrow has broadened and deepened over time as educational programs, statues, and regulations became more clear and specific.

Adult Gerontology Primary Care

Changes to the adult nurse practitioner (ANP) role have occurred over time as seen by the recent consensus model recommendation that the gerontology role merge with the ANP role by 2015 and further delineated the population focus by in-patient (acute care) or out-patient (primary care) status. The Adult Gerontology Nurse Practitioner-Primary Care (AGNP-PC) is the NP designated title that is discussed in this section. The AGNP-PC has a broad focus that includes the management of acute and chronic illness as well as preventative health care for the adult individual (AACN, 2010). They do not cover pediatric or obstetrical care services but can manage gynecological services for well women and those with acute (i.e. infections) and chronic (i.e. pelvic pain) diseases. The AGNP-PC is able to manage both genders so is often more versatile in their scope of practice. The competencies of the AGNP-PC are identified within seven domains according to AACN (2010) and include: management of health and illness, the nurse-patient relationship, teaching and coaching, maintaining a professional role, managing and negotiating health care delivery systems, providing quality care, and being culturally sensitive.

Some examples of services provided by the AGNP-PC include supportive care and management of cardio-vascular diseases like hypertension and heart disease, acute upper respiratory infections like colds and pneumonia, acute illnesses like flu and flu-like symptoms, gastro-intestinal disturbances such as reflux and inflammatory bowel, and endocrine disorders like hypothyroidism and diabetes to name a few.

The AGNP-PC is also acutely aware of and focused on health promotion and prevention of disease. In the primary care setting they often provide guidance on weight management, exercise, dietary and nutritional needs, smoking cessation, healthy environments, and wise alcohol consumption. Besides the physical needs of the patient the AGNP-PC is also aware of the importance of life-style choices that affect health so is a key player in promoting stress management, healthy personal relationships with family and friends, and psychological health.

Besides general practice and clinics the AGNP-PC can also function in a supervised role within any of the specialties. Usually the practice has a designated focus and the AGNP-PC works in collaboration with a physician. The services provided in these settings may be more specific to the nature of the practice and depend on training and/or state law in which they practice. For example, within a cardiology specialty the AGNP may do advanced cardiac monitoring and interpretation of cardiac tests or in a dermatology clinic preform biopsies, suturing, and cyrotherapy.

Because of the more intense training in gerontology the AGNP also manages elders in the primary care setting that may extend to homes, community centers, long term care facilities, and assisted living centers. Elderly patients are more likely to have chronic illness that create persistent and life changing demands on the person. The AGNP is uniquely qualified to manage the aging population as their foundational knowledge in the aging process brings an expanded understanding to the management of acute and chronic illness as well as preventative health care (AACN, 2010). The AGNP also brings knowledge about the effects of aging in the area of chronic disease and acute illness and adds a greater depth of understanding in prevention of falls, functional assessments and the performance of daily living tasks that include such things as independence in bathing, dressing, feeding, and managing house tasks. Besides the physical needs of the patient the AGNP is also aware of the importance of maintaining healthy personal relationships with family and friends, maintenance of cognition and psychological health. They can perform assessments, make management decisions and provide referrals where appropriate.

The AGNP has comprehensive knowledge about aging that makes them particularly in demand as health care providers as the demographics (i.e. aging baby boomers) in the United States changes. They also can provide independent or group practice management on those in long-term care facilities. Their focus is prevention of disease, management of acute and chronic health issues and compassionate care during death.

Family Nurse Practitioner

The specific competencies of the certified Family Nurse Practitioner (FNP) are identified to provide care to the family unit, as well as the individuals belonging to the family however the family chooses to define itself in the context of the community. The FNP has a broad knowledge and experience with people of all ages (AACN & NCHE, 2013). The FNP practices primarily in ambulatory care settings. Obtaining a relevant and thorough health history for patients of all ages and in all phases of the individual and family life cycle, allows for appropriate comprehensive or symptom-focused physical examinations on patients of all ages, including developmental and behavioral screening during physical system evaluations. Among the items assessed are conditions related to developmental delays and learning disabilities in all ages, women's and men's reproductive health (including but not limited to sexual health, pregnancy, and postpartum care), and problems of substance abuse and violence. Assessing the impact of an acute and/or chronic illness or common injury on the family as a whole¸ and distinguishing between normal and abnormal changes with aging are among the focused behaviors for the FNP.

FNPs are engaged in the diagnosis of health status using the diagnostic process of critical thinking, differential diagnosis, and the integration and interpretation of various forms of data. They identify signs and symptoms of acute and chronic physical and mental illness across the life span. Data from diagnostic tests and screening procedures are analyzed and synthesized to formulate comprehensive differential diagnoses, considering epidemiology, environmental and community characteristics, and life stage development, and behavioral risk factors.

The FNP acts to stabilize patients, minimizing physical and psychological complications, and maximizing the patient's health potential. Among the behaviors of this competency is to treat common acute and chronic physical and mental illnesses and common injuries in people of all ages to minimize the development of complications, and promote function and quality of life, to prescribe medications with knowledge of altered pharmacodynamics and pharmacokinetics with special populations such as infants and children, pregnant and lactating women, and older adults, make appropriate referrals to other health care professionals and community resources for individuals and families and assist families and individuals in the development of coping systems and lifestyle adaptations. Further, the FNP will perform primary care procedures, including, but not limited to, suturing, minor lesion removal, splinting, microscopy, and pap tests. The FNP applies research that is family-centered and contributes to positive change in the health of and health care delivery to families.

The FNP is also acutely aware of and focused on the practitioner-patient relationship that relates to therapeutic patient outcomes. Communication is the key to impart knowledge and associated psycho-motor skills to patients. They act in the role as a coach, and function to involve the skills of interpreting and individualizing therapies through the activities of advocacy, modeling, and tutoring to assist the child in assuming responsibilities for self-care and healthy behaviors in accordance with age and developmental readiness. The FNP demonstrates a commitment to the implementation, preservation, and evolution of the family nurse practitioner role, maintains current knowledge regarding state and federal programs for child and family health care. The FNP also monitors public issues that impact the delivery of health services for families and recognizes the influence of cultural variations on health practices (HRSA, 2002; AACN & NCHE, 2013).

Future Trends

Models of health care delivery in the United States are rapidly changing with the Affordable Care Act, growth in aging population, and chronic illnesses. Focus on the future of primary health care needs in all sectors of American population with the rapid transformation of health care gives rise to opportunities for the APRN to expand their practice and fulfill these needs. In addition to an expanded focus the educational training of the NP is also moving to a practice doctorate (DNP).

In conclusion, NPs continue to evolve in response to the health care needs of society and provide valuable care to some of the most vulnerable populations. The importance of NPs can no longer be questioned as they have become integral to delivering high quality health care.

References

Affordable Care Act. (n.d.). About the Law. Retrieved February 3, 2014, from http://www.hhs.gov/ healthcare/rights/.

Association of American Medical Colleges. (2010). The Impact of Health Care Reform on the Future Supply and Demand for Physicians Updated Projections Through 2025. Retrieved from https://www.aamc.org/download/158076/data/updated_projections_through_2025.pdf

American Association of Colleges of Nurses. (March, 2010). Adult-gerontology primary care nurse practitioner competencies. Retrieved from http://www.aacn.nche.edu/publications/.

American Association of Colleges of Nurses. (2013). Population focused Nurse Practitioner competencies: Family across the lifespan, Neonatal, Pediatric acute care, Pediatric primary care, Psychiatric-mental Health, Women's Health / Gender related. Retrieved February 12, 2014 from www.aacn.nche.edu/education-resources/Population.

American Academy of Family Physicians. (2014). Primary care: AAFP policies. Retrieved from http://www.aafp.org/about/policies/all/ primary-care.html.

American Academy of Nurse Practitioners. (2013a). The American Asssociation of Nurse Practitioners: Nurse practitioners in primary care. from http://c.ymcdn.com/sites/ www.nonpf.org/resource/resmgr/imported/ ACPCStatementFinalJune2012.pdf.

American Academy of Nurse Practitioners. (2013b). Historical timeline. from http:// www.aanp.org/about-aanp/historical-timeline.

American College of Nurse-Midwives. (2009). ACNM position statement - Midwifery certification in the United States. Retrieved February 3, 2014, from www.midwife.org

American Nurses Association. (1978). ANA funds certification program for two years: News areas added. *American Journal of Nursing*, *78*, 534-541.

APRN Consensus Work Group & the National Council of State Boards APRN Advisory Committee. (July 7, 2008). *Consensus Model for APRN regulation: Licensure, accreditation, certfication and education.* Retreived Feb 5, 2014, From https://www.ncsbn.org/4213.htm

Berg, M., Hawkins-Walsh, E., Gaylord, N., Lindeke, L., & Docherty, S. L. (2011). Emerging issues regarding pediatric nurse practitioner education in acute and primary care. *Journal of Pediatric Health Care, 25*(1), 62-66. doi: 10.1016/j.pedhc.2010.07.002.

Brown, M. A., & Draye, M. A. (2003). Experiences of pioneer nurse practitioners in establishing advanced practice roles. *Journal of Nursing Scholarship, 35*(4), 391-397.

Centers for Disease Control and Prevention (CDC). (2009). *The power of prevention: Chronic disease . . . the public health challenge of the 21st century.* Retrieved from http://www.cdc.gov/chronicdisease/pdf/2009-power-of-prevention.pdf.

Johns Hopkins Bloomberg School of Public Health, (2014). Definitions: What is primary care? Retreived from http://www.jhsph.edu/research/centers-and-institutes/johns-hopkins-primary-care-policy-center/ definitions.html.

Fontenot, H., & Hawkins, J. W. (2011). The evolution of specialists in women's healthcare across the life span: Women's health nurse practitioners. *Journal of the American Academy of Nurse Practitioners, 23*, 314-319.

HRSA, U.S. Department of Health and Human Services. (2002). Nurse Practitioner Primary Care Competencies in specialty areas: Adult, Family, Gerontological, Pediatrics, and Women's Health. U.S. Department of Health and Human Services Health Resources and Services Administration Bureau of Health Professionals Division of Nursing.

Kass-Wolff, J. H., & Lowe, N. K. (2009). A historical perspective of the women's health nurse practitioner. *Nursing Clinics of North America, 44*, 271-280.

Liu, N., Finkelstein, S. R., & Poghosyan, L. (2014). A new model for nurse practitioner utilization in primary care: Increased efficiency and implications. *Health Care Management Review, 39*(1), 10-20. doi: 10.1097/HMR.0b013e318276fadf.

Marecki, M. (2006). The past, present, ad future of the advanced practice role in women's healthcare. *Journal of Perinatal and Neonatal Nursing, 20*(1), 79-81.

Murphy, M. A. (1990). A brief history of pediatric nurse practitioners and NAPNAP 1964-1990. *Pediatric Health Care, 4*, 332-338.

National Association of Pediatric Nurse Practitioners. (2013). About NAPNAP - History. Retrieved 02/02/14, from http://www.napnap.org/aboutUs.aspx.

National Certification Corporation. (1999). NCC certification exams. Retrieved February 3, 2014, from http://www.nccwebsite.org/certification/exam-detail.aspx?eid=16

National Organization of Nurse Practitioner Faculties. (2012). Statement on acute care and primary care certified nurse practitioner practice 2012. From http://c.ymcdn.com/sites/www.nonpf.org/resource/resmgr/imported/ACPCStatementFinalJune2012.pdf.

National Organization of Nurse Practitioner Faculties. (2013). National Organization of Nurse Practitioner Faculties: Primary care and acute care certified nurse practitioners 2013. From http://c.ymcdn.com/sites/www.nonpf.org/resource/resmgr/consensus_model/acpcnpstatementfinal2013.pdf.

National Organization of Nurse Practitioner Faculties, & American Association of Colleges of Nurses. (2002). *Nurse practitioner primary care competencies in specialty areas: Adult, family, gerontological, pediatric, and women's health.* (HRSA 00-0532(P)). Rockville, MD: Retrieved from http://www.aacn.nche.edu/education-resources/npcompetencies.pdf.

National Research Council (1994). Defining primary care: An interim report. Washington, DC: The National Academies Press.

Naylor, M. D., & Kurtzman, E. T. (2010). The role of nurse practitioners in reinventing primary care. *Health Affairs, 29*(5), 893-899.

Nolte, E., & McKee, C. M. (2008). Measuring the health of nations: updating an earlier analysis. *Health Affairs*, *27*(1), 58-71.

O'Brien, J. M. (2003). How nurse practitioners obtained provider status: Lessons for pharmacists. *American Journal of Health-System Pharmacy*, *60*(22), 1-13.

Poghosyan, L., Lucero, R., Rauch, L., & Berkowitz, B. (2012). Nurse practitioner workforce: A substantial supply of primary care providers. *Nursing Economics, 30*(5), 268-294.

Reagan, P. B. & Salsberry, P. J. (2013). The effects of state-level scope-of-practice regulations on the number and growth of nurse practitioners. *Nursing Outlook, 61*(6), p.392-399. doi: 10.1016/j.outlook.2013.04.007.

Starfield, B., & Shi, L. (2002, June). Policy relevant determinants of health: an international perspective. *Health Policy*, *60*(3), 201-218.

U.S. Department of Health and Services. (2013). Human Title X: The national family planning program. Retrieved from http://www.hhs.gov/opa/pdfs/title-x-national-family-planning-overview.pdf.

U.S. Department of Health and Services. (2014). *Healthy People 2020.* Retrieved from http://www.healthypeople.gov/2020.

Walker, L., & Tinkle, M. (1996). Toward an integrative science of women's health. *Journal of Obstetric and Gynecologic Nursing*, *25*(5), 379-382.

World Health Organization. (2014). Primary health care. from http://www.who.int/topics/primary_health_care/en/.

In: Collaboration with the Advanced Practice Nurse ISBN: 978-1-63321-311-1
Editors: E.R. Giardino, R.G. Hanks and A.P. Giardino

Chapter 6

THE ACUTE CARE NURSE PRACTITIONER

Fran Stokes, DNP
Director Adult/Gerontology Acute Care Nurse Practitioner Program, University of Texas Health Science Center, Houston, TX, US
Acute Care Nurse Practitioner, ICU, Methodist Sugar Land Hospital, Sugar Land, TX
Consultant, NICHE Program, New York, US

ABSTRACT

Acute Care Nurse Practitioners (ACNP) are advanced practice nurses who provide care to patients with acute and complex conditions. They manage patients with specialized health care needs from critical care to discharge and facilitate the patient's transition to the community. ACNPs manage patients across the continuum of acute care services in both acute care inpatient and outpatient settings. The ACNP completes patient assessments, orders diagnostic and interventional procedures, has prescriptive privileges, and diagnoses complex clinical conditions. ACNPs treat patients in a variety of clinical practice settings including high and low acuity in-patient hospital units, as well as in the home. The ACNP scope of practice is based on the patient needs, rather than the setting in which the NP works (Bell, 2008; APRN Joint Dialogue Group Report, 2008) (APRN Consensus Work Group, 2008) This chapter addresses the development of the specialized ACNP role in advanced practice, what the ACNP does in clinical practice, the educational process, and scope of practice.

INTRODUCTION

Acute Care Nurse Practitioners (ACNP) provide care to patients with acute and complex conditions. They focus on the management of chronic illness, the care of acutely ill patients, and health promotion (Howie & Erickson, 2002). There are separate educational programs to become either a pediatric or an adult-gerontology acute care CNP. ACNPs manage patients with specialized health care needs from critical care to discharge and facilitate the patient's transition to the community. ACNPs manage patients across the continuum of acute care services in both acute care inpatient and outpatient settings. The ACNP completes patient assessments, orders diagnostic and interventional procedures, has prescriptive privileges, and diagnoses complex clinical conditions. ACNPs treat patients in a variety of clinical practice settings including high and low acuity in-patient hospital units, as well as in the home. The ACNP scope of practice is based on the patient needs, rather than the setting in which the NP works (Bell, 2008; APRN Joint Dialogue Group Report, 2008) (APRN Consensus Work Group, 2008).

The Pediatric and Adult-Gerontology Acute Care Nurse Practitioner

The APRN Consensus work group devised the LACE model (licensure, accreditation, certification, education) to bring continuity to APRN practice throughout the country and define the basics of advanced practice nursing through national guidelines for the licensure, certification, accreditation and education of advanced practice nurses (APRN Consensus Work Group, 2008). The work group recommended that ACNPs be educated broadly across the entire scope of adult, gerontology and pediatric practices (Cortes, 2012). The two population foci for the acute care nurse practitioner are pediatric and adult/geriatric. Prior to the LACE consensus model, the ACNP was certified as an adult ACNP rather than an adult/geriatric ACNP. Many adult acute care NP programs have converted traditional Adult ACNP programs to Adult-Gerontology Acute Care Nurse Practitioner (AGACNP-BC). Pediatric nurse practitioner programs are separated into primary care focus and an acute care focus to keep pace with the Consensus Model recommendations (Cortes, 2012). ACNPs can specialize after graduation in areas of Oncology, Cardiology, and Nephrology, to name but a few. The patient age focus of Adult-Gerontological ACNP programs include people ages of 18 years to the elderly (Reider-Demer, Zielinski, Carvajal, Anulao, & Van Roeyen, 2008).

ACNP Role: Historical Development

The role of Acute Care Nurse Practitioners (ACNP) started in the 1960s as pediatric and adult nurse practitioners emerged in clinical practice areas. There have been nurse practitioners (NPs) in acute care settings since the advent of the nurse practitioner role. A precursor to the current ACNP role started in the 1950s when Thelma Ingles, a professor of Medical Surgical Nursing at Duke University, met the Chairman of the Department of Medicine at Duke University, Dr. Eugene Stead, through department meetings and inpatient rounds. Ingles and Stead worked together in a mentor and student type relationship in the acute care hospital setting as Ingles learned more specific content and skills related to acute care practice. Ingles was so impressed by what she learned during one year of tutelage with Stead that she wanted to replicate her acute care focused educational experience with other nurses. In 1958, Ingles and Stead developed a curriculum for the Duke University nursing program for the inpatient setting. The new clinical role of nurse clinician in an acute care setting incorporated the nursing scope of practice with an advanced skill set for of the acute care focused nurse (Politt & Reesman, 2011). The skills taught in this nursing program included taking a patient's medical history and performing an associated physical examination, which were not the usual nursing practices. A Rockefeller Foundation grant enabled Duke University to develop the first nursing clinical specialty program. The first class began in 1958 with 5 nursing students. The program was one year in length and included weekly didactic content, clinical rotations, and research. Duke physicians lectured in the advanced nursing courses. Students spent six weeks in four mandatory specialty clinical areas of cardiology, respiratory, neurology and gastroenterology and then completed courses in two other clinical areas including obstetrics, pediatrics or psychiatry (Politt & Reesman, 2011).

The initial acute care nursing program at Duke University closed by 1962 as the program did not receive National League of Nursing (NLN) accreditation, apparently due to concerns about the strong medical influence over nursing practice (Holt, 1998; Politt & Reesman, 2011). Dr. Stead forged ahead with the acute care curriculum and developed a program which focused on military corpsman students and did not include nurses. In 1965, Stead and the Duke University Medical School admitted the first Physician Assistant class (Holt, 1998; Politt & Reesman, 2011).

Expansion of the ACNP Role

The ACNP role expanded as the need to enhance and support in-patient medical care arose. In the mid 1990s, concerns arose from outside of the medical community that the practice of resident physicians working 80 to 100 hours per week in impatient settings was placing patients in potentially harmful situations. The medical community determined that physician residents could not work more than 80 hours per week in hospital settings. The Accreditation Council for Graduate Medical Education (ACGME) placed an 80 hour per week limit on resident physician hours on duty (Accreditation Council for Graduate Medical Education, 2013). The restriction on resident work hours to 80 hours per week reduced the number of in-house physicians during all hospital shifts. The 80 hour cap made it necessary for academic medical centers and hospitals to hire more physicians, physician assistants, nurses, and other staff to compensate for the decreases in resident work hours (Block & Norton, 2007).

The influx of complex and acutely ill patients, coupled with reduced resident hours and fewer physicians caused a general shortage of medical staff to care for in-hospital patients. Academic medical centers sought a solution to the shortage of physicians to cover the medical needs of patients in acute care settings through the use of ACNPs in acute care settings (Block & Norton, 2007).

ACNP Education

ACNP educational programs are specific for the pediatric or adult-gerontology population. The level of education for ACNPs is at the masters or doctoral level. Most pediatric or adult-gerontology programs are at the master's level where the graduate receives a master of science in nursing (MSN) degree from an accredited university program. The

ACNP curriculum focuses on APRN competencies that as delineated by the American Association of Colleges of Nursing documents (Bell, 2008).

After the completion of the ACNP educational program, graduates are then eligible to take either the pediatric or adult-gerontological national certification examination. Most states require evidence of passing the national certification examination in the specific population that the ACNP student was educated (Bell, 2008; APRN Consensus Work Group, 2008; APRN Joint Dialogue Group Report, 2008).

Scope of Practice

The ACNP delivers comprehensive advanced nursing care to meet the specialized needs of patients experiencing critical, acute, and/or complex chronic health conditions. ACNPs may provide care is any clinical setting where there are patients with acute care needs. The ACNP acknowledges that acute, critical, and/or complex chronic illness care is dynamic and requires individualization to the specific needs of each patient (Bell, 2008). ACNPs are not certified to practice in primary care settings or in general hospital emergency departments. They practice in a number of clinical settings where patients have acute care needs. For example, the ACNP can work in a cardiac catheterization lab, all inpatient units, high acuity intensive care units (ICUs), and in a clinic that provides care to patients with acute care illnesses, to name a few practice sites.

Licensure, Scope of Practice, Certification, Credentialing and Hospital Privileges: Licensure

Individual State Boards of Nursing mandate licensure and scope of practice for ACNPs. The ACNP is a registered nurse and holds a current nursing license to obtain and maintain their advanced practice registered nurse (APRN) license, and adhere to RN regulations as well. Most states require that the ACNP hold national certification as an acute care nurse practitioner. States that do not require NPs to pass the national certification exam for acute care do require validation that the NP graduated from an accredited acute care masters in nursing program in order to meet state board of nursing certification requirements. It is incumbent upon each ACNP to determine specific State Board of Nursing requirements for both the RN and APRN License.

In most states, the ACNP must maintain national certification to work in the advanced practice role. The two national certifying bodies, the American Association of Critical Care Nurses (AACN) and the American Nurses Credentialing Center (ANCC), require the APN to recertify every 5 years. Each certifying body has specific continuing education requirements and guidelines for certification renewal.

ACNP Credentialing and Privileges

The ACNP must be credentialed and obtain hospital privileges to work as a nurse practitioner in a specific institution. Credentialing is part of the Joint Commission oversight and a process by which a hospital and its governing body gives the health care provider authority to provide patient care within the hospital setting (Hittle, 2010; Smolenski, 2005). The institution reviews the education, certification, training, skills, and licensure of the NP to determine if the clinician meets institution standards. Credentialing is granted on the hospital or institution level through established medical by laws. The process is also guided by the state boards of medicine and nursing as well as Medicare and Medicaid regulations at the state and federal level. While the state in which an ACNP practices may allow for independent or full practice, each health care institution may enact its own restrictions on ACNP practice.

The credentialing process vets the education, experience and background of the practitioner. ACNPs are usually credentialed through the medical staff office or department of medicine, however, credentials could also be obtained through the department of nursing, or even human resources. Individual institutions determine their own credentialing process.

Prescriptive authority requirements granted to ACNPs vary by state. Some states require the APRN to apply through the state board of pharmacy while others may grant prescriptive authority through the APRN licensure process granted through the state board of nursing. ACNPs in the acute care setting usually require a Drug Enforcement Administration (DEA) license for narcotic prescriptive authority. The employer and ACNP should research healthcare institutional requirements along with the requirements for state licensure, and prescriptive authority, and specific before applying to a specific institution.

Privileging

Privileging is a process in which the health care institution grants permission for the NP to provide specific aspects of patient care. Privileges usually encompass a list services and procedures the practitioner may perform in an institution. The institution grants permission for the NP to carry out specific tasks and responsibilities such as admitting patients, prescribing medications, and performing specific procedures. Within states, the NPs scope of practice as stated by the state Nurse Practice Act may allow certain patient care responsibilities, while a hospital may limit the NP to perform those same privileges within the hospital setting (Hravank, 2009; Hittle, 2010).

The NP application for privileges is reviewed by an institution's credentialing committee once an application is complete. Clinical procedures may require the NP to demonstrate competency to complete that procedure through a protocol check off process. For example, central line placement may require that a physician observe the practitioner to safely place 5 central lines before granting the privilege to perform the procedure. The hospital may set the criteria by which they grant privilege to perform specific clinical procedures. Procedures vary according the ACNPs role and requirements. For example, an ICU ACNP may require privileges to perform invasive procedures such as central line placement or intubation, while a cardiology ACNPs may need privileges to admit and discharge patients and administer conscious sedation for cardioversions.

ACNP Licensure, Collaboration and Independent Practice

The ACNP must be licensed and certified by the state in which she practices. State certification for advanced practice nursing requires a specific educational background, national certification as an acute care nurse practitioner in either an adult, adult/geriatric, or pediatric focus (APRN Consensus Work Group & National Council of State Boards of Nursing APRN Advisory Committee, 2008). State boards of nursing in each state dictate the terms of practice for the ACNP. Some states require a regulated collaborative agreement with a physician in order for the NP to provide patient care, while other states require a regulated collaborative agreement with a physician to provide patient care (American Association of Nurse Practitioners, 2013).

State legislatures dictate collaboration relationships between ACNPs and physicians, while other collaborative relationships are hospital or institution based. At least 15 states in the US passed legislation for independent practice which removes the need for a collaboration requirement with a physician (Vestal, 2013; AANP, 2013). Independent practice implies that the CNP may practice without the need to collaborate or have a physician supervise the CNPs practice. In states where ACNPs may practice independently, they practice under their own license, which includes state conferred prescriptive authority and DEA licensure.

ACNP Programs Abroad

ACNP programs abroad are designed and regulated individually in each country. There currently is no educational continuity internationally for ACNP programs. The lack of educational continuity abroad shows the need to apply a consistent education, licensing, credentialing and certification model around the world.

Practice Settings for the ACNP

ACNP graduates fill a variety of roles in acute care settings. Adult/Geriatric ACNPs (AGCNP) may work in most acute care environments that treat the adult and geriatric patient population. These areas include acute inpatient, intensive care units of all varieties, emergency departments, urgent care centers, skilled nursing facilities, rehabilitation facilities, and long term care environments. AGCNPs work in specialty practice areas such as cardiology, pulmonary, and oncology, acute care walk-in clinics and general adult emergency departments.

Both adult and pediatric ACNPs are utilized in high acuity transfer situations which include life flight, flight nursing, and in ground transport. The skill sets of ACNPs vary depending on the acute care area in which the ACNP works. Depending on specialization, ACNPs training occurs both in the master's program and during their post education clinical sites where they learn to intubate, manage ventilators, manage dialysis treatment, place central lines and perform other invasive procedures which are traditionally performed by medical/surgical residents, anesthesia personnel and surgeons. ACNPs are integral to procedure teams, rapid response teams and as first assist in some operating rooms (Daniele, Bova, LeGar, Smith, & Shortridge-Baggett, 2010; Kleinpell, Ely, & Grabenkort, 2008; Scherr, Wilson, Wagner, & Haughian, 2012; Schroeder, 2008; Sonday, Grecsedk, & Del Casino, 2010). Skills unique to specific acute care areas are enhanced after ACNPs graduate, pass national certification, gain state licensure to practice and are granted privileges as providers at their hospitals and sites of practice.

Current Issues in ACNP Nursing

Acute Care Nurse Practitioners are uniquely trained and adept in caring for the adult hospitalized patient (Klienpell, 1997). ACNPs address the care transitions of the acutely ill patient population. Acute care specialization has continued to develop due to an increasing inpatient census of patients spanning the age continuum a new need for specialization has had downstream affects for ACNPs. Today over 50% of patient admissions to acute care non specialty facilities are 65 years of age and older (NICHE, 2013).

Statistical predictions that by 2015, there will be a severe shortage of physicians in the United States of over 62,000 and estimated at 130,000 by 2025 (Dorio, 2013; Squiers, King, Wagner, Ashby, & Parmley, 2012). A physician intensivist shortage is also predicted (Klienpell, 1997). There are approximately 6,000 intensive care units in the US, and approximately 55,000 critically ill patients occupying beds in ICUs (Amba, 2011). Complicating matters are the number of aging elderly who are projected to utilize these services (SCCM, 2014).

The lower numbers of students enrolling into medical school programs is indicative of a physician shortage over the next 20 years (Cooper, 2004; Petterson et al, 2012). The growing need for highly trained and highly skilled practitioners for inpatient setting will not change over the next 40 years due to the increase in the number of the aging population and increased access to medical care for all age groups. The role of the NP in the acute care setting will become even more apparent as physician shortages are felt across the country and around the world.

As more ACNPs enter the realm of acute care, it will be important to further define scope of practice and defining outcome measures for metric comparison. Kapu and Kleinpell (2012) discuss the importance of outlining and defining NP associated metrics for outcome measurement and assessment. Doing so would help identify NP contributions to the healthcare team, to patients and employers. Defining metrics for NP related outcomes would also validate those same contributions and possibly point to yet untapped NPs as resources to create new and emerging roles for this valuable member of the healthcare team.

EFFECTIVENESS OF ACNP PRACTICE

The development and implementation of the ACNP role caused mixed emotions in the medical community regarding the skill and expertise of ACNPs to manage the care of acutely ill inpatients (Dorio, 2013). However, many physicians support the practice of specialty trained acute care nurse practitioners. There are a number of studies that address aspects of ACNP inpatient practice. Early studies evaluated the acute care role in comparison to medical and surgical resident's effectiveness and efficiency and evaluated ordering practices, safety, outcomes and length of stay. Later studies evaluated indirect outcomes of NP influence such as length of stay, glucose management and patient satisfaction (Hylka & Beschele, 1995; Larkin, 2003; Sidani, et al., 2006; Ettner, 2006).

It has been difficult to study the ACNP's direct impact on inpatient care due to a lack of randomized control trials (RCT) on the subject (Kleinpell, 2005) and difficulty in determining the cost of patient outcomes related to ACNP care as physicians often bill for inpatient care and services that the ACNP actually completed.

Larkin (2003) evaluated the substantial cost saving benefits of utilizing the ACNP in the acute care setting. In 1999, the University of Virginia Health System nurse practitioner model realized a $2.4 million savings in its first year. The success of the use of ACNPs in the program was attributed to NP skills, collaboration with physicians, and experience with applying evidence based practice (Larkin, 2003).

A study that looked at cost savings of an NP/MD practice model verses an MD or medical resident only practice model found that patient outcomes and cost containment over a four month period (Ettner, 2006). Findings showed that cost savings for the NP/MD model after adjustments for post discharge medical usage were an approximate and significant 978 dollars ($978) per patient. Overall, ACNPs in acute care settings are competent members of the healthcare team and are considered a valuable asset to patient care, team strength and safe patient outcomes.

ACNPs and Patient Satisfaction

Patient satisfaction studies of ACNPs in the acute care setting show that having nurse practitioners in units improves patient, nursing staff and physician satisfaction, while shortening length of stay and improving outcomes (Bruce & Steinke, 2006; Stanik-Hutt et al.,2013). Another study that compared perceptions of patients cared for by ACNPs and physician residents found higher levels of satisfaction with overall care and an increased level of physical, psychological and social functioning upon discharge with ACNPs (Sidani et al, 2006).

Van Oyen Force (2013) attributes a number of reasons that ACNPs achieve high satisfaction ratings to both similarities and differences between ACNPs and physicians/residents. Contributions to overall increased patient satisfaction are related to the ACNP spending more time reviewing charts, documenting and interacting with the patient, families and nurses. ACNP who are unit based are the mainstay for continuity. Physicians and residents often rotate assignments which make ACNPs invaluable to patient care continuity and patient flow (VanOyen Force, 2013).

ACNPs have a positive effect on patient satisfaction scores as well as nursing staff. Nursing staff rated ACNPs positively for ease of communication, ability to talk with the NP, and ability to create an environment of trust and non-judgment which can relieve the bedside nurse stress and improve satisfaction (Stanik-Hutt, et al, 2013; VanOyen-Force, 2013). Studies of physician perceptions of ACNPs found ACNPs to be reliable and an asset to the healthcare team because of their ability to spend more time with patients, and understand the diagnosis, treatment and evaluation processes involved in inpatient care. NPs also understand what to look for in changing levels of acuity, act on those changes and understand how to translate this information to the physician staff when indicated. When ACNPs are unit based either in ICU or on inpatient units, patient and family, staff and physician satisfaction is greatly enhanced.

Reimbursement and Billing for ACNP Services

There are a variety of ways in which ACNPs services are reimbursed through Medicaid, Medicare and private insurers. The reimbursement process is complicated and can be fraught with difficulty due to varying hospital Medical Staff By-Laws which can place restrictions on NP progress notes. Billing for ACNP services in the inpatient setting can be difficult and complicated. One of the reasons for this is the Centers for Medicare and Medicaid Services (CMS) rules and regulations which restrict billing by NPs in specific situations in the inpatient setting. One regulation is that NPs must have a supervising physician in the inpatient setting. Supervision is loosely interpreted by each hospital and each state (Buppert, 2009). There is incongruity from state to state and hospital to hospital adding to role, credentialing and licensure confusion. The variation in rules from state to state and hospital to hospital has an effect on direct work of NPs as recorded through the EMR

The second situation which confounds data collection can be contributed to the CMS rule and regulation for NP reimbursement in the inpatient setting (Buppert, 2009). This causes an indirect affect when considering using EMR data. The rule is that if an NP sees a patient and bills for the patient, then the NP will only be reimbursed 85% of the CMS reimbursement rate. Medicare uses 'Incident to' billing which states that the institution can receive 100% of the physician fee for NP services if: 1) the NP work is performed under the supervision and direction of the physician, 2) the physician is on site with the ACNP, 3) the physician treats the patient on the first visit, 4) the service be within the NP scope of practice in the state, and 5) the bill for service is submitted under the physician's provider identification number (IOM (Institute of Medicine), 2011). For the reason of Incident to billing, it makes fiscal sense to bill for NP services and care under Incident to billing. In order for the physician to bill when an ACNP delivers care to the patient, the physician must either sign the NP note with a statement verifying the patient was fully evaluated by the physician through a face to face encounter, or write a separate note with this same statement validating the face to face encounter with the patient. When the physician signs a statement such as this, s/he takes credit for the visit (Buppert, 2009).

DOCTOR OF NURSING PRACTICE AND THE ACNP

The purpose of the DNP degree for the ACNP is to enhance medical acumen coupled with systems thinking nursing skills in order to succeed and serve the ever growing number patients accessing healthcare. The focus of DNP education is to better understand and apply concepts of population healthcare with overlapping systems thinking.

The Doctor of Nursing Practice (DNP) Degree for advanced practice nurses is a natural extension for the progression of the ACNP degree plan. The DNP degree enables ACNPs nurses to address the ever increasingly complex practice roles, improve patient outcomes, and strengthen leadership skills to improve healthcare delivery. The second component involves specialty competencies. These are related to the competencies, content and practicum experiences for practice within a specialty area such as Acute Geriatric Care or Acute Pediatric Care. The competencies for NPs are derived from their core competencies for practice. An example of this would be the Acute Geriatric Care Nurse Practitioner core competencies.

The ACNP DNP graduate with a focus on patient care, should be able evaluate practice and system trends utilizing scholarly work in order to make recommendations regarding populations within their respective healthcare systems (AACN, 2014).

Role Issues/Conflicts

Role issues and conflicts related to ACNP practice have traditionally been related to situations where the NP role is new to an organization, unit or clinic. The misunderstanding of what an advanced practice nurse does in these environments can be challenging especially when staff have not worked with ACNPs. This usually stems from the lack of understanding of why they are now in this environment and what the APRN will be doing. When preparing to introduce the ACNP role into a new environment it is prudent to have a clear business plan in place which discusses billing, coding and procedures. One of the main reasons implementation and role confusion occurs when ACNPs are introduced is a lack of preparation by administration (Irvine et al., 2000). Appropriately preparing key stakeholders is a crucial step to success. Bringing the value of the role to each and every member of the healthcare team is important, especially physicians.

Conflicts can arise in acute care because of the complexities of adding a new provider into the billing, coding and reimbursement mix. Physicians do not always understand the benefits of adding an APRN and cannot understand the financial benefits. The regulations and rules of the Centers for Medicare and Medicaid have require the APRN to have a supervising physician. The reimbursement rate for APRNs is less than for physicians, as APRNs are reimbursed for their services at a lower rate even if the APRN fully manages the patient.

Role issues can be quickly dispelled by the appropriate support of physician staff and administration. However, role conflicts can and do occur when there are residents in the mix who overlap with the ACNP in the care of inpatients. Defining the role of ACNPs in these situations is important. ACNPs often can help residents learn procedures and help the residents learn how unit operations work and flow. Faculty attending physicians set the standards for practice in the ICU and on the floor where residents practice. When ACNPs and residents work together on a team, it is the physician attending who often assigns responsibilities to the team members which then prevents potential conflicts that arise from role confusion.

Conclusion

The roles of the ACNP are changing to be more population specific by adding the specialty foci of Geriatrics and Pediatrics to the Acute Care Nurse Practitioner education and certification. Although Pediatric NPs have been practicing in the inpatient setting, adjustments have been made to accommodate the acute care aspects of care for this patient population. These nurses will gain the education and training which will enhance their skills in the acute care arena.

ACNPs are found in all areas of healthcare. Increasing the number of ACNPs to all areas and specialty practice they will help decrease the access burdens felt by healthcare administrations and physicians. As ACNP doctorate level graduates merge into our societies, they will bring higher levels of clinical competence and new ideas to practice applications for our ever increasingly complex patient populations.

The ACNP role has proven to be a valuable member of the healthcare team in both inpatient and outpatient settings. Studies have shown that the clinical outcomes of ACNPs have proven to be similar to physicians and residents in the inpatient and ICU setting. They are skilled care coordinators and masters of communication with families and the healthcare team. They teach patients and staff in a way which resonates enabling the message to received and understood. The ACNP at the master's and doctorate level is the right application of this highly trained, educated and astute clinician to improve outcomes while cutting costs through decreased length of stay, while improving efficiency and effectiveness. ACNPs enhance patient, staff and physician satisfaction which has a positive effect on nursing and physician retention. Studies have supported the use of ACNPs to support the healthcare team in delivering safe and effective care. Healthcare and nursing must come together and realize that in order to sustain safe and appropriate care we must, as the healthcare team, change our old world view of advanced practice nurses and their roles in the future schema of healthcare.

References

AANP (2013). State Practice Environment. American Association of Nurse Practitioners [On-line]. Available: https://www.aanp.org/legislation-regulation/state-legislation-regulation/state-practice-environment

Accreditation Council for Graduate Medical Education. (2013). ACGME program requirements for graduate medical education in internal medicine. Accreditation Council for Graduate Medical Education [On-line]. Available: https://www.acgme.org/acgmeweb/Portals/0/PFAssets/2013-PR-FAQ-PIF/140_internal_medicine_07012013.pdf

American Association of Critical Care Nurses. (2014). Retrieved from http://www.aacn.org/

American Association of Nurse Practitioners. (2013). 2013 Nurse Practitioner State Practice Environment. State Nurse State Practice Acts And Administration Rules, 2012 [On-line]. Available: http://www.aanp.org/images/documents/state-leg-reg/stateregulatorymap.pdf

Amba, K. (2011). Acute care NPs have new opportunities in the virtual ICUs. *Nurse Practitioner World*. Retrieved from http://www.webnponline.wordpost/2011/10/27/ Nurse-Practitioner-World-News..

APRN Consensus Work Group & National Council of State Boards of Nursing APRN Advisory Committee. (2008). Consensus Model for APRN Regulation: Licensure Accreditation, Certification & Education. APRN Joint Dialogue Group Report.

APRN Consensus Work Group & National Council of State Boards of Nursing APRN Advisory Committee (2008). Consensus model for APRN regulation: Licensure, accreditation, certification & education National Council of State Boards of Nursing.

APRN Consensus Work Group. (2008). Consensus model for APRN regulation: Licensure, accreditation, certification & education.

Bell, L. (2008). AACN Scope and Standards for Acute and Critical Care Nursing Practice. Aliso Viejo, CA: American Association of Critical-Care Nurses.

Block, A. E. & Norton, D. M. (2007). Nurse labor effects of residency work hour limits. *Nursing economics*, 26, 368-373.

Bruce, K. & Steinke, E. (2006). The acute care nurse practitioner in hospital-basedpractice. *Red Orbit*. Retrieved from http://www.redorbit.com/news/health/539150/the_actue_care_ nurse_practitioner

Buppert, C. (2009). Billing issues for nurse practitioners who provide inpatient services.*Medscape*. Retrieved from http://www.medscape.com/viewarticle/705683_print

Cooper, R. (2004). Weighing the evidence for physician supply. *Annuls of InternalMedicine 141*, 705-714.

Cortes, T. (2012) Out of the ashes. Retrieved from http://hartfordinstittue.owrdpress.com/ 2012/0420/out-of-th-ashes/

Daniele, R. M., Bova, A. M., LeGar, M., Smith, P., & Shortridge-Baggett, L. (2010). Rapid Response Team Composition Effects on Outcomes for Adult Hospitalized Patients: A Systematic Review. *The JBI Database of Systematic Reviews and Implementation Reports*, *8*(24 Suppl), S269-286.

Dorio, G. (2013). Increasing the role of nurse practitioners in the inpatient setting. *KevinMD*. Retrieved from http://www.kevinmd.com/blog/2013/04/incrasing-role-nurse-practitioners-inpat..

Ettner, S. (2006). An alternative approach to reducing the costs of patient care? A controlled trial of the multi-disciplinary doctor-nurse practitioner (MDNP) model. *Medical Decision Making*, 26(1), 9-17.

Hittle, K. (2010). Understanding certification, licensure, and credentialing: A guide for the new nurse practitioner. *Journal of Pediatric Health Care*, *24*(3), 203-206.

Holt, N. (1998). "Confusion's Masterpiece": The development of the physician assistant profession. *Bulletin of the History of Medicine*, *72.2*, 246-278.

Howie, J. & Erickson, M. (2002). Acute care nurse practitioners: creating and implementing a model of care for an inpatient general medical service. *American Journal of Critical Care*, 11, 448-458.

Hravank, M. (2009). Credentialing and privileging for advanced practice nurses. *AACN Advanced Critical Care*, *20*, (1), 12–14.

Hylka, S. & Beschle, J. (1995). Nurse practitioners, cost savings, and improved patient care in the department of surgery. *Nursing Economics, 13*, 349-354.

IOM (Institute of Medicine). (2011). The Future of Nursing: Leading Change, Advancing Health Washington, DC: The National Academies Press.

Kapu, A. & Kleinpell, R. (2012). Developing nurse practitioner associated metrics for outcomes assessment. *Journal of the American Academy of Nurse Practitioners,00,* 1- 8.

Kleinpell, R. (2005). Acute care nurse practitioner practice: Results of a 5-year longitudinal study. *American Journal of Critical Care, 14*, 211-219.

Kleinpell, R., Ely, W., & Grabenkort, R. (2008). Nurse practitioners and physician assistants in the intensive care unit: An evidence based review. *Critical Care Medicine, 36*, (10), 2888-2897.

Larkin, H. (2003). The case for nurse practitioners. *Hospitals & Health Networks.* Retrieved from http://www.hhnmag.com/hhnmag/jsp/articledisplay.jsp?dcrpath=AHA/PubsNews

Morris, D. S., Reilly, P., Rohrbach, J., Telford, G., Kim, P., & Sims, C. A. (2012). The influence

Petterson, S. M., Liaw, W. R., Phillips, R. L., Rabin, D. L., Meyers, D. S., & Bazemore, A. W. (2012). Projecting US primary care physician workforce needs: 2010-2025. *The Annals of Family Medicine*, 10(6), 503-509.

Pollitt, P., & Reesman, K. (2011). Back to the beginning: The PA and NP professions each got a nudge from an MSN program at Duke. *Advanced healthcare NETWORK, for NPs & PAs, 2* (11), pg 37-39.

Reider-Demer, M., Zielinski, T., Carvajal, S., Anulao, K., & Van Roeyen, L. (2008). When is a pediatric patient no longer a pediatric patient?. *Journal of Pediatric Health Care*, *22*(4), 267-269.

Scherr, K., Wilson, D, Wagner J., & Haughian, M. (2012). Evaluating a new rapid response team: NP-led versus intensivist-led comparisons. *AACN Advanced Critical Care,* 23(1), 32-42.

Schroeder, J. (2008). Acute Care Nurse Practitioner: An advanced practice role for RN first assistants. *Association of peri-Operative Registered Nurses, 87*(6), 1205-1215.

Sidani, S., Doran, D., Porter, H., LeFort, S., O'Brien-Pallas, L. L., Zahn, C., & Sarkissian, S. (2006). Outcomes of Nurse Practitioners in Acute Care: An Exploration. *Internet Journal of Advanced Nursing Practice*, 8(1).

Smolenski, M. G. (2005). Credentialing, certfication, and competence: Issues for new and seasoned nurse practitioners. *Journal of the American Academy of Nurse Practitioners, 17*, (6), 201–204.

Sonday, C., Grecsedk, E., & Del Casino, P. (2010). Acute Care: Rapid response teams: NPs lead the way. *The Nurse Practitioner: The American Journal of Primary Health Care, 35*(5), 40-60.

Squiers, J., King, J., Wagner, C., Ashby, N., & Parmley, C. L. (2013). ACNP intensivist: A new ICU care delivery model and its supporting educational programs. *Journal of the American Academy of Nurse Practitioners*, *25*(3), 119-125.

Stanik-Hutt, J., Newhouse, R., White, K., et al. (2013). The quality and effectiveness of care provided by nurse practitioners. *Journal for Nurse Practitioners, 9*(8), 492-500.

Stanley, J., Crabtree M., Ackerman, M., et al. (2012). Adult-Gerontology Acute Care Nurse Practitioner Competencies. Retrieved from http://www.nonpf.org/.

VanOyen Force, M. (2013). Better Outcomes, Better Care. *Advanced Healthcare Network for NPs & PAs, 17(*2), 37-39.

Vestal, C. (2013). Nurse Practitioners Slowly Gain Autonomy. *Kaiser Health News*.Retrieved from http://www.kaiserhelathnews.org/stories/2013/july/19/stateline.

In: Collaboration with the Advanced Practice Nurse ISBN: 978-1-63321-311-1
Editors: E.R. Giardino, R.G. Hanks and A.P. Giardino

Chapter 7

PSYCHIATRIC-MENTAL HEALTH NURSING: A SPECIALTY IN TRANSITION

Linda Stafford*[1], *PhD, RN, CS and
Wanda Hilliard*[2], *MBA, MSN, APRN, PMHNP-BC
[1]UT School of Nursing, The University of Texas School Health Science Center at Houston, Houston, Texas, US
[2]Memorial Park Psychiatry, Houston, TX, US

ABSTRACT

Although previously functioning as a leader in advanced practice, the specialty of psychiatric- mental health nursing became internally focused around the mid-1990s due to tensions surrounding roles, titles, and certifying examinations. Much debate centered on the question of having more than one entry to advanced practice. The question arose as to whether there should there be a psychiatric mental health clinical nurse specialist (PMHCNS) or a psychiatric mental health nurse practitioner (PMHNP), or both. Through much work at the organizational level, momentum built toward educating a PMHNP workforce by 2000. The American Association of Colleges of Nursing (AACN), the International Society of Psychiatric Mental Health Nurses (ISPN), and the American Psychiatric Nurses Association (APNA) recognized changes in the practice front in PMH nursing, with its increased emphasis on prevention, primary care, and community-based treatment. Although much controversy surrounded the development of the PMHNP national certification exam by the American Nurses Credentialing Center (ANCC), the NP role is becoming the single entry to advanced practice. Although certified PMH clinical nurse specialists will be allowed to continue re-certification, the PMHCNS exam will retired at the end of 2014. The PMHNP will play a vital role in screening and treatment of individuals of all age groups, as well as provision of services to populations at risk, such as the homeless mentally ill and military veterans and their families. Additionally, the PMHNP offers valuable consultation services to nurses in emergency and primary care settings.

Psychiatric-Mental Health Nursing: A Specialty in Transition

It is estimated that mental illnesses and substance-related disorders cause more disability than most chronic medical diseases worldwide. They are believed to be second only to cardiovascular problems in contributing to the burden of disease in the US, occurring among one in four Americans (Institute of Medicine, 2006). Often subsumed under the rubric of *behavioral health* issues, mental disorders and substance abuse take a major toll in terms of human suffering, lost productivity, and financial cost to society on a global scale. Prompted by the effects of natural disasters, civil wars, poverty and other threats to mental health, the World Health Organization (WHO) developed an action plan within the past year. The WHO Comprehensive Mental Health Action Plan 2013-2020 addresses the role of mental health in achieving health for all people, irrespective of race, nationality, or income. The plan encompasses four major objectives. First, there is the need for a governance and effective leadership for mental health. The second objective speaks to the provision of comprehensive mental health care and social services in community settings. The next objective highlights the needed implementation of strategies for mental health promotion and preventive services. The fourth objective centers on the need to strengthen mental health evidence and research, as well as the utilization of information systems in mental health (WHO, 2013).

At the national level, *Healthy People 2020* (U.S. Department of Health & Human Services) has built on the work of previous agendas and recommended some new mental health priorities related to special populations (e.g. older adults and veterans). Thus, the complexity of needs requires a workforce prepared to deliver comprehensive primary care and mental health services in a seamless manner through interprofessional teams. Currently, the advanced practice psychiatric/mental health nurse is in a favorable position to be a key player in providing these services—perhaps, more than ever before.

Historical Perspective

The specialty of psychiatric/mental health (PMH) nursing was the first to develop generalist and specialty certification. As early as the 1950s, PMH nursing leaders recognized the need for advanced education to function at the specialist level (Critchley & Maurin, 1985). By 1947, eight master's level psychiatric nursing programs had been developed (Stuart, 2013); however the role of graduates of these programs was slow to be realized in the 1950s. Hildegard Peplau's landmark text, *Interpersonal Relations in Nursing*, was published in 1952 –although it had been completed in 1948. At that time there was no precedent for a nurse to publish a book that dealt with abstract psychiatric content without a physician co-author (O'Toole & Welt, 1989). However, once published, this book was to have a major impact on further development of the PMH clinical nurse specialist (CNS) role. As the PMH role was further refined into the 1960s and 1970s, practitioners became a valued resource in provision of direct patient care, clinical supervision, consultation, and mentoring of other nurses. Additionally, the PMHCNS functioned not as a physician extender, but as a health professional with both independent and complementary roles in the treatment of individuals with complex mental health problems (Dempsey & Ribak, 2012). Thus, the CNS role was seen as the entry into advanced practice PMH nursing until the mid-1990s.

The very first nurse practitioner (NP) program was conceived by Loretta Ford and a pediatrician, Dr. Henry Silver, at the University of Colorado's Schools of Nursing and Medicine, respectively. The focus of this program was on pediatric primary care, and its success led to the opening of other NP programs across the country. Unlike the development of the CNS role, the NP role was often conceptualized as a post-RN certificate program in its early days. However, federally funded educational grants awarded to graduate schools of nursing made it possible to prepare NPs at the master's level (Towers, 2005), thereby initiating the closure of certificate programs.

The 1990s witnessed considerable tensions in the specialty as to the merit of adding the NP role to advanced PMH practice, evidenced by a number of editorials and articles published in psychiatric nursing journals in that decade. For example, some critics saw this movement as a ploy to bolster sagging enrollments in PMH graduate programs (Lego, 1996). However, the influence of managed care could not be denied; the health care environment continued to shift toward a primary care, prevention, and community-based treatment focus. The American Association of Colleges of Nursing (AACN) supported this direction, placing an emphasis on preparing all advanced practice nurses (APNs) to be capable of practicing across various settings in provision of primary care (AACN, 1999; Bellack, Graber, O'Neil, Musham, & Lancaster, 1999).

Effect of the Consensus Model on Roles

At the organizational level, the Society for Education and Research in Psychiatric Nursing (SERPN), a division of the International Society of Psychiatric-Mental Health Nursing (ISPN), worked with the American Psychiatric Nurses Association (APNA) to collaborate as a single voice in response to the Consensus Model. The Advanced Practice Registered Nurse (APRN) Consensus Model was completed in 2008. A regulatory model providing definitions of APRN practice and recognized titles and specialties, the consensus model also addresses the relationships among licensure, accreditation, certification, and education. The APNA/ISPN coalition made several recommendations to facilitate implementation of the LACE model. A major recommendation is that the PMH NP with preparation across the lifespan be the one entry educational focus for mental health clinicians. The PMH NP will address mental illness diagnosis and treatment and mental health promotion (American Nurses Credentialing Center, 2011). The NP role with preparation across the life span will incorporate mental health promotion and mental illness diagnosis and treatment. Thus, the role of the psychiatric mental health clinical nurse specialist (PMHCNS) will soon be encompassed within the more recently developed role of the PMHNP. Although the PMHCNS exam will be retired by the end of 2014, certified PMHCNSs will be allowed to re-certify and continue to practice with appropriate continuing education (ANCC, 2011).

Some leaders in the mental health specialty have taken umbrage at the move to terminate the clinical nurse specialist role. They argue that this position heralds the end of not only of the PMHCNS role, but of many therapeutic modalities for patients, such as consultation-liaison nursing, individual, group, and family therapy. There is concern as to what is perceived as the "medicalization" of advanced practice nursing, with an emphasis on prescribing medications and very brief patient encounters (Dempsey & Ribak, 2012; Santos & Amaral, 2011). Others in the field have approached the controversy with less foreboding. Delaney (2009) opined that arguing about the value of one role over another was an unfortunate discussion platform at the beginning of the 21st century. Rather discussions should have centered on the economics that had been affecting psychiatric care, including the supply and demand for mental health practitioners. As Barker (2006) noted, discussions on the future of the specialty should not be on inherited roles, but for what services society needs advanced practice PMH nurses to provide.

The curricula for PMHNP programs include advanced pharmacology, physical assessment, physiology/pathophysiology, and specific PMH content, in addition to psychotherapeutic modalities (i.e., individual, family, and group). In addition to prescriptive practice, the PMHNP must be prepared to provide integrative and collaborative healthcare in a variety of settings. Finally, the PMHNP graduates must be eligible to sit for the certification examination provided by the ANCC, which became available in late 2000.

PMHNPs can practice autonomously in a wide variety of settings, dependent upon current state regulations. In 18 states, PMHNPs can assess and prescribe medications without physician supervision. In 21 states, these clinicians can assess and treat patients with a collaborative agreement with a physician. The other 12 states require that PMHNPs have physician supervision to provide patient care (APNA, 2014; AANP, 2014). Thus, in 39 states PMHNPs are allowed to practice with minimal supervision, to diagnose psychiatric disorders, provide psychotherapy, and prescribe psychotropic drugs as needed (APNA, 2014; AANP, 2014).

Growth of the PMHNP Role

A number of factors at the national level have contributed to the growth of the PMHNP role. The Affordable Care Act of 2010, years of underfunding of mental health programs, along with an increased occurrence and awareness of mental health disorders will continue to increase the demand for psychiatric and mental health services. As health care will continue to integrate both physical and mental health care, the challenge of preventive services and diagnosis will often occur in the primary care setting. Once a primary care practitioner determines that a patient may be manifesting a psychiatric disorder, a referral can be made to a PMHNP—who can treat, further assess, or appropriately refer the patient to another provider. This last decision is dependent on the complexity of problems presented, as well as the level of expertise of the individual PMHNP.

Future Trends

Affordable Care Act of 2010

The Patient Protection and Affordable Care Act (ACA) of 2010, which was signed into law on March 23, 2010, is the first comprehensive integrated healthcare insurance in the U.S. It is also the first major legislative healthcare policy passed since the establishment of

Medicare (Hofer, Abraham, & Moscovice, 2011). The ACA includes provisions for health care spending reform, an expansion of Medicaid, improved access to care, evaluation of patient outcomes with cost controls, along with improvements in the health care delivery system (Parker, Hernandez, & Wu, 2013). The goals of this legislation are aligned with the philosophy and practice skills of advanced practice psychiatric-mental health nursing, including the official organizations (APNA and ISPN).

Influence of Increased Knowledge of the Role of Genetics

Advances in the science of genetics are changing some attitudes and practices related to screening and treatment for mental disorders. In the future, a patient's complete genetic profile, including variants associated with neuropsychiatric disorders, will be available for utilization in treatment (Wilke & Dolan, 2011; Wilde, Mitchell, Meiser, & Schofield, 2013). If a patient so desires, clinicians will be able to personalize an individual's treatment plan based on genetic testing included in the comprehensive psychiatric assessment. Individuals and families will have questions and concerns regarding the heritability of certain mental disorders. Thus, understanding the role played by new knowledge in genetics will be critical to the role of the PMHNP.

Caring for Veterans and Military Personnel

PMHNPs are well equipped to provide patient care in a number of environments, based upon acuity and resources. Veterans returning from active duty are at risk for a variety of mental health disorders, including posttraumatic stress disorder (PTSD), mood and anxiety disorders, and substance-related disorders (Milanak, Gros, Magruder, Brawman-Mintzer, & Frueh, 2013). Veteran morbidity related to self-destructive and suicidal behavior has increased dramatically, sometimes leading to extended care, with ongoing medication management and other therapies (Stappenbeck, Hellmuth, Simpson, & Jakupeak, 2014). It has been reported that veterans with PTSD engage in more frequent risk-taking and suicidal behaviors than those without PTSD (James, Strom, & Leskela, 2014). In recent years, there is recognition of the alarming rate of suicides of veterans of Operation Enduring Freedom (OEF), Operation Iraqi Freedom (OIF), and Operation New Dawn (OND). Initial studies explored deployment factors, such as combat experience, cumulative days deployed, or number of deployments with equivocal results. As suicide ideation is a major focus of the Department of Veterans Affairs (VA) screening efforts, a prospective longitudinal study was completed in 2008 (LeardMann et al., 2013) which included data from current and former military personnel from all service branches.

Currently, PMHNPs assume an active role in V.A. hospitals and the rapidly growing Veteran Outpatient Centers. The National Death Index and the Department of Defense Medical Mortality Registry garnered data on death by suicide. The analysis of this study highlighted the critical role of suicidal screening in the veteran population. Results indicated that suicide risk was independently associated with male sex and psychiatric disorders, but not with military-specific variables such as deployment. The findings of this study support the need for mental health professionals, such as PMHNPs, to take an assertive role in screening and referral.

Services for the Homeless Population

Many opportunities exist to provide badly needed services, such as medication management, for homeless individuals in the community (Burda, Haack, Duarte, & Alemi, 2012). A systematic review (Roy, Crocker, Nicholls, Latimer, & Ayllon, 2014) noted that homeless adults with severe mental illness are victimized more than those adults with housing, but who also have a serious mental illness. Homeless adults with mental disorders also have more frequent encounters with the criminal justice system than other populations. These issues and the need for treatment of co-morbid health problems often lead to serious medical illnesses. Unfortunately, this population rarely seeks treatment until a life-threatening illness or incapacitation is the outcome (Zlotnick, Zerger, & Wolfe, 2013). Thus, the homeless mentally ill can benefit greatly from preventive healthcare services provided by PMHNPs.

Emergency Settings

Few healthcare settings challenge nurses and physicians more than an emergency department (ED) in a large urban area. In addition to frequent admissions of victims of vehicular trauma, other accidents, or physical/ sexual assault, the presentation of individuals with psychiatric and substance abuse-related symptoms is well documented (Williams, Jelinek, Rogers, Wenban, & Jacobs, 2000; Larkin, Claassen, Emond, Pelletier, & Camargo, 2005; Nicholls, Gaynor, Shafiei, Bosanac, & Farrell, 2011). A recent trend is the addition of PMHNPs to provide assessment and intervention services in hospital emergency departments, both in the U.S. and abroad. There appear to be a number of positive outcomes related to this practice, including reduced waiting time for patients, improved coordination of care, and increased sensitivity for mental health issues among staff (Wand & White, 2007). In evaluating PMHNPs in the ED, patient participants in an Australian qualitative study reported that they received a number of benefits. They specifically identified support, understanding, and a focus on solutions rather than problems in their encounters with the PMHNPs (Wand, White, Patching, Dixon, & Green, 2011). In this particular study, the therapeutic use of self was embedded in the theoretical framework that guided activities of the nurse practitioners. Participants in the study were pleased with longer consultations and a greater quantity of health teaching provided by the PMHNPs.

Conclusion

The Affordable Care Act of 2010 is intended to improve the psychiatric and mental health care components of population health. Additionally, partnerships from public and private sectors, as well as changes in the current clinical delivery system are required to meet the goals and objectives of the World Health Organization and make the vision of improved mental health care a reality. Interprofessional collaborative decision-making is essential to the quality of outcomes for patients. Evidence supports that utilization of PMHNPs result in an increase in the availability of mental health services for populations in need, which leads to an improvement in population health (Gilfedder, Barron, & Docherty, 2010). The role of the PMHNP continues to evolve and is a model of the flexibility and expertise needed to adapt to the challenges of the ever changing health care system.

References

American Association of Colleges of Nursing (1999). A vision of baccalaureate and graduation education: The next decade. *Journal of Professional Nursing, 15,* 59-65.

American Nurses Credentialing Center (2011). Consensus Model for APRN regulations, frequently asked questions. Available at: http://www.nursecredentialing.org/APRN-FAQ.aspx.

Barker, P. (2006). Mental health nursing: The craft of the impossible. (*Journal of Psychiatric and Mental Health Nursing, 13,* 385-387.

Bellack, J. P., Graber, D. R., O'Neil, E. H., Musham, C., & Lancaster, C. (1999). Curriculum trends in nurse practitioner programs: Current and ideal. *Journal of Professional Nursing, 15,* 15-27.

Burda, C., Haack, M., Duarte, A. C., & Alemi, F. (2012). Medication adherence among homeless patients: A pilot study of cell phone effectiveness. *Journal of the American Academy of Nurse Practitioners, 24* (11): 675-681. Doi:10.1111/j.1745-7599.2012.00756.x

Critchley, D. L. & Maurin, J. T. (1985). *The clinical nurse specialist in psychiatric mental health nursing.* New York: John Wiley & Sons.

Dempsey, A., & Ribak, J. (2012). The future of the psychiatric mental health clinical nurse specialist: Evolution or extinction. *Nursing Clinics of North America* (47): 295-304.

Gilfedder, M., Barron, D., & Docherty, E. (2010). Developing the role of advanced nurse practitioners in mental health. *Nursing Standard, 24,* (30), 35-40.

Hofer, A. N., Abraham, J., & Moscovice, I. (2011). Expansion of coverage under the Patient Protection and Affordable Care Act and primary care utilization. *Milbank Quarterly, 89,* (1), 69-89.

Institute of Medicine (2006). Improving the Quality of Health Care for Mental and Substance-Use Conditions: Quality Chasm Series, Washington, DC: National Academy Press.

James, L. M., Strom, T. Q., & Leskela, J. (2014). Risk-taking behaviors and impulsivity among veterans with and without PTSD and mild TBI. *Military Medicine (4)*: 357-363.

Larkin, G. L., Claassen, C. A., Emond, J. A., Pelletier, & Camargo, C. A. (2005). Trends in U.S. emergency department visits for mental health conditions, 1992-2001. *Psychiatric Services 56,*671-677.

LeardMann, C. A., Powell, T. M., Smith, T. C., Bell, M. R., Smith, B., Boyko, E. J., Hoge, C. W. (2013). Risk factors associated with suicide in current and former military personnel. *Journal of the American Medical Association, 310,* 496-506.doi:10.1001/jama.2013.65164

Milanak, M. E., Gros, D. R., Magruder, K. M., Brawman-Mintzer, O., & Frueh, B. C. (2013). Prevalence and features of generalized anxiety disorder in Department of Veteran Affairs primary care settings, *Psychiatry Research, 209* (2): 173-179.

NCSBN, National Council of State Boards of Nursing Advanced Practice Consensus Model (2009). Available at: https://www.ncsbn.org/index.htm.

Nicholls, D., Gaynor, N., Shafiei, T., Bosanac, P., & Farrell, G., (2011). Mental health nursing in emergency departments: The case for a nurse practitioner role. *Journal of Clinical Nursing, 20,* 530-536. doi: 101111/j.1365-2702.2010.03504.x

Parker, R. M., Hernandez, L. M., & Wu, V. Y. (2013). Advancing a shared conversation to enhance health care enrollment in the United States—a timely opportunity and challenge for health literacy. *Journal of Health Communication 18* (9): 1021-1023.

Roy, L., Crocker, A. G., Nicholls, T. L., Latimer, E. A., Ayllon, A. R. (2014). Criminal behavior and victimization among homeless individuals with severe mental illness: A systematic review. *Psychiatric Services.* doi: 10.1176/appi.ps.201200515

Santos, J. C., & Amaral, A. F. S., (2011). Effectiveness of psychiatric mental health nurses: Can we save the core of the profession in an economically constrained world? *Archives of Psychiatric Nursing, 25* (5): 329-338.

Stappenbeck, C. A., Hellmuth, J. C., Simpson, T., & Jakupeak, M. (2014). The effects of alcohol problems, PTSD, and combat exposure on nonphysical and physical aggression among Iraq and Afghanistan ware veterans. *Psychological Trauma: Theory, Research, Practice, and Policy, 6* (1), 65.

Towers, J. (2005). After forty years. *Journal of the Academy of Nurse Practitioners. 17,* 9-13.

U.S. Department of Health and Human Services. Office of Disease Prevention and Health Promotion. Healthy People 2020. Washington, DC. Available at http://www.cdc.gov/nchs/healthy_people/hp2020.htm. Accessed [4/15/2014].

Wand, T. & White, K. (2007). Examining models of mental health service delivery in the emergency department. *Australian and New Zealand Journal of Psychiatry, 41,* 784-791.

Wand, T., White, K., Patching, J., Dixon, J., & Dixon, T. (2011). An emergency department-based nurse practitioner outpatient service: Part I, participant evaluation. *International Journal of Mental Health Nursing, 20;* 392-400.

Wilde, A., Mitchell, P. B., Meiser, B., & Schofield, P. R. (2013). Implications of the use of genetic tests in psychiatry, with a focus on major depressive disorder: A review. *Depression and Anxiety, 30* (3), 267-275.

Wilke, R. A., & Dolan, M. E. (2011). Genetics and variable drug response. *Journal of the American Medical Association, 306* (3), 306-307.

Williams, A. G., Jelinek, G. A., Rogers, I. R., Wenban, J. A., & Jacobs, I. G. (2000). The effect on hospital admission profiles of establishing an emergency department observation ward. *The Medical Journal of Australia 173,* 411-414.

World Health Organization (2013). Mental health action plan 2013-2020. http://www.who.int/mental_health/publications/action_plan/en/index.html.

Zlotnick, C., Zerger, S., & Wolfe, P. B. (2013). Healthcare for the homeless: What we have learned in the past 30 years and what's next. *American Journal of Public Health. 103* (S2), S199-S205.

In: Collaboration with the Advanced Practice Nurse
Editors: E.R. Giardino, R.G. Hanks and A.P. Giardino
ISBN: 978-1-63321-311-1

Chapter 8

The Certified Nurse-Midwife in Advanced Practice Nursing

Mary Traub[1], APRN, CNM, MS and Lisa Hollier[2], MD, MPH
[1]Instructor and Director, Midwifery Section
[2]Professor, Maternal-Fetal Medicine, Department of Obstetrics & Gynecology
Baylor College of Medicine, Houston, TX, US

Abstract

The role of the certified nurse-midwife (CNM) is presented in this chapter especially for someone who may be considering this profession. The rich history is presented as a foundation for the profession. In discussing the CNM of today, a comparison is made of the different midwifery roles including the CNM, the certified midwife, the certified professional midwife, and the unlicensed lay midwife. Currently there is an ongoing movement to standardize the roles of Advanced Practice Registered Nurses (APRN) which includes the CNM and would provide for standardization nationally for licensure, accreditation, certification, and education.

The specifics of the role of the CNM including the Scope of Practice, model of care, collaboration with physicians and other staff, and prescriptive authority are discussed. Practice settings typical for midwifery are presented including the group model of care, CenteringPregnancy®. A comprehensive discussion related to CenteringPregnancy® is provided with inclusion of significant research that has improved patient outcomes. Also included is a look into the future of the role of the CNM with innovative care and the vision as noted by the American College of Nurse-Midwives.

Introduction

The role of the Certified Nurse-Midwife (CNM) is a very exciting Advanced Practice Registered Nurse (APRN) role. Someone interested in pursuing a career as a CNM needs to carefully consider what it takes to be a CNM. This chapter will assist the reader to understand the opportunities and challenges that may be experienced as a CNM and appropriately guide them in their decision.

This chapter begins with the rich history of midwives which goes back to the Old Testament of The Bible. It then follows the centuries of progression of the midwifery role from about the 13th Century to current time. Included is information about how midwives learned their profession prior to the onset of modern medicine, along with the struggles they faced. There are different classifications of midwives by today's standards which are compared. The variety of training and yet the similarity in name has created some confusion throughout the years as to who midwives are, how they are trained, and what skills they have.

There is discussion regarding the Consensus Model for APRNs as it relates to the CNM. The Consensus Model is a much needed standardization to provide for more consistency nationally in the areas of licensure, accreditation, certification and education. Although the goal for implementation of recommended changes is in 2015, many of the states have a significant amount of work to accomplish in order to meet the standards that have been established through the Consensus Model (APRN Joint Dialogue Group Report, 2008).

The CNM specific role recognizes that the CNM practices the art and science of midwifery which are influenced by training as a registered nurse and training as a nurse-midwife. Nurse-midwifery practice is based on standards and core competencies developed by the American College of Nurse-Midwifery and are listed within this chapter.

Midwifery supports collaborative practice in which communication is a key aspect of that process as excellent communication enables the CNM and physician along with other team members to provide the highest level of care possible. It is appropriate for the CNM to strive to work to the fullest extent allowed by the APRN license and midwifery certification. Midwifery collaborative management includes consultation, collaboration, and referral.

CNMs have numerous opportunities related to practice settings and the range of clinical care opportunities in private, public, and academic institutions. Those opportunities also include teaching, administration, and other non-patient care options. Midwife means with woman, and whatever the setting, the personalized approach should be evident. Perseverance, patience, and professionalism are three essential characteristics of an excellent midwife. These characteristics are in addition to clinical competence and the ability to work well both alone and within a team.

This chapter describes the CenteringPregnancy® model of group prenatal care. Research outcomes related to CenteringPregnancy® are presented. CenteringPregnancy® group prenatal care is both the present and the future for prenatal care. The Center for Children and Women is presented as an example of an innovative care delivery system which utilizes the CenteringPregnancy® model of care. Within this clinic collaboration is essential to providing high quality care for women and children. It provides a concrete example of what to expect within the CNM role.

The vision for the future from the American College of Nurse-Midwives is presented and focuses on the potential for role autonomy, growth in the number of CNMs, increased presence at deliveries, and improved outcomes for pregnancy.

It is the goal of the authors that you will be able to better understand the role of the CNM and share the excitement of working in a team setting to improve care and outcomes for the women we care for while at the same time growing professionally.

HISTORICAL PERSPECTIVE

Midwives have been attending births for centuries and are mentioned numerous times throughout the Bible. Perhaps the best known scripture is Genesis 35:17 "And it came to pass, when she was in hard labour, that the midwife said unto her, Fear not thou shalt have this son also" (The Holy Bible,Genesis 35-17, n.d.).

Universities offered medical education in the 13th century to train physicians to care for the sick. From the 14th to the 17th century women were often seen as "healers" (Ehrenreich & English, 1973) and commonly practiced midwifery. The personal experience of childbirth was considered a prerequisite for the practice of midwifery. Particularly in European countries, midwives and women healers were thought to be witches, often placed on trial, and subjected to being burned at the stake or other types of torture. It was felt that their healing was related to satanic powers. Illness was thought to be caused by witchcraft (Ewell, 1990). Colonial midwives were generally held in high esteem in the 17th century, however, they were also accused of practicing witchcraft if there were birth defects or stillbirth. By the 18th century there were more formally trained physicians and the profession was dominated by men. Wealthy women sought the educated physicians but the outcomes were not better from what was being provided by midwives providing care at home. During this time women were considered intellectually inferior to men (Litoff, 1982). A wide range of providers continued into the 19th century with those educated as physicians unable to meet the health needs of the population.

The 1879 supplement to Howard's Domestic Medicine titled *Midwifery and the Diseases Peculiar to Women*, clearly supported of the profession of midwives, although that was not true in all circles. "…it is the circumstances by which this reputed mysterious art is surrounded that impresses us with a seriousness and diffidence with which, in our other medical labors, we had not to contend" (Howard, 1879, p 70). The thought was that all women should be educated and knowledgeable related to childbirth. Midwives were recognized for their "patience in attendance" (Howard, 1879) with laboring women and at birth. In fact, Dr. James Ewell, who was a physician in the early part of the 19th Century and wrote on the complaints peculiar to women and children, (Ewell, 1990) expressed his opinion about the increased presence of men practicing midwifery by stating, "…a source of serious evils…an imposition upon the credibility of women, and upon the fears of their husbands—as a means of sacrificing delicacy, and consequently virtue—a robbery of many of the good common women [midwives] of their employment and support" (Howard, 1879, p 71). On the occasion when it was necessary to call a physician at that time, the practice was for the physician to "discover something wrong" (Howard, 1879) and then he would skillfully set everything right and would be applauded while the midwife was condemned. Ewell also noted that midwifery did not require any particular skill, superior knowledge, or sleight of hand, but rather the patience of waiting and not interfering with a natural process (Howard, 1879).

The early 20th century brought more strict licensing and regulation for physicians. Thus, the midwives who were delivering about 50% of babies were being driven out of practice. Women were then recruited as nurses to provide care to patients (Ehrenreich & English, 1973). It was at this time that the wealthy were choosing to have their babies delivered in hospitals by physicians. The poor people including immigrants and blacks utilized midwifery services rather than accepting charity and also many of them preferred a female birth attendant (Litoff, 1982). At this time there was increased interest in medical education and it was noted that there was a high rate of infant mortality at 124 deaths per 1000 live births. In addition, maternal deaths related to childbirth were the second highest cause of death in women of childbearing age. Many references can be found about the midwife problem (Litoff, 1982). The Bellevue School for Midwives was established in 1911 in New York City. There was also increased interest nationally in educating midwives. The goal was to reduce the infant and maternal mortality, which was accomplished following the improved education for both physicians and midwives. Midwifery births continued to decline as more women were seeking medical intervention (Litoff, 1982). "In the 1920's midwifery was allowed to exist only if it was attached to nursing and under the auspices of medical supervision and control. Those compromises made nearly a century ago still influence current-day philosophical interprofessional, and practical issues" (Burst, 2005, p 21). There was some promise for midwifery as the Maternity Center Association of New York City and the Frontier Nursing Service in Kentucky began two of the earliest schools of nurse-midwifery in the United States (Litoff, 1982). Frontier Nursing Service now known as Frontier University is the oldest school of nurse-midwifery and continues to operate today. Review of records at Frontier reported 8596 midwifery births with a puerperal death rate of 9.1 per 10,000 live births compared to the national death rate of 34 per 10,000 births during the same period (1925-1954) (Burst, 2005, p 130).

More formal organization and structure for the practice of nurse-midwifery was badly needed and continued to be developed to around the middle of the 20th century. At that time nurses with a public health background studied midwifery and became nurse-midwives. In 1955 as a result of the work of an organizational committee, the American College of Nurse-Midwifery was established. The first definition of nurse-midwifery adopted by membership of the college was in 1962. "Nurse-Midwifery is an extension of nursing practice into the area of management of care of mothers and babies throughout the maternity cycle so long as progress meets criteria accepted as normal." That definition was changed in 1978 to the definition that is current today. "A Certified Nurse-Midwife (CNM) is an individual educated in the two disciplines of nursing and midwifery, who possesses evidence of certification according to the requirements of the American College of Nurse-Midwives" (Burst, 2005).

In the 1960s only 2 states recognized the practice of nurse-midwifery. This resulted in midwifery graduates entering teaching, supervisory, administrative or consultative positions. But there was great effort made for hospital privileges and the landscape changed going into the 1970s when there was increased demand for midwives. Although women who preferred out of hospital deliveries sought the services from lay midwives, the demand for certified nurse-midwives increased as they became an accessible option for women. Midwifery educational programs became more prevalent (Burst, 2005). An official joint statement was issued in 1971 by the American College of Obstetricians and Gynecologists (ACOG), the Nurses Association of the American College of Obstetricians and Gynecologists (NAACOG), and the ACNM that recognized and supported the education of nurse-midwives. Recognition was for the practice of nurse-midwifery within "teams of physicians, nurse-midwives, obstetric registered nurses and other health personnel…directed by a qualified obstetrician-gynecologist…for the complete care and management of uncomplicated maternity patients" (American College of Nurse-Midwives, American College of Obstetricians and Gynecologists & Nurses Association of the American College of Obstetricians and

Gynecologists, 1971). Midwives began to enter into private practice often with physicians. Women sought care from the midwives because of the relationship established with the midwife, which included extensive teaching and a commitment to be present with the woman throughout labor and promotion of a normal childbirth experience. The 1980s saw increased opportunities for CNMs working in a variety of positions including private and public practice, outpatient and inpatient, and even out of hospital birth. More education programs opened in the 1990s. A goal was set in 1995 to increase the number of CNMs from about 5,000 to 10,000 by 2001 by the ACNM. The goal was nearly met with just over 9,000 CNMs that had ever been certified. It was at this time that managed care was influencing health care, and midwives were seldom included in policy discussions which limited the option of utilizing a CNM for care for many women.

Interest developed to look at standards for non-nurse professional midwives. Direct-entry programs were established and the first graduates completed their programs in 1997. Although direct-entry midwives are certified by the same testing process as CNMs, they face limited practice opportunities. Direct-entry midwives are licensed as certified midwives (CM) in five states where they are authorized to practice. Unfortunately few hospitals will credential CMs. They are generally regulated by midwifery boards established by the individual states (Varney, 2015).

Comparison of Types of Midwives

There are three types of certified midwives. The certified nurse-midwife (CNM), certified midwife (CM), and certified professional midwife (CPM). The CNM and CM are very similar in that they both require a graduate degree which has been determined to be important by many, with the primary difference that the CNM has a nursing degree in addition to the graduate degree. The professional association for both is the ACNM. Both CNM and CM are certified by passing the same exam, which is known as The National Certification Examination in Nurse-Midwifery and Midwifery. CNMs and CMs need to recertify every 5 years. Their clinical requirements are essentially the same and they must clinically meet the core competencies which are listed later in this chapter. CNMs are licensed in all states plus the District of Columbia. CMs are licensed only in New Jersey, New York, and Rhode Island, with authorization to practice in Delaware and Missouri. Both can be regulated by Midwifery Boards, the Board of Medicine and the Department of Health. CNMs additionally can be regulated by the Board of Nursing. CNMs and CMs can deliver in hospitals, birth centers, and homes.

CPMs are professionally associated with Midwives Alliance of North America (MANA) and National Association of Certified Professional Midwives (NACPM). Their certifying agency is the North American Registry of Midwives (NARM). No college degree is required, but they must be educated in the profession of midwifery or complete an apprenticeship by working with an experienced preceptor. The preceptor must have at least 3 years of experience and delivered 50 babies. They are required to recertify every 3 years. Their clinical skills must meet core competencies of MANA. CPMs are illegal in 12 states (Williams & Choen & Thomas, 2015) their licensure is managed by the Department of

Health, Board of Medicine, or Midwifery Board. Deliveries occur in an out of hospital setting.

A lay midwife is someone who is neither certified nor licensed. They learn their skills by working with other midwives and generally do not have formal education. They do deliveries outside of the hospital and are considered illegal in some states (American College of Nurse-Midwives, 2011).

Consensus Model

The Consensus Model as a regulatory model is currently being incrementally implemented and thus is still a work in progress with the goal for full implementation in 2015. The Consensus Model was developed by a work group of Advanced Practice Registered Nurses (APRN) and endorsed by professional organizations representing most of the APRN organizations. Those specific to certified nurse-midwives were the Accreditation Commission for Midwifery Education (ACME), the American College of Nurse-Midwives (ACNM), the American Midwifery Certification Board (AMCB), and the Association of Women's Health, Obstetric, and Neonatal Nurses (AWHONN). The National Council of State Boards of Nursing (NCSBN) also had representation on this work group. This Consensus Model includes "the essential elements: licensure, accreditation, certification and education (LACE)." Through implementation of this model we can anticipate improved consistency in all of the areas covered under LACE. We anticipate that the profession of the Certified Nurse-Midwife (CNM) will be regulated in the future by the standards from the Consensus Model. CNMs licensed to practice should expect to continue their present practice as there would be a grandfathering provision (Report: Consensus Model for APRN Regulation: Licensure, Accreditation, Certification & Education. 2008) In 2010 the ACNM noted that current educational programs were meeting the required separate graduate courses in health assessment, physiology/pathophysiology and advanced pharmacology within their curriculums for ongoing certification by the AMCB. They also reiterated that licensure would be by the boards of nursing as opposed to the boards of medicine. Licensure would require a national recognition of the profession, and would require that "educational standards and practice competencies must exist, be consistent, and must be nationally recognized by the profession" (Report: Consensus Model for APRN Regulation: Licensure, Accreditation, Certification & Education. 2008, p 13). The identified characteristics which would be used to develop the core competencies, and standards for education and practice are "national in scope; inclusive; transparent; accountable; initiated by nursing; consistent with national standards for licensure, accreditation, certification and education; evidence-based, and consistent with regulatory principles". (Report: Consensus Model for APRN Regulation: Licensure, Accreditation, Certification & Education. 2008. p 13). Licensure would still be the responsibility of the board of nursing of the state in which the graduate plans to practice. Licensing of an APRN/CNM would be "as independent practitioners with no regulatory requirements for collaboration, direction or supervision" (The APRN Consensus Workgroup & the APRN Joint Dialogue Group members, 2008). Certification would be accomplished by standardized testing that is shown to measure knowledge in the appropriate specialty as well as the basic requirements. The certification needs to be granted by a national organization such as the AMCB for CNMs.

The Consensus model recommends that accreditation of midwifery education programs would be by the U.S. Department of Education (USDE) and/or the Council for Higher Education Accreditation (CHEA). This would be determined based on if the program meets the established requirements noted in the specialty of education. Ongoing programmatic review would be required to verify that they are continuing to meet previously established requirements and adapting newer requirements as assurance of quality education (The APRN Consensus Workgroup & the APRN Joint Dialogue Group members, 2008).

Within education, the APRN/CNM would be required to complete comprehensive graduate level courses in physiology/pathophysiology, health assessment, and pharmacology. The level of formal education would be at the master's or doctoral level or post-graduate certificate at an accredited institution. The Consensus model plan is that the student would be educated in the previously mentioned areas and also related to specific population groups. All of this would be intended to prepare the CNM for practice including "responsibility and accountability for health promotion and/or maintenance as well as the assessment, diagnosis, and management of patient problems, which includes the use and prescription of pharmacologic and non-pharmacologic interventions" (The APRN Consensus Workgroup & the APRN Joint Dialogue Group members, 2008).

The Consensus Model suggests standardization of the APRN title for Advanced Practice Nurses. The model identifies the four recognized roles for advanced practice nurses that would be eligible to be licensed as APRNs. They are the Certified Nurse-Midwife, the Certified Nurse Practitioner, the Certified Registered Nurse Anesthetist, and the Clinical Nurse Specialist. The model identifies specific Population Foci which include Family-Individual across Lifespan, Adult Gerontology, Neonatal, Pediatrics, Women's Health/Gender Related, and Psychiatric-Mental Health (The APRN Consensus Workgroup & the APRN Joint Dialogue Group members, 2008).

Full information about all aspects related to the Consensus Model for APRN Regulation: Licensure, Accreditation, Certification and Education can be accessed at ncsbn.org which is the website for the National Council of State Boards of Nursing (The APRN Consensus Workgroup & the APRN Joint Dialogue Group members, 2008).

Ongoing barriers related to implementation of the Consensus Model for CNMs are outlined in a 2011 paper from ACNM. Although the Consensus Model clearly supports autonomous practice, "state legislatures and regulatory boards in many states continue to have regulatory requirements for collaboration, direction, or supervision of APRNs" (Midwifery in the United States and the Consensus Model for APRN Regulation, 2011, p 2). The recommendation is to eliminate these regulations through appropriate legislation. Likewise, the Consensus Model supports regulation by Boards of Midwifery, Boards of Nurse-Midwifery, or Boards of Nursing, however in many states the Board of Medicine maintains some control over the practice of APRNs/CNMs. CNMs provide care in "women's health/gender related" population focus area which meets the requirement of providing care in one or more of the established groups (Midwifery in the United States and the Consensus Model for APRN Regulation, 2011). Clearly there are still issues that need work related to the Consensus Model and the implementation of the model, but it is an appropriate step in the right direction related to the regulation of licensure, accreditation, certification, and education. A summary of where each state's progress is regarding meeting the key components related to the Consensus Model, including APRN Title, Roles, License, Education, Certification, Independent Practice and Independent Prescribing, show 7 states meeting all of the requirements, 13 states at 75-96% of requirements, 20 states at 50-71% of the requirement, and 10 states at less than 50%. The primary areas of not meeting the key components are related to independent practice and independent prescribing (NCSBN, 2013).

Scope of Practice

The Scope of Practice for CNMs according to the ACNM "encompasses a full range of primary health care services for women from adolescence beyond menopause. These services include primary care, gynecologic and family planning services, preconception care, care during pregnancy and childbirth and the postpartum period, care of the normal newborn during the first 28 days of life, and treatment of male partners for sexually transmitted infections. Midwives provide initial and ongoing comprehensive assessment, diagnosis and treatment. They conduct physical examinations; prescribe medications including controlled substances and contraceptive methods; admit, manage and discharge patients; order and interpret laboratory and diagnostic tests and order the use of medical devices. Midwifery care also includes health promotion, disease prevention, and individualized wellness education and counseling. These services are `provided in partnership with women and families in diverse settings such as ambulatory care clinics, private offices, community and public health systems, homes, hospitals and birth centers" (American College of Nurse-Midwives, 2011).

Scope of practice is also detemined by legal jurisdiction, institutional policies, and individual experience, education, and training. The practice of midwifery falls along a continuum of direct physician management as the most restrictive and independent practice and collaborative management as the least restrictive. Relative to the institution, CNMs usually need to be credentialed and the specific competencies stated for practice in that setting. The institutional bylaws also set forth specifics such as the ability to admit a patient (Williams & Cohen & Thomas, 2015).

CNM Specific Role

Model of Care

A CNM is educated in the art and science of midwifery as a nurse and a midwife. The entry level to practice currently requires a Master's degree with interest by some of increasing that to requiring a DNP. However, that is not clearly supported by the ACNM at this time. Nurse-midwifery practice is based on standards and core competencies.

"Midwifery practice as conducted by certified nurse-midwives (CNMs) ...is the independent management of women's health care, focusing particularly on pregnancy, childbirth, and the post partum period, care of the newborn, and the family planning and gynecologic needs of women. The CNM...practices within a health care system that provides for consultation, collaborative management, or referral as indicated by the health status of the client" (American College of Nurse-Midwives, 2012). The Core Competencies for Midwifery

Practice are listed in detail in Appendix A. They are essential guidelines that assist in understanding what the basic skills are of a new graduate from an accredited midwifery education program. Additionally, they are guidelines used by employers, and consumers. Policy can be based on what is listed within the Core Competencies.

Standards for the practice of midwifery have been developed by ACNM and clarify the foundation for midwifery.

The Standards for practicing midwifery

Standard I. Midwifery care is provided by qualified practitioners.

Standard II. Midwifery care occurs in a safe environment within the context of the family, community, and a system of health care.

Standard III. Midwifery care supports individual rights and self-determination within boundaries of safety.

Standard IV. Midwifery care is comprised of knowledge, skills, and judgment that foster the delivery of safe, satisfying, and culturally competent care.

Standard V. Midwifery care is based upon knowledge, skills, and judgments which are reflected in written practice guidelines and are used to guide the scope of midwifery care and services provided to clients.

Standard VI. Midwifery care is documented in a format that is accessible and complete.

Standard VII. Midwifery care is evaluated according to an established program for quality management that includes a plan to identify and resolve problems.

Standard VIII. Midwifery practice may be expanded beyond the ACNM core competencies to incorporate new procedures that improve care for women and their families.

Standards are from the ACNM Document Standards for the Practice of Midwifery, Division of Standards and Practice, 2011. P 1-3.

Collaboration

Midwifery supports collaborative practice among and between all of the members of the health care team. A number of widely used communication methods employed to facilitate collaboration are utilized both in the inpatient and outpatient settings. SBAR (Situation-Background-Assessment-Recommendation) is an acronym for reporting a handoff of a patient in a structured manner and focuses on what is absolutely necessary to ensure patient safety. SBAR is initiated by the person currently providing care to the patient. Other communication methods include TeamSTEPPS to improve communication for the benefit of the patient. TeamSTEPPS includes a huddle of team members at predetermined times to give an overview of particular concerns for the day and may include information specific to the individual patient or any environmental or situational concerns. The purpose is to increase awareness of all team members regarding any concerns to increase safety for the patient. In addition, in the situation where there is concern regarding something that is being done, any member can say "I need clarification" and that is a message to stop and reevaluate what is happening at the time. Although there are many other similar methods, these are the ones used most recently practiced by the authors of this chapter.

In midwifery, collaborative management consists of 3 levels which are consultation, collaboration, and referral. The first level is consultation in which the CNM presents a patient to another provider or team member with the intention of getting advice or an opinion regarding the patient's care. In this case, the primary management is the responsibility of the CNM. The second level is collaboration in which the CNM presents a patient to another provider usually as a result of preexisting or new complications. This patient is managed by the CNM/MD team. A discussion related to appropriate management and plan of care may result in the CNM continuing to care for the patient or may result in the patient being transferred to the collaborating provider. The third level of collaboration is if a patient is referred to another provider for the management of a particular problem or complete management of care. The responsibility for this patient is with the physician. It is possible that a patient may be referred back to the CNM following appropriate management/resolution of the problem for which she was referred. These levels of collaborative management are further addressed in a Position Statement from the ACNM regarding collaborative management (American College of Nurse-Midwives, 2013).

An important distinction is between collaborative management and a collaborative agreement. "The ACNM opposes requirements for signed collaborative agreements between physicians and CNMs as a condition for licensure, reimbursement, clinical privileging and hospital credentialing, or prescriptive authority as such requirements, in practice, interfere with effective coordination of care" (American College of Nurse-Midwives, 2011). However, state and institutional policies must be followed and individual states may have such requirements for collaborative practice and collaborative agreements. The ACNM supports independent midwifery care within the scope of practice and utilization of collaborative management.

In 2011, ACNM and ACOG developed a joint statement of policy addressing the practice relations between obstetrician-gynecologists and certified nurse-midwives. The policy statement noted that "...care is most effective when it occurs in a system that facilitates communication across care settings and among providers. Ob-GYNs and CNMs/CMs are experts in their respective fields of practice...who may collaborate ...based on the needs of their patients. Quality of care is enhanced by collegial relationships characterized by mutual respect and trust, as well as professional responsibility and accountability" (American College of Nurse-Midwives & American College of Obstetricians and Gynecologists, 2011). Both organizations recognize differing positions on home birth.

In 2012 an entire issue of Obstetrics and Gynecology Clinics of North America was devoted to the subject of collaborative practice in obstetrics and gynecology. That journal was prefaced with a statement co-authored by Dr. Richard Waldman from ACOG and Holly Powell Kennedy from ACNM. Together they recognized the growing shortage of obstetric health care providers and predicted that an increase in the number of midwives would be part of the solution in conjunction with a redesign of the maternity care system. Waldman and Powell noted that the previous two years had been utilized to "improve our collaborative intelligence" (Waldman & Kennedy, 2012, p. 1) at the same time they were "focused on improving the relationship between ACOG and ACNM" (Waldman & Kennedy, 2012). They also sought articles describing collaborative practices and published a number of the responses. This collaborative effort was a major step toward the future.

The seventh edition of *Guidelines for Perinatal Care by the American Academy of Pediatrics and ACOG* stated that, "A qualified physician or certified nurse-midwife or certified midwife should attend all deliveries. Collaborative practice involving a multidisciplinary team is encouraged. ...team members work together, utilizing mutually agreed upon guidelines and policies that define the individual and shared responsibilities of each member. ...The concept of a team guided by one of its own members and the acceptance of shared responsibility for outcomes promote shared accountability. Facilitation of communication among health care providers is essential for the provision of safe, quality care" (American Academy of Pediatrics & The American College of Obstetricians and Gynecologists, 2013, p. 24).

Prescriptive Authority/Credentialing

Prescriptive authority comes with its own issues related to APRNs and CNMs. These issues are not limited to CNMs, but impact all of the APRN professionals. As of 2013, fewer than 50% of the states authorize independent prescribing for APRNs (NCSBN, 2013). State regulations determine what is needed in the majority of states that require written collaborative agreements. The regulations specify delegation requirements, the classes of drugs that can be prescribed, the relationship that needs to exist between the physician and the CNM including the number of CNMs to whom a physician may delegate prescriptive authority, and the type of quality assurance that is required for prescriptive authority. CNMs require authority for prescribing from their board of nursing, the state, and may require an individual DEA number for controlled substances.

Credentialing is related to the authorization to practice in a particular facility. Before being hired into a position, most employers will make the CNM aware of the requirements that are needed to proceed with practice in a particular facility or with an entity. This may include a delineation of the request to perform specific procedures for which the CNM must provide documentation of appropriate education and training, particularly those procedures that are considered outside the core competencies of the midwifery program.

Practice Settings/Care Provided

Decision regarding the practice setting in which a CNM chooses to practice is made based on the individual's preference. There are multiple options. Midwives are trained as primary care providers who can provide care across the lifespan of women, generally, beginning in adolescence and continuing beyond menopause. While many think of midwifery as only providing care during the childbearing years, or more specifically during pregnancy, midwifes can provide care to women across the lifespan This includes caring for women with peri and post-menopausal problems, gynecologic problems, and routine well-women examinations.

Midwives partner with women to provide high quality personalized care. Midwives care for many women in private practice settings where the CNM may partner with an Obstetrician/Gynecologist to provide well-woman screenings, preconception counseling, contraceptive and medication management, diagnostic tests and procedures, and treatment of sexually transmitted infections. They also provide prenatal care many times offering the option of group prenatal care. When necessary, midwives can consult, collaborate, or refer patients to a physician colleague for services that may be beyond their scope of practice. CNMs also provide care to laboring women either in the hospital, in hospital birth centers, free standing birth centers, or at home. Most CNM births occur in hospitals.

It is within the CNM scope of practice to provide care for newborn for the first 28 days of life. However, many CNMs refer newborn care to nurse practitioners or physicians. CNMs also manage postpartum follow up visits including family planning. As part of their practice, some CNMs provide surgical assistance to physicians for surgical procedures on their patients such as cesarean delivery, or gynecologic surgery.

The same services listed above may also be provided in a public health setting providing care to the underinsured or underserved populations. CNMs consistently involve their patients in their care by providing education and helping them understand what to expect. They formulate the plan of care with their patient while addressing her particular needs. Although CNMs do not provide primary care services to men, CNMs are able to provide care to male partners of their patients who have been diagnosed with sexually transmitted infections. Expedited partner therapy is supported by the Centers for Disease Control and Prevention, and is legal in many states. Expedited partner therapy allows the provider to treat the partner without performing any type of examination.

CNMs may choose to provide any range of the clinical care mentioned above for their patients. Some prefer working only in the clinic setting; while others prefer working in the hospital setting, and a high percentage prefer full scope midwifery providing care for all of the needs of women across the life span. There are many clinical care options for CNMs with physicians in specialized areas such as reproductive endocrinology and infertility, sexual dysfunction, and dysplasia. New midwives often seek to join a practice team which is supportive of his/her developing skills.

From an academic perspective, CNMs can teach in midwifery programs or work with medical students and residents in medical schools. They can also teach in undergraduate and graduate nursing programs. CNMs are leaders in healthcare, and can work as administrators, with insurance companies, in quality systems and information technology, as well as many other areas of healthcare administration.

Midwives are entrepreneurs that can own their own birth centers and women's health care practices. As the owner of a practice, the CNM can work as manager, administrator, care provider, and educator. In addition, the entrepreneurial midwife can oversee all aspects of coding and billing activities that are then submitted to third party payers. CNMs need to form collegial relationships for outside referrals for their patients that may need them.

In whatever clinical setting, the characteristic of midwifery care is that of being very personalized for each woman. For example, if the CNM evaluates a woman for the first time at the time of delivery, she does everything possible to identify what it is that the woman is seeking from her birth experience and how she wants the process to precede. The CNM recognizes that it is the woman and her family's birth experience, not that of the CNM. Midwives support birth as a natural process and recognize that even historically, midwives remained patient and allowed the birth process to proceed with minimal intervention. The CNM has a multitude of pain management options available for the patient including epidural analgesia, medications for cervical ripening, and induction of labor, as well as antibiotics. The CNM skillfully practices the art and science of midwifery drawing from his/her nursing and midwifery background.

CENTERINGPREGNANCY® AS A MODEL OF PRENATAL CARE

One of the most exciting changes to prenatal care in the last 10 years is the development of CenteringPregnancy® by Sharon Schindler Rising, CNM. In videos and articles on the CenteringPregnancy® website, www.centeringhealthcare.org, Ms. Schindler describes how she developed the idea for CenteringPregnancy®. She saw many patients every day in her practice and found that she was frequently repeating herself in the process of providing education about pregnancy. This repetition was causing her to run behind, keep patients waiting, and feel frustrated about what was happening. It was then that she began her development of what has grown to become widely recognized as CenteringPregnancy® group prenatal care.

CenteringPregnancy® brings groups of 8-12 women together to receive their prenatal care. The women are generally placed into groups with others who are due in the same month. Thus, their concerns and interests are likely to be similar. Groups include both nulliparous and multiparous women and both find benefit in the education and support provided by the group. Typically group sessions are 2 hours in length with time for assessment, education and some unstructured time for casual conversation. Other support facilitators are invited to participate in the group sessions to bring the information to the women. Included are social workers to facilitate discussion on domestic violence, nutritionists to facilitate discussion of good eating habits, lactation consultants to facilitate discussion on breastfeeding, and pediatric providers to establish the important link for ongoing care. In fact, Centering Healthcare Institute also offers CenteringParenting® to begin where CenteringPregnancy® ends. In subsequent pregnancies, women often choose to return to group as they continue to learn and often have become the experts offering advice to other pregnant women. Lab draws and immunizations can also be done within the group setting.

CenteringPregnancy® has 3 major components: health assessment, education, and support. In taking the history, the CNM or other licensed provider inquires about particular problems or concerns. With the permission of the patient, the concerns are brought to the group for further discussion. The provider performs the health assessment, including fundal height measurement and evaluation of fetal heart rate. The patient is empowered by participating in the assessment, measuring her own blood pressure and weight, and then logging the values into her CenteringPregnancy® notebook. The patient then adds other information such as the gestational age, fundal height, and fetal heart rate. During the check in time and the health assessment time, the CNM shares with the patient any pending lab or diagnostic test results. Two facilitators (typically the CNM and a co-facilitator, such as medical assistant) lead the educational activities of the group. Although there is a curriculum plan for each of the 10 sessions, the group has the flexibility to address emerging issues raised by participants. If curriculum material is not covered in one session, it can be covered in a subsequent session. Provider facilitated group health care allows more time to explore important health topics. Women experience the component of support through the stability of the group and the sense of community. Women are more involved in their care and become empowered by the group interactions.

Group prenatal care has been associated with improved pregnancy and neonatal outcomes. In a prospective matched cohort study comparing women receiving group prenatal care to women receiving traditional individual care, birth weight was greater for infants of women in group versus individual prenatal care (P < .01). Among those children born preterm, infants of group patients were significantly larger than infants of individual-care patients (mean, 2398 versus 1990 g, P < .05). There were no differences in number of prenatal visits or other risk characteristics (patient age, race, prior preterm birth) (Ickovics, 2003). A subsequent randomized controlled trial conducted at university-affiliated hospital prenatal clinics had similar findings. Women assigned to group care were significantly less likely to have preterm births compared with those in standard care: 9.8% compared with 13.8% (OR 0.67, 95% CI 0.44-0.99, P=.045). Effects were strengthened for African-American women: 10.0% compared with 15.8% (odds ratio 0.59, 95% confidence interval 0.38-0.92, P=.02). Women in group sessions were less likely to have suboptimal prenatal care (P<.01), had significantly better prenatal knowledge (P<.001), felt more ready for labor and delivery (P<.001), and had greater satisfaction with care (P<.001). Breastfeeding initiation was higher in group care: 66.5% compared with 54.6%, P<.001. There were no differences in costs associated with prenatal care or delivery (Ickovics & Kershaw & Westdahl & Magriples & Massey & Reynolds, 2007).

The degree of fidelity to the CenteringPregnancy® model has been associated with the degree of success. CenteringPregnancy® has 13 Essential Elements which are required to achieve the benefits from this care model. The Essential Elements are:

1. Health assessment occurs within the group space.
2. Participants are involved in self-care activities.
3. A facilitative leadership style is used.
4. The group is conducted in a circle.
5. Each session has an overall plan.
6. Attention is given to the core content, although emphasis may vary.
7. There is stability of group leadership.
8. Group conduct honors the contribution of each member.
9. The composition of the group is stable, not rigid.
10. Group size is optimal to promote the process.
11. Involvement of support people is optional.
12. Opportunity for socializing with the group is provided.
13. There is ongoing evaluation of outcomes.

Recent research indicates that greater process fidelity was associated with significantly lower odds of both preterm birth and intensive utilization of care. Greater content fidelity was associated with lower odds of intensive utilization of care. These findings suggest that adequate training, including training clinicians in facilitative leadership, plays an important role in achieving improved outcomes for women (Novick & Reid & Lewis & Kershaw & Rising & Ickovics, 2013).

The IHI (Institute for Healthcare Improvement) Triple Aim is a framework developed by the Institute for Healthcare Improvement that describes an approach to optimizing health system performance. It is IHI's belief that new designs must be developed to simultaneously pursue three dimensions, which we call the "Triple Aim":

- Improving the patient experience of care (including quality and satisfaction);
- Improving the health of populations; and

- Reducing the per capita cost of health care (Institute for Healthcare Improvement, 2014)

The Centering Healthcare Institute website states the following regarding how they feel that CenteringPregnancy® meets the U.S. Triple Aim goals.

Centering is Better Care
Centering is a team approach to care that actively engages patients in goal setting, skill-building, and peer support. Provider facilitated group health care allows more time to explore important health topics. The model includes three components of care: assessment, learning, and community building.

Centering is Better Health
Centering is an evidence-based innovation that has been nationally recognized by leading healthcare experts because of the improved outcomes for important maternal child health factors including preterm birth rates, low birth weight rates, small for gestational age, breastfeeding rates, and immunization rates.

Centering is Lower Cost
Through improved outcomes, Centering delivers great value to the healthcare system. In 2012, the reduction in preterm births alone through Centering saved over $40 million (Centering Healthcare, n.d.).

Centering Healthcare Institute (CHI) provides assistance and training in establishing the system changes necessary to implement the CenteringPregnancy® model of care. CHI provides the expertise through the Model Implementation Plan, a well-designed and comprehensive process, to help practice sites to adopt this model of group care. Because model fidelity is so important to outcomes, medical sites that chose to offer the program must be approved by the Centering Healthcare Institute. Training is provided at various locations throughout the country. The approval process is detailed on their website: www.CenteringHealthcare.org. The staff at Centering Healthcare Institute are always willing to provide advice and support to prospective institutional clients (Centering Healthcare, n.d.).

FUTURE TRENDS/INNOVATIVE CARE

Collaboration among provider types is facilitated by an understanding of and respect for the unique training and skill sets of the provider groups. This understanding may be developed by interdisciplinary education, providing opportunities to build relationships and shape teamwork from early in training. The Accreditation Council on Graduate Medical Education currently requires that Obstetrics & Gynecology residents learn to work on interdisciplinary teams (ACGME Program Requirements for Graduate Medical Education in Obstetrics and Gynecology, 2008).

One model providing the opportunity for interprofessional training is The Center for Children and Women in Houston, Texas, which opened in August of 2013. The Center is a patient and family-centered medical home providing comprehensive care for women and children under one roof. The medical home model with emphasis on comprehensive, coordinated primary care can achieve improvement in healthcare outcomes. With the most successful implementation of this model, the financial incentives are aligned to promote the provision of the highest quality of care and the reduction in unnecessary testing, emergency room utilization and hospitalization for conditions that can be managed as an outpatient.

One of the key components of the medical home initiative is that care is provided by a team of professionals including advanced practice nurses—both certified nurse-midwives and nurse practitioners. APRNs are integral to the design of The Center for Children and Women and were involved from the conceptualization through the implementation phases. The certified nurse-midwives and the Ob/Gyns are all faculty at Baylor College of Medicine and medical students, as well as residents in Pediatrics and Obstetrics/Gynecology also receive training at the facility. Dental students, nursing students, and APRN students will all learn together. Classrooms and collaborative workspaces in The Center for Children and Women were designed specifically for group educational endeavors. A Cochrane meta-analysis on interdisciplinary education reported that interdisciplinary education results in improvement in the working culture, including collaborative team behavior, reduction in clinical errors, and patient satisfaction (Reeves, n.d.).

The physicians and certified nurse-midwives practice side-by-side in clinic and determine which patients are seen by each provider type. The physicians and certified nurse-midwives utilize the same protocols and workflows, reducing variability in patient care. Physicians are continuously available for consultation and referral. Many patients are co-managed due to the nature of the practice environment.

The new clinical model utilizes CenteringPregnancy® along with the traditional model to provide prenatal care. The early decision to incorporate CenteringPregnancy® allowed the facility design and construction to be tailored to optimize success of the group model.

All staff for The Center for Children and Women were presented with basic information regarding the CenteringPregnancy® model of care so they could understand how their role would fit in the care delivery. More detailed training (a two day Level I Facilitators Workshop) was presented by the Centering Healthcare Institute and was attended by providers, key OB staff and other support staff and administration.

We believe that the interprofessional education and the practice environment will prepare the next generation of providers for success in collaborative practices.

Vision for the Future from the Perspective of ACNM

The ACNM has established goals for the future of midwifery.

- CNMs/CMs will achieve full autonomy in practice and equitable reimbursement by 2015.
- There will be 1000 newly certified CNMs/CMs per year by 2015.
- Support the provision of high-quality maternity care and women's health services by CNMs and CMs as reflected in the ACNM mission statement.

- Ensure the organizational effectiveness and efficiency of ACNM through the volunteer structure and national office.
- Position ACNM and its members to be leaders in efforts to reduce infant mortality and improve maternal health globally by 2015 (American Colleges of Nurse-Midwives, 2011).
- CNMs/CMs will attend 20% of births in the United States by the year 2020 (American College of Nurse-Midwives, 2013).

These goals are excellent goals with the 1st one partially met related to equitable reimbursement. This has in part been accomplished through the Affordable Care Act (ACA), that reimbursements are equitable. The ACA is striving to reimburse for outcomes. "Medicaid reimbursement for CNM care is mandatory in all states. Congress set their Medicare payment under Medicare at 100% of physician rates recognized the value of CNM services by. The majority of states also mandate private insurance reimbursement for midwifery services" (American College of Nurse-Midwives, 2013). However, according to the 2013 Education Report, "we are still less than halfway to attaining our goal of 1,000 new certificants per year." The reasons for this are multifactorial and include limited availability of clinical sites, and availability of program spaces nationally is about 900 as of 2012; however those spaces are not filled. Although more students enter each year, it is taking some of them longer than initially planned to graduate due to requirements needed or those seeking DNP or part-time education (American College of Nurse-Midwives, 2013).

In 2012 the ACNM Board of Directors approved an updated Vision, Mission, and Core Values as listed below:

- Vision: Advancing the health and well-being of women and newborns by setting the standard for midwifery excellence.
- Mission: ACNM works to establish midwifery as the standard of care for women. We lead the profession through education, clinical practice, research, and advocacy.
- Core Values:
  - Excellence
  - Evidence-Based Care
  - Formal Education
  - Inclusiveness
  - Woman-Centered Care
  - Primary Care
  - Partnership
  - Advocacy
  - Global Outreach (American College of Nurse-Midwives, 2012)

CONCLUSION

Although involved in the care of women for many centuries, midwives can anticipate further growth in the presence and role of the CNM. This chapter traced the historical role to the present day role with attention given to the Consensus Model as a regulatory model on the future development of nurse-midwifery. Current aspects of the CNM regulations, role, and scope of practice were presented.

The examples of the CenteringPregnancy® model of care along with The Center for Children and Women describe innovative practice settings for the delivery of quality care to women. The chapter described many aspects of the role of the certified nurse-midwife from education to certification and practice settings. The chapter concludes with the goals established by the ACNM for the future along with an updated Vision, Mission, and Core Values statement.

References

ACGME. (2008, January 1). ACGME Program Requirements for Graduate Medical Education in Obstetrics and Gynecology.

American Academy of Pediatrics and The American College of Obstetricians and Gynecologists. (2013). *Guidelines for Perinatal Care, seventh edition.*

American College of Nurse-Midwives. (2010). *ACNM Future Focus.* American College of Nurse-Midwives. (2011, September 24). *Standards for the Practice of Midwifery.* American College of Nurse-Midwives. (2011, December). Collaborative Agreement between Phsycians and Certified Nurse-Midwives and Certified Midwives. *Position Statement.*

American College of Nurse-Midwives. (2011, August). Comparison of Certified Nurse-Midwives, Certified Midwives, and Certified Professional Midwives. American College of Nurse-Midwives. (2012). Core Competencies for Basic Midwifery Practice.

American College of Nurse-Midwives. (2012, April). Mission, Vision, and Core Values.

American College of Nurse-Midwives. (2013, May). Collaborative Management in Midwifery Practice for Medical, Gynecologic and Obstetric Conditions. *Postion Statement.*

American College of Nurse-Midwives. (2013). *Midwifery Education Trends Report 2013.*

American College of Nurse-Midwives. (2013, August 6). News Release. *American College of Nurse-Midwives Supports Legislation to Improve Medicaid Reimbursement.*

American College of Nurse-Midwives and American College of Obstetricians and Gynecologists. (2011, February). Joint Statement of Practice Relations Between Obstetrician-Gynecologists and Certified Nurse-Midwives/Certified Midwives. *College Statement of Policy.*

American College of Nurse-Midwives. (December 2011). Definition of Midwifery and Scope of Practice for Certified Nurse-Midwives and Certified Midwives. *Position Statement.*

American College of Nurse-Midwives, American College of Obstetricians and Gynecologists, and Nurses Association of the American College of Obstetricians and Gynecologists. (1971). Joint Statement on Maternity Care, 1971. *Joint Statement.*

APRN Joint Dialogue Group Report (2008). Consensus Model for APRN Regulation: Licensure, Accreditation, Certification & Education APRN Joint Dialogue Group Report.

Burst, H. V. (2005, March/April). The History of Nurse-Midwifery/Midwifery Education. *Journal of Midwifery & Women's Health*, 129-137.

Centering Healthcare. (n.d.). Retrieved January 2014, from centeringhealthcare.org.

Ehrenreich, B., & English, D. (1973). Witches, Midwives, and Nurses. A History of Women Healers. New York: The Feminist Press.

Ewell, J. H. (1990). Retrieved January 2014, from Our Family Genealogy Pages: http://www.ewellfamily.org/genealogy/getperson.php?personID=I3479&tree=ewellcombo

Howard, H. (1879). *Supplement to Howard's Domestic Medicine, Midwifery and the Diseases Peculiar to Women.* Philadelphia, PA: Hubbard Brothers.

Ickovics J, K. T. (2003). Group prenatal care and preterm birth weight: results from a matched cohort study at public clinics. *Obstetrics & Gynecology.*

Ickovics, J., Kershaw, T., Westdahl, C., Magriples, U., Massey, Z., Reynolds, H., et al. (2007). Group Prenatal Care and Perinatal Outcomes-A Randomized Controlled Trial. *Obstetrics & Gynecology. Institute for Healthcare Improvement.* (2014). Retrieved February 2014

Litoff, J. (1982, November/December). The Midwife Throughout History. *Journal of Nurse-Midwifery, 27*, 3-11.

Midwifery in the United States and the Consensus Model for APRN Regulation. (2011).

NCSBN. (2013). *Major Components of the Consensus Model by State.*

Novick, G., Reid, A., Lewis, J., Kershaw, T., Rising, S., & Ickovics, J. (2013). Group prenatal care: model fidelity and outcomes. *Am. J. Obstet. Gynecol.*, 209(2):112.e1-6.

Reeves S, Z. M. (n.d.). Interprofessional education: effects on professional practice and health care outcomes. *Cochrane Database Syst. Rev. 2008; (1):CD002213.*

The APRN Consensus Workgroup and the APRN Joint Dialogue Group members. (2008, July 7). *Consensus Model for APRN Regulation: Licensure, Accreditation, Certification & Education. The Holy Bible. Genesis 35:17.* (n.d.).

Varney, H. (2015). *Varney's Midwifery* (Fifth ed.). (T. L. King, M. C. Brucker, J. M. Kriebs, J. O. Fahey, & H. Varney, Eds.) Burlington, MA: Jones & Bartlett Learning.

Waldman, R., & Kennedy, H. P. (2012). Preface: The Long and Winding Road to Effective Collaboration. *Obstetric and Gynecologic Clinics of North America.*

Williams, D. R., Cohen, S. R., & Thomas, C. R. (2015). *Varney's Midwifery* (Fifth ed.). (T. L. King, M. C. Brucker, J. M. Kriebs, J. O. Fahey, & H. Varney, Eds.) Burlington, MA: Jones & Batlett Learning.

APPENDIX A

Core Competencies for Basic Midwifery Practice

I. Hallmarks of Midwifery

The art and science of midwifery are characterized by the following hallmarks:

A. Recognition of menarche, pregnancy, birth, and menopause as normal physiologic and developmental processes
B. Advocacy of non-intervention in normal processes in the absence of complications
C. Incorporation of scientific evidence into clinical practice
D. Promotion of woman- and family-centered care
E. Empowerment of women as partners in health care

F. Facilitation of healthy family and interpersonal relationships
G. Promotion of continuity of care
H. Health promotion, disease prevention, and health education
I. Promotion of a public health care perspective
J. Care to vulnerable populations
K. Advocacy for informed choice, shared decision making, and the right to self-determination
L. Integration of cultural humility
M. Incorporation of evidence-based complementary and alternative therapies in education and practice
N. Skillful communication, guidance, and counseling
O. Therapeutic value of human presence
P. Collaboration with other members of the interprofessional health care team

II. Components of Midwifery Care: Professional Responsibilities of CNMs and CMs

The professional responsibilities of CNMs and CMs include but are not limited to the following components:

A. Promotion of the hallmarks of midwifery
B. Knowledge of the history of midwifery
C. Knowledge of the legal basis for practice
D. Knowledge of national and international issues and trends in women's health and maternal/newborn care
E. Support of legislation and policy initiatives that promote quality health care
F. Knowledge of issues and trends in health care policy and systems
G. Knowledge of information systems and other technologies to improve the quality and safety of health care
H. Broad understanding of the bioethics related to the care of women, newborns, and families
I. Practice in accordance with the ACNM Philosophy, Standards, and Code of Ethics
J. Ability to evaluate, apply, interpret, and collaborate in research
K. Participation in self-evaluation, peer review, lifelong learning, and other activities that ensure and validate quality practice
L. Development of leadership skills
M. Knowledge of licensure, clinical privileges, and credentialing
N. Knowledge of practice management and finances
O. Promotion of the profession of midwifery, including participation in the professional organization at the local and national level
P. Support of the profession's growth through participation in midwifery education
Q. Knowledge of the structure and function of ACNM

III. Components of Midwifery Care: Midwifery Management Process

The midwifery management process is used for all areas of clinical care and consists of the following steps:

A. Investigate by obtaining all necessary data for the complete evaluation of the woman or newborn.

B. Identify problems or diagnoses and health care needs based on correct interpretation of the subjective and objective data.
C. Anticipate potential problems or diagnoses that may be expected based on the identified problems or diagnoses.
D. Evaluate the need for immediate intervention and/or consultation, collaborative management, or referral with other health care team members as dictated by the condition of the woman, fetus, or newborn.
E. In partnership with the woman, develop a comprehensive plan of care that is supported by a valid rationale, is based on the preceding steps, and includes therapeutics as indicated.
F. Assume responsibility for the safe and efficient implementation of a plan of care that includes the provision of treatments and interventions as indicated.
G. Evaluate the effectiveness of the care given, recycling appropriately through the management process for any aspect of care that has been ineffective.

IV. Components of Midwifery Care: Fundamentals

A. Anatomy and physiology, including pathophysiology
B. Normal growth and development
C. Psychosocial, sexual, and behavioral development
D. Basic epidemiology
E. Nutrition
F. Pharmacokinetics and pharmacotherapeutics
G. Principles of individual and group health education
H. Bioethics related to the care of women, newborns, and families
I. Clinical genetics and genomics

V. Components of Midwifery Care of Women

Independently manages primary health screening, health promotion, and care of women from the peri-menarcheal period through the lifespan using the midwifery management process. While the woman's life is a continuum, midwifery care of women can be divided into primary, preconception, gynecologic, antepartum, intrapartum, and post-pregnancy care.

A. Applies knowledge, skills, and abilities in primary care that include but are not limited to the following:
   1. Nationally defined goals and objectives for health promotion and disease prevention
   2. Parameters for assessment of physical, mental, and social health
   3. Nationally defined screening and immunization recommendations to promote health and to detect and prevent disease
   4. Management strategies and therapeutics to facilitate health and promote healthy behaviors
   5. Identification of normal and deviations from normal in the following areas:
      a. Cardiovascular and hematologic
      b. Dermatologic
      c. Endocrine
      d. Eye, ear, nose, and throat

   e. Gastrointestinal
   f. Mental health
   g. Musculoskeletal
   h. Neurologic
   i. Respiratory
   j. Renal
6. Management strategies and therapeutics for the treatment of common health problems and deviations from normal of women, including infections, self-limited conditions, and mild and/or stable presentations of chronic conditions, utilizing consultation, collaboration, and/or referral to appropriate health car services as indicated.

B. Applies knowledge, skills, and abilities in the preconception period that include but are not limited to the following:
   1. Individual and family readiness for pregnancy, including physical, emotional, psychosocial, and sexual factors including
      a. Non-modifiable factors such as family and genetic/genomic risk
      b. Modifiable factors such as environmental and occupational factors, nutrition, medications, and maternal lifestyle
   2. Health and laboratory screening
   3. Fertility awareness, cycle charting, signs and symptoms of pregnancy, and pregnancy spacing

C. Applies knowledge, skills, and abilities in gynecologic care that include but are not limited to the following:
   1. Human sexuality, including biological sex, gender identities and roles, sexual orientation, eroticism, intimacy, and reproduction
   2. Common screening tools and diagnostic tests
   3. Common gynecologic and urogynecologic problems
   4. All available contraceptive methods
   5. Sexually transmitted infections including indicated partner evaluation, treatment, or referral
   6. Counseling for sexual behaviors that promote health and prevent disease
   7. Counseling, clinical interventions, and/or referral for unplanned or undesired pregnancies, sexual and gender concerns, and infertility
   8. Identification of deviations from normal and appropriate interventions, including management of complications and emergencies utilizing consultation, collaboration, and/or referral as indicated

D. Applies knowledge, skills, and abilities in the perimenopausal and postmenopausal periods that include but are not limited to the following:
   1. Effects of menopause on physical, mental, and sexual health
   2. Identification of deviations from normal
   3. Counseling and education for health maintenance and promotion
   4. Initiation or referral for age/risk appropriate periodic health screening
   5. Management and therapeutics for alleviation of common discomforts

E. Applies knowledge, skills and abilities in the antepartum period that include but are not limited to the following:
   1. Epidemiology of maternal and perinatal morbidity and mortality
   2. Confirmation and dating of pregnancy
   3. Promotion of normal pregnancy using management strategies and therapeutics as indicated
   4. Common discomforts of pregnancy
   5. Influence of environmental, cultural and occupational factors, health habits, and maternal behaviors on pregnancy outcomes
   6. Health risks, including but not limited to domestic violence, infections, and substance use/abuse
   7. Emotional, psychosocial, and sexual changes during pregnancy
   8. Anticipatory guidance related to birth, breastfeeding, parenthood, and change in the family constellation
   9. Deviations from normal and appropriate interventions, including management of complications and emergencies
   10. Placental physiology, embryology, fetal development, and indicators of fetal well-being

F. Applies knowledge, skills, and abilities in the intrapartum period that include but are not limited to the following:
   1. Confirmation and assessment of labor and its progress
   2. Maternal and fetal status
   3. Deviations from normal and appropriate interventions, including management of complications, abnormal intrapartum events, and emergencies
   4. Facilitation of physiologic labor progress
   5. Measures to support psychosocial needs during labor and birth
   6. Labor pain and coping
   7. Pharmacologic and non-pharmacologic strategies to facilitate maternal coping
   8. Techniques for
      a. administration of local anesthesia
      b. spontaneous vaginal birth
      c. third stage management
      d. performance of episiotomy repair of episiotomy and 1st and 2nd degree lacerations

G. Applies knowledge, skills, and abilities in the period following pregnancy that include but are not limited to the following:
   1. Physical involution following pregnancy ending in spontaneous or induced abortion, preterm birth, or term birth
   2. Management strategies and therapeutics to facilitate a healthy puerperium
   3. Discomforts of the puerperium
   4. Self-care
   5. Psychosocial coping and healing following pregnancy
   6. Readjustment of significant relationships and roles

7. Facilitation of the initiation, establishment, and continuation of lactation where indicated
8. Resumption of sexual activity, contraception, and pregnancy spacing
9. Deviations from normal and appropriate interventions including management of complications and emergencies

VI. Components of Midwifery Care of the Newborn

Independently manages the care of the newborn immediately after birth and continues to provide care to well newborns up to 28 days of life utilizing the midwifery management process and consultation, collaboration, and/or referral to appropriate health care services as indicated.

A. Applies knowledge, skills, and abilities to the newborn that include but are not limited to the following:
   1. Effect of maternal and fetal history and risk factors on the newborn
   2. Preparation and planning for birth based on ongoing assessment of maternal and fetal status
   3. Methods to facilitate physiologic transition to extrauterine life that includes but is not limited to the following:
      a. Establishment of respiration
      b. Cardiac and hematologic stabilization including cord clamping and cutting
      c. Thermoregulation
      d. Establishment of feeding and maintenance of normoglycemia
      e. Bonding and attachment through prolonged contact with neonate.
      f. Identification of deviations from normal and their management.
      g. Emergency management including resuscitation, stabilization, and consultation and referral as needed
   4. Evaluation of the newborn:
      a. Initial physical and behavioral assessment for term and preterm infants
      b. Gestational age assessment
      c. Ongoing assessment and management for term, well newborns during first 28 days
      d. Identification of deviations from normal and consultation, and/or referral to appropriate health services as indicated
   5. Develops a plan in conjunction with the woman and family for care of the newborn for the first 28 days of life, including nationally defined goals and objectives for health promotion and disease prevention:
      a. Teaching regarding normal behaviors and development to promote attachment
      b. Feeding and weight gain including management of common breastfeeding problems
      c. Normal daily care, interaction, and activity including sleep practice and creating a safe environment
      d. Provision of preventative care that includes but is not limited to
         (1) Therapeutics including eye ointment, vitamin K, and others as appropriate by local or national guidelines

(2) Testing and screening according to local and national guidelines
(3) Need for ongoing preventative health care with pediatric care providers

e. Safe integration of the newborn into the family and cultural unit
f. Appropriate interventions and referrals for abnormal conditions:
(1) Minor and severe congenital malformations
(2) Poor transition to extrauterine life
(3) Symptoms of infection
(4) Infants born to mothers with infections
(5) Postpartum depression and its effect on the newborn
(6) End-of-life care for stillbirth and conditions incompatible with life

g. Health education specific to the infant and woman's needs:
(1) Care of multiple children including siblings and multiple births
(2) Available community resources

(American College of Nurse-Midwives. 2012)

In: Collaboration with the Advanced Practice Nurse ISBN: 978-1-63321-311-1
Editors: E.R. Giardino, R.G. Hanks and A.P. Giardino

Chapter 9

THE ROLE OF THE NURSE PRACTITIONER IN CONVENIENT CARE CLINICS

Julie Lindenberg[1], DNP, APRN, FNP-BC, DCC and Kiley Black[2], MSN, ANP
[1]The University of Texas School Health Science
School of Nursing at Houston, TX, US
[2]Clinics, Standards & Medical Education, KTarget, Minneapolis, MN, US

ABSTRACT

This chapter provides a summary of the autonomous role the nurse practitioner (NP) holds in the relatively new clinical arena of the convenient care industry. The chapter describes the history of convenient care clinics (CCCs), services provided and patient utilization patterns. Clinical regulations and standards are discussed as related to NPs, medical doctors (MDs) and physician assistants (PAs) as well. The chapter presents the NP impact on patient care as it relates to access, cost, patient satisfaction, quality and safety and clinical educational opportunities for family nurse practitioner (FNP) and doctor of nurse practitioner (DNP) students. Finally, it concludes with a look at the current and future trends of services provided in this field of advanced practice nursing.

INTRODUCTION

The concept of convenience and utilization of highly trained nurses to provide accessible health care has been around since the 1890's when Lillian Wald opened the famous Henry Street Settlement to provide care for low-income residents (Henry Street, 2014); however, convenient care clinics can trace their roots back to Minneapolis, MN. One day in 1999 Rick Krieger's son developed an ear infection. Rick was unable to schedule an appointment with the child's pediatrician, which left the emergency room as the default place to obtain treatment. Frustrated with the wait time and cost of a conventional ER visit, Rick, along with partners Douglas Smith, MD, Steve Pontius and Kevin Smith, RN, FNP, developed a medical model that could provide low-cost, high quality health care for low acuity problems such as ear infections and sore throats (K. Smith, personal communication, February 1, 2014).

The provider of choice for these facilities was and remains nurse practitioners. In-store clinics, operated by QuickMedx, soon began opening their doors in retail locations such as grocery stores, pharmacies and big box retail chains. Initially, these clinics had a very limited list of services and only accepted cash for payment. Known as "disruptive innovators," in the healthcare industry, this consumer-driven model of health care quickly became a novel way to deliver basic health care in a convenient setting. Today, clinic operators consist of hospitals and health systems and corporations. Many of the larger retail clinics have formed affiliation with medical systems and physician groups to enhance collaboration and serve as a referral network system for patients (Hanlon, 2007). In addition, insurance companies became very interested in the convenient care model as they repeatedly demonstrated cost savings to their insured. CCCs evolved to forming contracts with these companies while still accepting cash payments for visits.

SERVICES AND UTILIZATION

CCCs by nature are designed to occupy small spaces and provide basic medical care. A few large centers have radiology equipment but most do not. CCCs are relatively large users of point of care (POC) tests, clinical chemistry and immunoassay tests and vaccines, with vaccines accounting for a considerably greater share than POC tests. Prices for services provided at CCCs are readily available to patients at the clinic. Providers discuss what impact, if any, any additional services will have on the ultimate cost to the patient.

While it's difficult to gather statistical data regarding volume of clinic visits given this information is considered proprietary, since its inception, CCCs continue to have high utilization rates from patients. CVS, the corporate owner of MinuteClinic, reached a new milestone of 18 million patient visits by end of the year 2013 (CVS, 2014). RAND originally published a 2008 article that characterized the patient groups and clinical complaints most likely to be seen at retail clinics, prior to 2007 (Mehrotra, 2009). An update to that research in 2012 reveals how patient traits and visit reasons have changed; nationally, visits to retail clinics increased fourfold from 2007 to 2009, and shifts in use showed:

- Patients over the age of 65 increasingly sought care from retail clinics. The proportion of visits made by seniors increased from 7.8% (pre-2007) to 18.9% (from 2007 to 2009). Approximately 85% of those visits were for vaccinations.
- Acute care visits made up a smaller proportion of overall visits, dropping from 78.2% of visits to 52.2%.
- The proportion of preventive care visits doubled over the same period, from 21.8% of visits to 47.3% (Mehrotra, 2012).

REGULATIONS AND STANDARDS

Regulation of CCCs currently varies from state to state. In some states, clinics are licensed as physician practices and are therefore subject to regulations developed by the state Board of Medicine.

EXHIBIT 5

Reasons For Visits To A Retail Clinic, 2000–06 And 2007–09

Reason	Time period		Age group, 2007–09 visits only		
	2000–06 (N = 1.35 million)	2007–09 (N = 8.89 million)	<18 years (n = 1.77 million)	18–64 years (n = 5.77 million)	≥65 years (n = 1.35 million)
Preventive care	21.8%	47.5%	40.2%	41.2%	85.2%
Vaccine	19.7	40.8	26.9	35.9	81.8
Other preventive care[a]	2.1	6.7	13.3	5.2	3.3
Acute care	78.2	51.4	59.6	57.7	12.9
Upper respiratory infections	27.4[b]	18.7[b]	5.7	5.3	1.4
Bronchitis	—[b]	—[b]	1.7	5.8	1.3
Sinusitis	—[b]	—[b]	3.8	13.4	2.7
Pharyngitis	21.2	11.7	21.3	10.9	1.0
Otitis externa	12.7[b]	7.4[b]	2.3	1.7	1.2
Otitis media[c]	—[b]	—[b]	13.0	4.2	0.7
Urinary tract infections	3.5	2.5	0.3	3.8	0.3
Conjunctivitis	4.6	2.8	3.8	2.9	0.7
Allergy	2.1	2.0	1.5	2.4	0.7
Other acute care	8.9	6.5	6.2	7.4	2.9
Chronic disease[d] care	0.1	1.1	0.2	1.2	1.9

Source: Author's analysis. From: Copyrighted and published by Project HOPE/*Health Affairs* as Mehrotra, A., and Lave, J., Visits to retail clinics grew four-fold from 2007 to 2009, although their share of overall outpatient visits remains low, Health Aff (Millwod). 2012, 31, 9, 2123-2129. The published article is archived and available online at www.healthaffairs.org.

Note: Not all percentages sum to the total because of rounding. The classification of the visits is based on the principal diagnosis associated with each visit. [a]For example, sports physicals and blood pressure screenings. [b]Because pre-2007 data were based partly on reason for visit as opposed to postvisit diagnosis codes, some diagnoses with similar presentation are combined. Comparable data from 2007-09 are combined to ease comparison across columns. We combined upper respiratory infections, bronchitis, and sinusitis. We also combined otitis media and otitis externa. [c]Includes otalgia. [d]For example, asthma, hypertension, or diabetes.

Other requirements related to licensing and physician supervision also vary, as do rules regarding the scope of practice of NPs. The convenient care industry adheres to all state regulations regarding practice issues for the advanced practice nurse.

In 2006, the American College of Nurse Practitioners adopted a resolution in support of CCCs and their role in improving access to care. Later in that year, the American Academy of Family Physicians (AAFP) and American Medical Association published a set of principles and guidelines addressing CCC operations and the quality of care delivered.

While developed more as a preventive measure to ensure high quality of care rather than as a reaction to perceived quality shortfalls, they form the basis of a model that can be utilized broadly throughout the emerging CCC sector. Many of the leading CCC organizations have embraced these types of standards, which include, but are not limited to:

- Having a well-defined scope of clinical services, consistent with the state scope of practice laws
- Having standardized protocols derived from evidence-based practice guidelines to ensure quality of care
- Having established arrangements by which NPs and PAs have direct access to and supervision by MDs, as consistent with state laws
- Having established protocols for ensuring continuity of care with primary care providers (PCPs) within the local community and encouraging patients to establish care with a PCP

- Having an established referral system with specialists or other facilities for appropriate treatment if the patient's conditions or symptoms are beyond the scope of services provided by the CCC
- Having an established electronic medical record as a means of communicating patient information and facilitating continuity of care (Dolan, 2007)

Standardized protocols assist providers in clinical decision making at most CCCs; however, these protocols are used as a tool or guideline and are not intended to replace the critical thinking or the providers' clinical judgment. For example, the leading CCCs' guidelines are grounded in evidence-based medicine and guidelines published by the major medical bodies such as the American Academy of Pediatrics and the AAFP (Hansen-Turton, 2007).

Most of the clinics are incorporating rigorous quality assessments into their evaluative structures. Both internal and external reviews are being built in, including formal chart review by collaborating physicians and peer-review by NPs. Credentialing of NPs and thorough work history is established as well as a process for ensuring adequate experience level to work in an independent role (Hansen-Turton, 2007).

In 2006, a trade organization, the Convenient Care Association (CCA), was created in order to enable store-based health clinics to share best practices, establish common standards of operation, and develop professional relationships with the medical community and health care providers. The CCA has implemented other quality and safety standards for the industry, in addition to those already mentioned; these include:

- Assuring provider credentialing, licensing, training, experience and background checks
- Collecting aggregate data on selected quality and safety outcomes
- Collecting data on patients' perceptions of care and engagement with the model
- Providing health promotion and disease prevention education to patients to maximize the impact of the patient encounter
- Providing a visit summary and discharge instructions and educational materials to the patient at each encounter
- All CCA members agree to pursue a third-party certification or accreditation of their choice to demonstrate their adherence to these standards (CCA, 2010).

All CCA members are in compliance with applicable OSHA, CLIA, HIPAA, and ADA standards. All CCA members follow Centers for Disease Control and Prevention (CDC) guidelines. All CCA members establish emergency response procedures to ensure the patients in need of emergency care can be transported to an appropriate setting as quickly as possible.

In addition, the CCA has established a Clinical Advisory Board to provide input and guidance on the creation of national, industry-wide quality standards for store-based health clinics.

Some standards may include peer and physician review, and the collection of patient outcomes and satisfaction at store-based health clinics (Kalorama, 2013). CCA membership includes over 95% of clinics in operation.

The CCA has implemented an independent certification program for CCA members; all clinics that are members of the CCA are either certified or accredited by a third party.

NP Impact on Care

CCCs improve patient access to care, in fact, some hospital systems report their CCCs are the largest entry point into their healthcare system (Mehrotra, 2008). Forty percent or more of CCC patients report they would have gone to the emergency room, an urgent care center or forgone treatment altogether if there had not been a CCC available, according to one study (CCA, 2010). Families who reported not getting or delaying needed medical care were 2.5 times more likely to have used CCCs compared to families without such problems (Bukata, 2010). The top reasons for choosing CCCs over other providers includes: more convenient clinic hours (64%), more convenient location (62%), no appointment necessary (53%), and no usual source of care (34%) (Bukata, 2010).

CCCs help to lower health care costs. CCCs are more cost-effective for basic healthcare needs than physicians' offices, urgent care clinics and emergency rooms. This is possible because CCCs provide high-quality care by certified NPs or PAs. CCCs are affordable to the insured (43%), underinsured (30%) and uninsured (27%) alike (Bukata, 2010).

Total costs for episodes of care (including prescriptions received, any testing, and follow-up visits) for three conditions (urinary tract infection, upper respiratory infection, and otitis media) were lower at CCCs compared to urgent care clinics by an average of 30%, physician offices (34%), and emergency departments (80%) (Mehrotra, 2009). The cost of receiving care for a strep throat at a CCC is less than one third of what it costs at an emergency room (CCA, 2010). In another study conducted by Blue Cross and Blue Shield of Minnesota, CCC visits were found to cost consumers half as much as physicians' appointments for similar conditions (CCA, 2010). There was no increase in the use of prescription drugs at CCCs and the percentage of patients who had any follow-up appointments after their first visit was almost identical at CCCs, urgent care clinics, and physician offices.

CCCs may reduce health care costs by providing preventive care (e.g., influenza vaccine) and facilitating earlier access to care. CCCs demonstrate significant cost savings for both consumers and third party payers. All evidence points to the clinics as being a cost-effective addition to health care delivery. A RAND Corporation study said about 17% of all visits to hospital emergency departments across the US could be treated at CCCs or urgent care centers, potentially saving $4.4 billion annually in health care costs (Price, 2010). CCCs report high patient satisfaction. Patients who use CCCs are satisfied with their visit. According to a 2013 Kalorama survey entitled "Retail Clinics: Consumer Attitudes," 91% of respondents who had used a CCC were either satisfied or very satisfied.

Gallup's leading research on customers and customer engagement found that the nation's largest and most comprehensive manager of CCCs rank among the top 10 percent of all organizations globally in engaging their customers (Clinician1, 2010). The same operator received the highest satisfaction ratings from more than 9-out-of-every-10 patients; compared to the typical company in Gallup's database that receives the highest satisfaction from just 1-in-every-three patients. More than 9-out-of-every-10 patients strongly felt that the NP or PA spent enough time with them, and similar number strongly felt that the NP or PA carefully listened to them and explained things to them in a way that was easy to understand.

Consumers have expressed high levels of satisfaction with the services provided by NPs, PAs, and physicians in CCCs, as well as the convenience of the CCC model (Hansen-Turton, 2007).

CCCs provide high-quality care. Quality care and quality assurance are critical to the long-term survival of the convenient care industry. Ateev Mehrotra, a policy analyst at the RAND Corporation found that on the quality side, the care provided at CCCs is very similar to what is found at physician offices and urgent care centers, and in some cases, even superior to what is found in emergency departments. Mehrotra and his colleagues also found that antibiotic prescribing rates at the three sites they researched were equivalent. CCC providers are unlikely to overprescribe, because any prescription that is made outside of standard clinical indications must be backed up by an explanation of the clinical reasoning behind that decision. In other studies, the quality of care provided by NPs in CCCs has been repeatedly shown to be equivalent to, or better than, comparable settings. On 14 quality measures, compliance at the CCCs, physician offices, and urgent care centers averaged between 61-64%, compared to only 55% in the emergency departments (Bukata, 2010).

CCCs have a return visit rate comparable with standard medical offices; the care is high quality and does not generate additional follow up utilization (Rohrer, 2012). Quality scores and rates of preventive care offered are similar for CCCs as for other delivery settings (Mehrotra, 2009). CCCs had a 92% compliance with quality measure for appropriate testing of children with pharyngitis vs. HEDIS average of 75%; they also had an 88% compliance score for avoidance of antibiotic prescribing in children with upper respiratory infection vs. HEDIS average of 83% (Jacoby, 2010).

Another study by the RAND Corporation easily dispelled the myth that CCCs disrupt the relationship between the primary care provider (PCP) and the patient. In fact, only 39% of the CCC patients in their study had a PCP; thus, because most CCC patients lack a usual source of care, they have no primary care relationship to disrupt (Mehrotra, 2009).

CCCs demonstrate a strong safety record. The industry's track record on patient safety is compelling, and the companies and health systems that run the clinics have taken steps internally to ensure their policies and procedures are beyond reproach. Each clinic also has policies and procedures to identify any untoward event. Records are routinely reviewed by audit committees, and in states where there are statutory or regulatory requirements for physician collaboration or supervision, these oversight physicians review records on an ongoing basis. As of a 2011 review, not a single malpractice suit had been filed against a provider in the CCCs (Miller, 2011).

Clinical Opportunities for the NP Student

According to the Bureau of Labor Statistics, the annual number of NP graduates is declining by 4.5% every year, while the annual number of PA graduates is projected to fall 25% by 2020. Approximately 80% of NPs practice in primary care, whereas only 44% of PAs currently practice in primary care (Hansen-Turton, 2007). According to the AAFP, both NPs and PAs remain important contributors to the primary care workforce and should not be neglected in workforce projections or in the designing of effective interdisciplinary teams. Approximately 6000 NPs graduate from schools of nursing on an annual basis, and of this number 53% are FNPs (Miller, 2011).

There are approximately 5000 NPs working in CCCs (CCA, 2010). NPs with a family primary health care background are the most sought after by the convenient care industry, because they are credentialed and licensed to care for patients of all ages. Most CCCs prefer that FNPs they hire have a minimum of one year experience before applying for a position.

The benefit to the student in the CCC setting is that they gain the understanding of the importance of the clinical patient/consumer and financial business metrics. Additionally, the opportunity will expose the student to a career path that includes leadership opportunities.

NPs who have earned a DNP degree are taught to see health care from a broader perspective. When employed by CCCs, DNPs help the industry give greater attention to population-based health care (Ford, 2011). The DNP may function as an aid to expanding health care services to CCC patients. As CCCs become more main stream, academia has integrated convenient care into advanced nursing curricula, and creating partnerships between schools of nursing and convenient care operators. The DNP student has research opportunities in the CCC practice environment and can complete the DNP capstone project in the setting.

A major CCC operator in conjunction with the National Organization of Nurse Practitioner Faculties has sponsored a new program to support the clinical education of NPs. The program includes a Preceptor Web Portal containing web-based resources that clinical preceptors use to promote education for NPs nationwide (http://www.nonpf.org/?page=84).

CURRENT AND FUTURE TRENDS

Current trends in CCCs continue to focus on acute care needs and vaccinations. Several clinic operators offer services geared towards chronic disease management, preventive care and lifestyle behavior changes (i.e. weight management and smoking cessation). In addition, they cater to specific ages and/or disease processes, such as the aging adult and offer injection services for infertility patients. Diabetes management is one disease process where CCCs are making significant inroads. With recent technological advances, the ability to perform a point-of-care hemoglobin A1C test, LDL cholesterol and urinary microalbumin testing are now readily available in CCCs. Combined with blood glucose measurement, patients can complete 4 out of 5 key diabetes screening/management goals. In fact, a study conducted by Reid et al. found that retail clinics do not disrupt preventive health care and diabetes management (Reid, 2012).

Another consideration is the impact the Affordable Care Act will have on CCCs. With an expected increase in number of insured individuals in the United States and the projected shortage of PCPs, many patients will find their way to CCCs for diagnosis and treatment of many chronic diseases. Walgreen's announced in April 2013 that they were getting into the chronic care 'business.' Per Sandra Ryan, then Chief Nurse Practitioner Officer, "All the retail clinics have historically done screenings, but until now, we have never initiated treatment or officially made diagnoses of these conditions. The big difference now is people can come in and the NPs can diagnose their condition, treat them, coordinate their care and work with their primary care physician (PCP). If they don't have a PCP, and they wish to be treated and followed by us, we will do that" (Merchant Medicine, 2014). One example is hypertension evaluation. Previously, diagnosis and treatment was initiated and maintained in the PCP office. However, in partnership with national laboratory vendors, CCCs have the ability to obtain a comprehensive laboratory analysis on patients in order to properly prescribe anti-hypertensive medication. The same holds true for hyperlipidemia.

Another example of expanded service for chronic disease is asthma management. Given that this disease process is protocol driven, it is a natural progression for CCCs to provide care for this patient population. In addition to medication management of asthma, the NP can administer nebulizer treatments to treat mild asthma exacerbations.

A newer area of focus for CCCs centers on initiating behavioral change for lifestyle issues including weight management and smoking cessation. RediClinic, in conjunction with Dr. David Katz of the Yale Prevention Center, developed the Weigh Forward program. The lifelong weight control program includes ten weekly visits with the CCC clinicians and is available seven days a week in a convenient, food oriented location of the grocery store (Buhler, 2011). Other clinic operators have followed suit.

One interesting link is the fact that most, if not all CCCs perform biometric screenings, which includes BMI, waist circumference, glucose and cholesterol measurements. If a patient has abnormal results, the nurse practitioner can check for diabetes start a patient on a statin, refer directly to the weight loss program and refer the patient to a PCP.

Finally, CCCs, because of their convenience, have recognized the need to accommodate specific patient populations, such as the older adult. With updates to the Centers for Medicaid and Medicare Services (CMS), all new Medicare patients are now eligible for a 'Welcome to Medicare' one-time visit. During this visit, patients are evaluated for BMI, blood pressure, have a simple eye test and most importantly, receive counseling on topics such as depression risk, vaccinations, home safety, preventive health screenings and advanced directives (http://www.medicare.gov/coverage/your-medicare-coverage.html). Another area of interest for CCCs is collaborating with pharmacy benefit programs to provide injection teaching for their patients currently receiving medications for conditions such as infertility, rheumatoid arthritis, and coagulopathy.

CONCLUSION

CCCs have been successful, to a large extent, because they have routinized and simplified the basic delivery of health care. Nurse practitioners are the backbone of the clinicians who provide care to the clients who use CCC services. Service offerings of CCCshave remained focused and target only a specific population of health care consumers. To be successful in the mission of delivering care that is convenient and accessible, staying within the 15-20 minute no appointment visit times and providing cost–effective care will have to remain the mainstays of the industry. The Accenture report predicted the growing number of CCCs would create $800 million in savings annually in overall healthcare expenditures by 2015 and add capacity for 10.8 million patient visits per year nationally (Zamosky, 2013). To that end, nurse practitioners are a main reason for the continued and growing success of the CCC model in the provision of healthcare services.

REFERENCES

Buhler, J. (2011). Weight loss through RediClinic Weigh Forward program. Retrieved from http://www.examiner.com/article/weight-loss-through-rediclinic-weigh-forward-program.

Bukata, R. (2010). Wal-Mart medicine. *Emergency Physicians Monthly.* Retrieved from http://www.epmonthly.com/archives/features/wal-mart-medicine/

Clinician1 Editors. (2010). New study on Take Care Clinic satisfaction. Retrieved from http://clinician1.com/posts/article/new_study_on_take_care_clinics_satisfaction.

Convenient Care Association. (2010). Increasing access. Retrieved from http://www.ccaclinics.org.

Convenient Care Association. (2010). Reducing costs for consumers and third-party payers. Retrieved from http://www.ccaclinics.org.

Dolan, W. A. (2007). Update on store-based health clinics. *Report of the Council on Medical Service, CMS Report* 5-A-07.

Ford, J. (2011). *The DNP in retail health: Can a degree impact an industry?* Retrieved from http://www.advancweb.com.

Hanlon, M. (2007). The emergence of the convenient care clinic. *Gizmag.* Retrieved from http://www.gizmag.com/go/7068.

Hansen-Turton, et al. (2007). Convenient care clinics: The future of accessible health care. *Disease Management,* 10(2), 61-73.

Henry Street Settlement (2014). *Our history.* Retrieved from http://www.henrystreet.org/about/history/

Jacoby, R., et al. (2010.) Quality of care for 2 common pediatric conditions treated by convenient care providers. *American Journal of Medical Quality,* 26, 53-58.

Kalorama Information Survey. (2013). *Retail clinics: Consumer attitudes results of the 2013 Kalorama Information Survey.* Retrieved from http://www.kaloramainformation.com/Retail-Clinics-Consumer-7479194/

Mehrotra, A., et al. (2008). A comparison of patient visits to retail clinics, primary care physicians, and emergency departments. *Health Affairs,* 27(5), 1271-1282.

Mehrotra, A., et al. (2009). The costs and quality of care for three common illnesses at retail clinics as compared to other medical settings. *Annals of Internal Medicine,* 151(5), 321-328.

Mehrotra, A. and Lave, J. (2012). Visits to retail clinics grew four-fold from 2007-2009, although their share of overall outpatient visits remains low. *Health Affairs,* 2123-2129.

Merchant Medicine. (2014). News: Take Care expands services. Retrieved from http://www.merchantmedicine.com/News.cfm?view=156.

Miller, K. (2011). Retail clinics: A promise made is a promise kept. *The Journal for Nurse Practitioners,* 7(1), 51-54.

Price, W. T. (2010). *Urgent care clinics carve out a key health care niche.* Retrieved from http://usatoday30.usatoday.com/money/industries/health/2010-10-10-urgent-care-expansion_N.htm.

Reid, R., Ashwood J., Friedberg M., Weber, E., Setodji, C., and Mehrotra, A. (2012). Retail clinic visits and receipt of primary care. *The Journal of General Internal Medicine,* 28 (4):504-12.

Rohrer, J. E. and Angstman, K. B. and Garrison, G. (2012). Early return visits by primary care patients: A retail nurse practitioner clinic versus standard medical office care. *Population Health Management,* 15, 1-4.

Wilson, A., et al. (2010). Retail clinic versus office setting: Do patients choose appropriate providers? *The American Journal of Managed Care,* 16(10), 753-758.

Zamosky, L. (2013). *Retail clinic growth sparks new partnership in San Diego*. Retrieved from http://www.californiahealthline.org/features/2013/

In: Collaboration with the Advanced Practice Nurse ISBN: 978-1-63321-311-1
Editors: E.R. Giardino, R.G. Hanks and A.P. Giardino

Chapter 10

THE INTERFACE OF CASE MANAGEMENT AND CARE COORDINATION WITH ADVANCED PRACTICE NURSING

Janet Treadwell, PhD, RN, MSN, CCM, CPHQ
Texas Children's Health Plan, Houston TX, US

ABSTRACT

Case Management and Care Coordination fulfill an important role in family and team-based care. Care coordination is a common theme in new models of care delivery as it helps to improve clinical and financial outcomes. Advanced practice nurses must understand the relevance of case management and care coordination in order to equip them with an appreciation of how these key concepts are utilized in a collaborative framework of care. Elements of the case management process, explained in this chapter, set expectations for what should be included in service provision with an emphasis on the importance of the individualized plan of care. Theory and models from nursing, social work, and systems theory, provide framework for the process of case management and care coordination. Legislation and Technology are also addressed due to the great influence of both upon the future of care coordination.

GROWING IMPORTANCE OF CASE MANAGEMENT AND CARE COORDINATION

Fragmentation and lack of care coordination in primary and acute care practices put individuals at unnecessary clinical and financial risk. The lack of communication, facilitation and planning present in the United States healthcare system presents financial, clinical and ethical concern. Care coordination forms the framework of support to bring together necessary information with knowledge of best practice and consideration of individual preferences. The Patient Protection and Affordable Care Act specifically mentions care coordination and indicates its necessary inclusion in new models of care delivery (2010). Collaboration and coordination across all services and health care providers are in place in acute care, primary care, and managed care models. This chapter is intended to expand awareness of care coordination, the role of the case manager, and how care coordination has application within the practice of the Advanced Practice Nurse. All healthcare professionals can benefit from understanding the professional role of the case manager and the tools of technology and influence of policy upon the profession. Case managers possess the skills and expertise to conduct and facilitate care coordination, integral to ensuring effective and quality implementation of a comprehensive plan of care. The importance of care coordination for children extends to the health of the family recognizing the physical and emotional stressors of being a family inclusive of a child with special healthcare needs (Cousino & Hazen, 2013; Hudy et al., 2006. The National Association of Professional Geriatric Care Managers has identifies the expanding number of home-based care coordination programs as a professional issue for nursing (2013). Delivery of care programs are of prime importance to maximize the independence and autonomy of elders (2013). It is evident that care coordination is important for national healthcare programming given that 80% of older adults have one chronic condition and almost 50% have multiple chronic conditions (Battersby et al., 2007). Viewing the need for care coordination from an economic perspective, the 15% of Medicare enrollees with chronic conditions and functional limitations using long-term services and supports account for one-third of Medicare spending (Komisar & Feder, 2011).

The subject of care coordination has relevance to Advanced Practice Nurses (APN) for overall continuity of care and delivery of family-centered care. Understanding definitions, key concepts, theory support, and structure of case management and care coordination will improve interprofessional collaboration, and assimilation of care coordination into practice. Knowledge of the benefits that care coordination provides to families is important to support self-management of patients and self-advocacy efforts. Care coordination takes on both a financial and clinical importance as new delivery models include provisions for effective care coordination as part of the reimbursement structure. Discussion of the role of case management in various settings, should inform ways to implement effective features within the systems of care of advanced practice.

Relational to the advanced practice registered nurse (APRN), it is important to understand the role of case managers and others on the coordination team as part of patient-centered care. In many clinical situations the APRN collaborates with the case manager to find resources and support communication across numerous providers. In other instances the APRN collaborates with the case manager to promote care planning and barrier dissolution, and in other cases, the APRN is active member of the care coordination team in roles such as home visits for assessment and prevention of potentially preventable emergency room visits. No matter the intersect, the interplay of care coordination and case managers is important to practice as the healthcare environment moves to accountable care.

DEFINITIONS AND DIFFERENCES

The Case Management Society of America (CMSA), is a certification entity for professional case managers, and defines case management as:

> "a collaborative process of assessment, planning, facilitation, care coordination, evaluation, and advocacy for options and services to meet an individual's and family's comprehensive

> health needs through communication and available resources to promote quality cost effective outcomes " (CMSA, 2010, p. 6).

The terms case management, care coordination, case manager, care managers, care coordinators, health coach, and patient navigator pose confusion to both consumers and health care professionals. Case managers are health care professionals who conduct the services and functions of case management and care coordination using knowledge of their specialty area combined with an understanding of the case management process. These individuals most frequently additionally hold a license as a registered nurse or social worker. Case managers may perform services in a facility, practice or as an independent small business. Often the case manager is lead of a care coordination team comprised of multiple individuals with varying roles and functions focused on a particular type of case management such as Medical, Behavioral Health, Managed Care, Worker's Compensation, Transition, Rehabilitation, or Geriatric.. Case managers interface with nurse practitioners in clinical settings to improve patient outcomes through recommendations for the modification of treatment plans and prescribing patterns. Case managers may contact APNs and physicians within a health plan's network to suggest drug selection and use, preferred formularies, potential polypharmacy and changes in dosage for a particular patient; or give treatment recommendations.

Care coordination is a team effort, not one person's responsibility. In fact, it is a responsibility of the entire healthcare delivery team and the patient/family. Communication and coordination with the patient/family and all care providers delivering components of care to a child is both an ethical and professional responsibility of all health professionals. Creation of links with community and educational resources, and driving focus to the patient-centered plan of care often falls to a case manager. The case management role performs oversight and connection in the context of benefits and patient/ family preferences as well as the practitioner team through care coordination.

The Agency for Healthcare Research and Quality defines care coordination as:

> "the deliberate organization of patient care activities between two or more participants (including the patient) involved in a patient's care to facilitate the appropriate delivery of health care services. Organizing care involves the marshalling of personnel and other resources needed to carry out all required patient care activities, and is often managed by the exchange of information among participants responsible for different aspects of care (Markowitz, 2004)"

Professional case managers perform the intervention approaches of care coordination independently or as part of a team due to their expertise across the continuum and in family/patient-centered care. The foundational element of care coordination is maintaining the client as the central focus of care while ensuring all other participants are duly involved and informed of needs of preferences of the client and the plan of interventions. Promotion of central coordination eliminates duplication of services and connects the patient/family to needed services for their child. Care coordination has gained recognition in importance over recent years. As an example, the promotion of effective communication and coordination of care is one of the National Quality Forum's six priorities, chosen due to their impact on health outcomes (National Quality Forum, 2013). The American Nurses Association (2012) sites care coordination as a core professional standard and competency and the U.S. Department of

Health and Human Services established the importance of care coordination in its' National Quality Strategy and the Institute of Medicine has gone on record with the assertion care coordination could save up to $240 billion in healthcare system savings (American Nurses Association, 2010). The National Committee for Quality Assurance (NCQA) defines care coordination as a function that "supports information-sharing across providers, patients, types and levels of service, sites and time frames."

The Case Management Process

Providing a structural approach to case management is the case management process. This process is constructed as a framework to assisting individuals (clients) and families through the care and habilitation process to achieve maximum health care outcomes. Table 1 shows the case management process. This model involves an iterative profess of planning, intervention and monitoring as re-assessments and plan adjustments result from evaluations made during the course of the relationship.

Table 1: The Case Management Process

1. Identification and selection of individuals who benefit from program services
2. Assessment and problem identification
3. Development of a case management plan
4. Implementation and coordination of the plan
5. Evaluation of changes in the person's needs/preferences and progress
6. Follow-up to extend, modify, or close the plan.

The term integrated case management addresses the assessment phase of the process. In integrated case management there is recognition of the interconnectedness of physical health, behavioral health, and environmental/systems of care which need to be considered in developing an individualized plan of care (Kathol, Perez, & Cohen, 2010). From the perspective of a whole person/family, this approach recognizes one cannot separate the interplay between medical and emotional beings (patient and caregivers) when developing a plan to identify needs and preferences that encompasses access, quality, safety, and efficiencies. Using an integrated approach for assessment paired with diagnoses specific evidenced based guidelines provides a solid foundation for development of interventions and self-management strategies.

Identification and Selection

Identification of individuals who could benefit from services can be a challenge. Methods of identification are dependent on the setting/employer of the case manager. As an example, a discharge planner in a hospital setting may connect with an insurance company case manager to facilitate equipment hand-off to a pediatric primary care setting. During a well-child visit, identification of failed developmental screen may precipitate action by an office-based care coordinator to facilitate therapies and further testing as well as link the child with community supports and services. Subsequent to an occupational accident, a case manager may be called in to coordinate treatments, specialist and vocational rehabilitation. All healthcare professionals can consider themselves identifiers, the awareness of how to connect the individual with a case manager is often the missing element. The case manager linked to a person's benefits is typically the most efficient contact from the perspective of the care practitioner.

Screening tools can help in the assessment process. An example is the Child Adolescent Needs and Strengths (CANS) tool which captures parent/caregiver stress levels in addition to providing a resiliency picture of the child/adolescent. This is important to ensure the child and care giver(s) receive support and resources to achieve the highest level of functioning possible. Another screening tool is the Children with Special Healthcare Needs Screen which can identify areas for further in-depth assessment (see Table 1).

Table 1. Tools used for Pediatric Screening for Special Healthcare Needs

Child Adolescent Needs and Strengths (CANS): http://www.dhs.state.or.us/caf/safety_model/procedure_manual/ch04/ch4-section6.pdf CSHCN Screener: http://www.childhealthdata.org/docs/cshcn/cshcn-screener-cahmi-quickguide-pdf.pdf Parents' Evaluation of Developmental Status (PEDS): http://www.Pedstest.com Modified Checklist for Autism in Toddlers (MCHAT): http://www.mchatscreen.com Ages & Stages Questionnaires (ASQ): http://agesandstages.com/

Table 2. Adult Screening Tools for Case Management Services

Uniform Comprehensive Assessment Tool (UCAT) http://www.okdhs.org/NR/rdonlyres/D8BE9DC5-F9DC-405A-9267-53A32D08EF51/0/UCATAssessorManual_asd_05022011521l.pdf Adult Needs and Strengths Assessment (ANSA) https://myshare.in.gov/FSSA/pmo/dmha---survey/ATRproviders/Shared%20Documents/INATR%20Forms/ANSA%20Resources/ANSA---Comp4302009.pdf. Daily Living Activities-20 http://www.thenationalcouncil.org/galleries/resources---services%20files/DLA%20Sample.pdf. Level of Care Utilization Scale (LOCUS) http://communitypsychiatry.org/publications/clinical_and_administrative_tools_guidelines/LOCUS2010.pdf. *for older adults:* The Geriatric Depression Scale http://consultgerirn.org/uploads/File/trythis/try_this_4.pdf Confusion Assessment Method http://consultgerirn.org/uploads/File/Confusion%20Assessment%20Method%20(CAM).pdf

Adult screening tools screen for impact on activities of daily living, safety, barriers to care access, physical needs (inclusive of nutrition) and available support networks. Cultural and linguistic preference and transportation barriers are important elements of adult assessment. Behavioral health assessment is important in case management planning as many adults with chronic medical conditions also have behavioral health conditions in addition to many individuals with behavioral health as a primary diagnosis.

Health care insurers identify individuals who qualify for potential program inclusion by using referrals from practitioners or from analytic reporting obtained from claim information. Predictive modeling programs enable case manages to outreach to individuals that appear, based upon health services use history, to need coordination services. Programs for case management are most often voluntary. This means a request for participation is made to the child/family, to explain the available program and services, as well as who will be interfacing with the family. Initial contact with a family is most often telephonic, although may come in written format as well. Care coordination staff ask for a verbal or written consent of participation from the responsible individual. Some health promotion or disease management programs are considered 'opt-out,' meaning that any person meeting the program inclusion criteria receives information and reminders or calls unless a person requests not to be included in a program.

Assessment

The initial assessment goal is to obtain a comprehensive and accurate baseline describing the person across a holistic set of domains. The process is extremely important and can be time consuming. Clear expectations should to be set with the client/family explaining the importance of this foundational activity. The individualized evaluation includes information that will outline future frequency, mode and time of contacts, and is inclusive of defining cultural and religious preferences, literacy screening, and assessment of barriers to function and treatment engagement.

The initial assessment is an essential part of the process as it is extremely comprehensive and begins establishing the relationship of trust integral to optimal success. Assessment information is gained from a variety of sources including the client/family, current health care providers, records of past health care experiences, work or school educational plans (as applicable) and assessment of the community offerings of available services. Items included in the assessment cover domains inclusive of medical and psychosocial areas that best describe an individual as well as questions to gauge specific needs and preferences of the client/family that may arise from cultural or spiritual beliefs.

Understanding of the usual source of care, access to care, current self-management practices, and overall health status further enables understanding of the whole person. The National Committee for Quality Assurance (NCQA) offers some guidance as to the content of case management assessments (Table 3). Supplementing the assessment information are assessment tools which may be initiated by the case manager, a primary care practitioner, or specialist.

Table 3. Contents of Typical Case Management Assessment

- Assessment of clients' health status, including condition-specific issues
- Documentation of clinical history, including medications
- Initial assessment of the activities of daily living
- Initial assessment of mental health status, including cognitive functions
- Initial assessment of life-planning activities
- Evaluation of cultural and linguistic needs, preferences or limitations
- Evaluation of visual and hearing needs, preferences or limitations
- Evaluation of caregiver resources and involvement
- Evaluation of available benefits within the organization and from community resources
- Development of an individualized case management plan, including prioritized goals, that considers the clients' and caregivers' goals, preferences and desired level of involvement in the case management plan
- Identification of barriers to meeting goals or complying with the plan
- Facilitation of member referrals to resources and follow-up on process to determine whether the member acts on the referral
- Development of a schedule for follow-up communication with clients
- Development and communication of member self-management plans for clients

(Source; NCQA, 2013).

The assessments conducted as part of the case management process can provide a more robust picture of the patient to the APRN, important in the quest to attain true patient-centered care. Use of the team concept, using open communication and mutual respect enables the exchange of vital information focused on the shared patient goals while preventing redundant inquiry, thus improving efficiencies for the advanced practice nurse in the primary care or behavioral health role.

PROBLEM IDENTIFICATION AND CARE PLAN DEVELOPMENT

The assessment information results in a shared care planning session as part of team-based care. The case manager, healthcare professionals, and family support work as a team in the planning phase. The team creates clinical (medical/behavioral), social service, environmental and wellness goals, as applicable to the client. Inclusion of the medical/behavioral home practitioners optimally occurs in real time during a case conference. The shared care plan that is developed is given (or available online) to the client/family, the primary practitioner, and specialists or ancillary care providers as applicable. The team-created care plan creates a unified document to support coordination and consistency for service and to reach the client's goals.

To give an idea of the content of a care plan, one can review the results of The National Initiative for Children's Healthcare Quality and the Center for Medical Home Improvement collaborative. This workgroup met to develop both content and explanation of a comprehensive care plan for children with special healthcare needs (http://www.medicalhomeinfo.org/downloads/pdfs/ComprehensiveCarePlanning.pdf). The document contains sample forms with topical areas of importance, stressing the need for a plan of care whether in paper copy format, contained on a memory stick or accessible through the internet. The care plan content areas are applicable across age spans.

Implementation and Coordination

In a team-based model of care, a designated care coordination member employs a process of implementing activities to address barriers and prioritized goals as well as performs ongoing assessment and documentation to monitor the quality of care and services provided. Feedback is given to the team, preferable in an electronic feed to the medial record or through a patient portal. During interim evaluation of the care plan, the case manager adjusts interventions upon information drawn from the client/caregivers and all care providers to ensure goals are addressed with interventions. Case managers review and update care plans as needed based on condition changes but no less frequently than on a semi-annual basis. In many programs, an onsite visit to the client for face-to-face assessment is made on a semi-annual or annual basis with other contacts made telephonically or through email. Home visitation programs exist for specific vulnerable populations with varying home visitation frequency and program duration. Practitioners need to clarify the type and frequency of care coordination service delivery. Resources for developing a Family Centered Coordination (Table 5) are available to share with the entire team.

An area where APRN's have successfully employed the care coordination model is in transitional care interventions (American Nurses Association, 2012). Providing home visits to ensure understanding and competence of the patient/caregivers in the home environment after an inpatient acute or rehabilitation stay. Utilizing clinical skills for medication reconciliation, assessment of physical status, and successful understanding of the treatment plan accommodating family needs and preferences, can avoid unnecessary readmissions and improve patient clinical outcomes.

Evaluation and Follow Up

Movement toward goal achievement is important to intervention modification and program evaluation on a client-specific and overall program basis. Evaluation assesses movement outlined in the plan of care and determines the impact of care coordination and care interventions on outcomes (Table 5).

Table 4. Goal Evaluation Measures of Patient-Centered Plan

- Goal achievement
- Adherence to medication/treatment regimen(s)
- Barriers to compliance with practitioner appointments
- Development of self-management skills
- Nutritional and cognitive status
- Psychosocial status
- Satisfaction with current services (equipment, professional)
- Adequacy of work/school provision to meet needs
- Changes in self-reported health status
- Days missed school or work
- Changes in frequency of emergency room or hospital use
- Activation of community connections

Table 5. Resources for Family Centered Coordination Approach

Teamwork and communication Module PS 103 http://app.ihi.org/lms/coursedetailview.aspx?CourseGUID=3e37eb4a-4928-4d8b-976e-3a2a1a5f2c08&CatalogGUID=6cb1c614-884b-43ef-9abd-d90849f183d4 Patient and Family Centered Care PFC 101 http://app.ihi.org/lms/coursedetailview.aspx?CourseGUID=8eb52137-21d7-4b30-afcd-fd781de6d6d5&CatalogGUID=6cb1c614-884b-43ef-9abd-d90849f183d4 Writing the IFSP: National Dissemination Center for Children with Disabilities http://ifspweb.org/ Tools to Foster the Collaboration with Patient and Family Advisors http://www.ipfcc.org/tools/downloads-tools.html

The case manager established, measurable case management goals, which promote evaluation of the access, cost and quality of the care provided to the child to facilitate measures of goal achievement that directly result from the case management interventions.

Within a practice setting or care coordination program, outcomes can drive changes to the program or refinement of processes. Case managers use their goal directed patient/family-centered practice to not only evaluate each individual but the overall program they are delivering on a population management basis to identify patterns to maximize clinically positive, cost-effective outcomes. This evaluation includes aggregate reporting of health outcomes, results of client satisfaction surveys, cost analysis, visit success rates, and care plan adherence. Outcomes are frequently then compared to national benchmarks such as the Kids Inpatient Database (http://www.hcup-us.ahrq.gov/kidoverview.jsp) or the Centers for Disease Control and Prevention Chronic Disease Calculator (2009).

Case Closure Criteria

How long does a client remain in case management? Care coordination needs may end due to death, disease/condition improvement, or upon demonstration of self-management. Case closure may also occur due to change in insurance coverage, or a geographic move. A client/ family may always refuse or terminate services. The case manager documents the rationale for case closure and client health status when closing a case.

Models and Theory

Theories and Models of Practice for Case Management and Care Coordination

Care coordination has value for transition across services and as an organizing framework to support best practice. It is especially significant when addressing clients with multiple chronic conditions. According to a white paper published by the Partnership to Fight Chronic Disease, one in fifteen children in the United States has a chronic disease (Thorpe, 2013). Additionally, it is known that significant in-person interaction between the individual and care manager is associated with reduced hospital admissions and Medicare spending (Nelson, 2012). Care coordination addresses the need for education and support of clients and their families through alignment of both treatment and communication using the structure of an evidenced-based model. In addition professional education and health system knowledge, case managers use theory and evidenced-based practice to support families across the continuum of care.

The Chronic Care Model

Wagner's Chronic Care Model (Figure 1) is a useful visual tool for care coordination as it demonstrates the wider influences to client health. Wagner's model supports an informed and activated patient (child/family) coupled with a prepared and proactive practice team. The model defines the influences of the community and the healthcare system on ultimate patient outcomes. In care coordination this relates to negotiating with employers, interacting with schools, and identifying neighborhood and state resources for a specific client. Wagner's model is easily applied in team-based medical home models and has evidence of improved delivery of care to recipients when adopted by practitioners (Coleman, Austin, Brach, & Wagner, 2009).

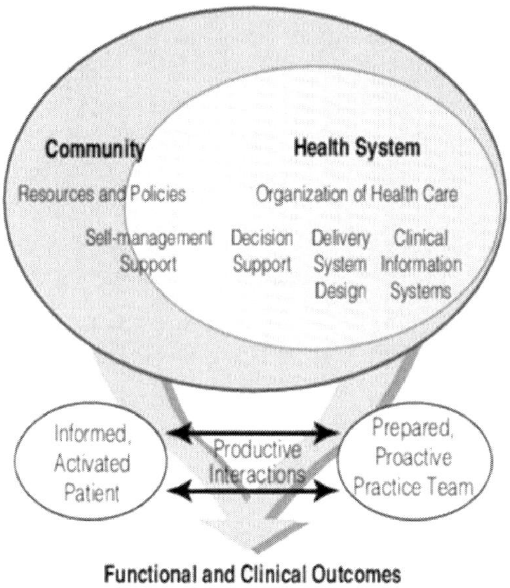

Wagner, EH. Chronic Disease Management: What Will It Take to Improve Care for Chronic Illness? Effective Clinical Practice. 1998;1:2-4. (used with permission).

Figure 1. Chronic Disease Management.

Continuum of Healthcare Model

The Case Management Society of America (CMSA) supports a continuum model of health care. Focusing on a patient centered model of case management delivery, the case management process is viewed within a circular model of financial, ethical and legal, social support and care providers. The philosophy targets optimum client wellness and function through communication, advocacy, education, resource identification, and facilitation of services to benefit the client, support system, healthcare delivery system and reimbursement (CMSA Standards of Practice for Case Management, 2010).

Nursing and Social Work Theories of Case Management

The case manager draws upon the applicable theories as a basis for practice. General System's theory, surveying relationships in the universe, and critical theory, is presented in nursing literature as a useful case management model. The nursing theory of Sister Calista Roy, stressing adaptation and Dr. Jean Watson's Caring Science theory (Roussel, 2011) also can be applied to case management practice. Social work theory supporting case management emphasizes a biopsychosocial perspective including strengths-based theory, use of learning theory, psychoanalytic theory, role theory and social network theory (Brandell, 2010). The social work perspective of case management unites concepts of community and the individual into a practice structure.

Roles of the Case Manager

Case management roles may vary depending on the program. The CMSA Standards of Practice describes the role of the case manager and use of evidence-based guidelines in practice (2010). The case manager is challenged to minimize fragmentation, navigate care transitions and work in interprofessional teams. The roles of planning care and improving patient safety also fall to the case manager. A hospital-focused professional case management organization, the American Case Management Association, adds the element of resource utilization to the role of case management through their Standards of Practice indicating the case manager utilizes resources prudently and balances cost and quality to insure the best outcomes (American Case Management Association, 2013).

Case managers lead the care coordination teams which may include: registered nurses, social workers, experienced parent partners, community health workers, educational specialists, and often dieticians in addition to the primary care medical home (pediatrician or advanced practice nurse) and specialist healthcare professionals. Interprofessional collaboration defines the supporting culture of the care coordination team with an emphasis on clear communication, professional accountability, shared decision-making and mutual trust across all roles on the team. This collaboration results in cooperative interaction achieving improved outcomes from teamwork as opposed to a singular practitioner approach (McDonald et al, 2007).

Team-based care coordination provides a contribution to individual and population. The triple aim of improving the quality and experience of care as well as overall cost through developing efficiency and effectiveness through coordination is a team responsibility (http://www.ihi.org/offerings/Initiatives/TripleAim/Pages/default.aspx). The team approach requires valuing the opinions and experience of the client/family and other team members. The goal is effective communication pertinent clinical information and treatment preferences across all professional types. This means the coordination organizes care to avoid duplication, support safe transfers and care transitions. Use of evidenced based guidelines across the team delivers consistency and expectations to the client. Team training in guidelines as well as resources and culture build is necessary. Care coordination requires interaction among all roles as each person on the team has a unique expertise to add to the child's success and resiliency build.

Ethics

There is an obligation in all models of case management and care coordination to behave in a moral and ethical manner. All healthcare professionals are responsible to a code of professional conduct (nursing, social work, physician) and team members responsible to ethical standards of their affiliated employer. Training for care coordination teams includes areas of: confidentiality, client respect, cultural competency, disclosure of conflicts of interest, and acknowledgement of self-determination. Underscoring the primary obligation to the client, principles of beneficence, non-malfeasance, autonomy (respecting right to choose), and justice and fidelity (follow through) align to care coordination practice (http://ccmcertification.org/sites/default/files/downloads/2012/41%20-%20Ethics%20issue%20brief.pdf). Ethical dilemmas do arise for the case manager due to issues of benefits versus cost, policies and regulations that require administrative review and documentation.

The care coordination team promotes self-advocacy of the client by encouraging decision-making and self-management. Education about choices and the promotion of shared decision-making assists the client. The care coordination team is responsible for advocating on behalf of the client, facilitating access to needed services, and addressing barriers/disparities that may occur during care coordination (http://www.preventioninstitute.org/tools/focus-area-tools/health-equity-toolkit.html).

Impact of Policy and Legislation on Case Management and Care Coordination

National Policy

On a national level, policy most recently impacting care coordination is the Patient Protection Affordable Care Act (www.HealthCare.gov/laresources/index.html). The Affordable Care Act (ACA) impacts individuals through removal of lifetime financial limits, the facilitation of 2.5 million young adults in maintaining access to coverage (by being able to stay on their parents insurance plan), and the emphasis of care coordination within the language of the bill specific to models of care, care transitions, and access to needed services. The ACA also contained provisions for the Centers for Medicaid and Medicare Strategies (CMS) to implement an Innovation Center. The Innovation Center supports research into new health care models that strengthen quality and support innovative strategies to address chronic disease and vulnerable populations. Care Coordination aligns to the Affordable Care Act goal of improved population management using value-based strategies inclusive of care coordination (Llewellen, 2013). Section 3025 of the Affordable Care Act added section 1886(q) to the Social Security Act establishes the Hospital Readmissions Reduction Program to reduce hospital payments based on excessive readmissions (http://www.cms.gov/Medicare/Medicare-Fee-for-Service-Payment/AcuteInpatientPPS/FY-2012-IPPS-Final-Rule-Home-Page-Items/CMS1250103.html). Effective beginning 2012, facilities must coordinate safe discharges or not be paid for that readmission. CMS has also established an Improving Care Transitions program in Medicaid. An item missing in the ACA, relevant to care coordination is definition of the qualifications of the people providing the coordination services. Clarification is necessary to protect the public from inexperienced or uninformed people engaging in care coordination activity at the potential financial and safety risk of children.

There are many important pieces of national legislation that impact coordination of health care. The Health Insurance Portability (HIPAA) removes the preexisting condition requirement from health coverage and protects the privacy of health information by requiring security measures of people and entities that hold health information. This includes anyone conducting care coordination activity. Healthcare information needs to be shared between healthcare providers associated with client care coordination. Case managers often take on the responsibility of facilitating communication between care practitioners. Specifically, the George Washington University School of Public Health and Health Services (SPHHS) research of healthcare information sharing indicates information on treatments and screening does not require additional consent across providers to aid in seamless care for children (Perna, 2013).

Federal legislation addressing care coordination for children includes Medicaid and State Children's Health Insurance Programs statutes and the associated State Waiver programs. Medicaid, CHIP, and Waiver recipients are all eligible for case management services. Most private commercial plans also have case management capability that may be requested. Total well-being of a child involves school and health, which the Individuals with Disabilities Education Act (IDEA), No Child Left Behind Act (NCLB), Section 504 of the Rehabilitation Act, and Assistive Technology Act (ATA) address in combination of education and health programs and rights.

It is important that APRNs understand care coordination and the law that can be leveraged in communication with school administration when advocating for children who need assistance. Often school services do not provide certain levels of support without advocacy from the health system. The Individuals with Disabilities Education Act (IDEA) provides school district funding to support education of children with disabilities. This includes free public education in the least restrictive setting for the child. The No Child Left Behind Act (NCLB) addresses the accountability of special education programs to protect students with disabilities (Yell, Katsiyannas, & Shiner, 2006). The Office of Special Education Programs (OSEP), provides oversight to these programs. This includes Parent Training and Information Centers (PTI) in every state to supports projects providing information and technical assistance to families of children with disabilities.

The case manager needs to be aware of ADA provisions to inform clients of the process and requirements of accommodation to enable school/work success. *Section 504 of the Rehabilitation Act,* requires schools to provide a free appropriate public education to students with a physical or mental impairment that limits life activities. This includes educational aids that assist in language and communication. The Americans with Disabilities Act (ADA) also requires that daycare and schools have to make reasonable modifications for children with disabilities. These laws are supported by the Assistive Technology Act (ATA) which enables the provision of devices including wheelchairs, communication devices, durable medical equipment, lifts, accessibility adaptations for both home and school, and equipment to help in recreation and study (e.g. magnifiers, reachers, large keyboards). The American Disabilities Act (ADA) supports all adults and children in provision of reasonable accommodation in the workplace of school.

Case managers and the care coordination team will reference policy and specific legislation as necessary when developing a child's plan of care or interacting with teacher or school boards. Familiarity with policy helps support the developmental needs of a child in areas of both health and education. Since over one in three children were covered through a federal benefit program in 2012, the public health insurance benefit provisions are an important component of coordinating children's health services (Sebelius, 2013). Although coverage and qualifications vary from state to state, benefit provisions exist for the child's plan of care. Children with commercial health coverage have like program provisions which can be referenced through the insurance carrier.

Certification of Care Coordinators or Case Managers

Professional certification is another national issue. The point at issue is how Americans define those who call themselves a care coordinator or case manager. Although certification is presently available to qualified professionals seeking to evidence their experience and understanding of case management and care coordination, one does not have to have national certification to call themselves a case manager. While The Accredited Care Management Association adopted a position statement proclaiming that nurses and social workers should attain case management certification by the year 2016, there is not strength to enforce such a goal. An example of entities providing education and examination for certification include: the Case Management Society of America, American Case Management Association, the American Association of Managed Care Nurses, the American Nurses Credentialing Center Nursing Case Management credential, and the American Academy of Case Management. Individuals who perform non-professional care coordination services as part of a team should demonstrate competency through certificate completion of a Community Health Worker program or from Patient Advocate training, indicating education and understanding of family-centered care coordination. Legislative action in state and federal venues will be required to settle this area of ambiguity.

State Policy

Differences exist at the state level in regards to special programming and resources. State waivers offering richer benefit packages are available in some states. Specific information on care in specific states can be found through the National Academy for State Health. The national strategy includes improved screening for children and programming for older adults to enable them to live in the community. Individualized care planning and cross systems planning is promoted within state Health and Human Services Commissions to utilize all resources and be as family centered as possible. State policy supports technology infrastructure to facilitate improved coordination long term. Those strategies are essential during natural disasters when coordination needs to extend beyond a local community and perhaps even state. States have acknowledged addressing the health and developmental needs citizens requires linkage across communities and monitoring of those referrals just as satisfaction and cost outcomes are measured. States are engaging public and private managed care organization partners to provide evidence of those outcomes.

Payment for Care Coordination services is a changing area although the Centers for Medicaid and Medicare Services did approve, for 2014, reimbursement supporting care management "outside the routine office interaction to promote high quality care and efficiency" in Medicare for physicians and non-physicians. State adoption into Medicaid will be an issue to follow across states. Care planning and consultation of the team also requires time, effort and a corollary reimbursement from payers.

Multistate licensure is another state issue impacting care coordination. Case Managers as healthcare professionals license within a state. Nurses and Social Workers as a case manager must hold a license in a state where the client lives. It is common for case managers living near state borders to have patients in multiple states. Case managers must hold a license in every state in which they provide care to patients and families. Acquiring a license in each state is administratively and financially burdensome. Twenty-four states, per the Multi-State Licensure National Council of State Boards of Nursing, have agreed to a compact that would recognize nursing licensure across states. Movement in all states is necessary to protect case managers. There is a belief that interest in the advancement of telemedicine (which transcends state lines) and physician action to move their licensing to multi-state status will add strength to this issue, compelling adoption in additional states over the next few years. The goal is an integrated care coordination infrastructure to deliver optimal pediatric health care. A framework for high performing pediatric care coordination draws attention to all levels within the health care system and across community sectors (Antonelli, McAllister, & Popp, 2009). Program and workforce infrastructure to provide the number of case managers, education, policy support, and financing is also important at the state level (Antonelli et al, 2009).

Advocacy

There is a difference between gaps in coordination of services and a lack of programming or coverage for a service. The care coordination team, in concert with the family and health professionals should be able to address communication and coordination in care and services between insurance coverage, waiver offerings, and community services. When holes in coverage or benefits exist that impair continuity of care or adequate healthcare provision, advocacy groups become essential in initiating changes to existing policy or working on new policy creation. This requires a strong voice, that of an advocacy organization. A resource for advocacy groups Comes from Health Access. An additional example of a national organization in addition to those found at Health Access is Family Voices, an organization that helps families make informed decisions and works to influence public policy.

Advocacy groups inform public policy and give hope to families. Care coordination teams pointing clients to advocacy groups connect them with a voice of experience. Individuals or families sharing the same or similar diagnoses and circumstances can be immensely important to families trying to cope with the health needs and life balance. Tips on arranging furniture and supply storage can help families improve their day. Training on advocacy is even provided by groups such as Parent to Parent. State chapters of the national Parent to Parent organization will also identify a match of experienced support parents that can help with both needed information and emotional support. Another two great resources can be found through the sites of the National Center for Medical Home Implementation and The Maternal and Child Health Library at Georgetown University. The Medical Home site has resources for parents and practitioners on care plans, shared decisions and family inclusion. The Georgetown University is a place for disease- specific focused on providing coordinated support for family-centered care.

Successful advocacy involves social media and grassroots efforts. To be effective in our communities, advocating for our clients, we need to support good policies. Letters, emails, or calls to a state or federal legislator, or testifying at a state committee can make a difference. Legislators understand and relate when they can hear a real story about how policy affects the health and family life of someone in their community. Case managers and entire care coordination team may be called to work with the media in telling the story of how coordination decreases fragmentation, improves clinical and financial outcomes of care and increases family satisfaction.

Case Management, Care Coordination and Transition

Care Transition

Transition of care or care transitions occur when there is movement of patients from one health care practitioner or setting to another based upon change in an individual's condition and need. Care transitions are not limited to inpatient discharges. Transition occurs during a move between units (intensive care to medical surgical floor); between facilities (acute care to skilled nursing facility); across health states (curative care to hospice); in the change of health practitioners (pediatric to adult setting), or across care settings to the home environment. Not surprisingly, transitions often place the very old and very young most at risk. Care coordination must be in place to secure next-step appointments, medication reconciliation, understanding of dietary needs, and likelihood of the receiving environment and caregivers to support adherence to a plan of care. In the case of elders, diminished mobility, sensory ability (inability to see labels or clearly hear instructions), and frequently depression may lead to poor outcomes related to non-compliance. It is said 66% of medication errors occur during transition (Santell, 2006).

However, transitional care programs are applicable to all populations and are increasingly being seen in advanced in research due to the potential impact on quality of care and economic spend (Taylor, 2013). Language barriers and health literacy are areas of risk during transition that are specifically addressed by the case manager. Cultural preferences are another important consideration to keep in mind when developing a plan of care for an individual to follow at home. Examples of adult care coordination and transition programs include:

Adult Comprehensive and Transitional Care Management Programs	
Care Management Plus (CMP)	Better Outcomes for Older Adults through Safe Transitions (Project BOOST)
State Programs	The Bridge Model
Guided Care	Care Transitions Intervention (CTI)
Home Based Primary Care (HBPC)	Interventions to Reduce Acute Care Transfers (INTERACT II)
Improving Mood-Promoting Access to Collaborative Treatment (IMPACT)	Re-engineered Discharge (RED)
Program of All-inclusive Care for the Elderly (PACE)	Transitional Care Model (TCM)

One reason transitional care is becoming important in the healthcare industry is due to economic performance measures associated to transitions from inpatient to home. Continuity of care is the goal of the care coordination team when developing effective discharge planning whether to home, a rehabilitation setting, or even another acute care environment. Inadequate coordination during handoffs has resulted in readmissions and poor health outcomes for patients. With the purpose to improve quality outcomes through continuity and communication across transitions, the National Transition of Care Coalition (NTOCC) was established, in 2008, to guide the quality and provide tools for transition management. Providing tools for health care professionals, families, and informing legislators on policy needs, this organization is focused on quality care. In 2008, the NTOCC workgroup developed Transition of Care Measures for practitioners and organizations, to guide the reporting of outcomes and to use in structuring intervention programs.

Regulation and Policy Implications on Care Transitions

The Committee on Healthcare Quality in America, formed by the Institute of Medicine, reported on morbidity and mortality resulting from poor transitions in their sentinel publication, *Crossing the Quality Chasm.* This paper gained much publicity on the American healthcare system and also made recommendations for improvement. Among them, was the need for care coordination and improved transitions to impact safety and effectiveness (Institute of Medicine, 2001). The Committee continues its' quality charge and oversight today, looking at safe and efficient care transitions. As an example, in 2013 they formed a subcommittee on Improving the Health, Safety, and Well-Being of Young Adults (ages 18-26). This workgroup is researching the issues of chronic condition care and lack of access to health care for young adults moving to the adult care community. This transition places these individuals at risk for poor health care outcomes (http://www.iom.edu/Activities/Children/ImprovingYoungAdultHealth.aspx).

In April 2011, Centers for Medicare and Medicaid Services (CMS) announced the development of the Community-Based Care Transition Program (CCPT) (http://innovation.cms.gov/initiatives/CCTP). CCPT was created by Section 3026 of the Patient Protection and Affordable Care Act (PPACA) to link acute-care hospitals with high readmission rates to community based organizations for outreach at discharge. In a similar show of support for quality care, the Department of Health and Human Services agreed to use

$1 billion in PPACA funds in the Partnership for Patients program which uses coordination to reduce millions of preventable injuries and complications. Public and private entities are creating coordination programs to impact factors associated with readmissions for patients of all ages. The Hospital Readmissions Reduction Program and the Improving Care Transitions Program has potentially significant financial impacts for hospitals and has caused an increase in attention on the development of transitional care management programs in an attempt to reduce hospital readmission rates. Consumers are being asked to participate in that program through satisfaction survey response. Hospitals commonly use the Hospital Consumer Assessment of Hospital Providers and Systems for their accreditation reporting to provide data on patient perception. There is an inclusion of how hospitals perform during transition in the 2014 measures signifying the rising importance by both regulatory and accrediting entities on care transitions (Centers for Medicare and Medicaid, 2013): These questions are:

- The hospital staff took my preferences and those of my family into account when deciding what my health care needs would be when I left the hospital.
- When I left the hospital, I had a good understanding of the things I was responsible for in managing my health.
- When I left the hospital, I clearly understood the purpose for taking each of my medications.

Delivering education and providing a specific contact for questions has been used as an effective transition intervention for many facilities. Frequency and delivery of that connection varies by program. The Veterans Health Administration used a program with Veterans diagnoses with chronic heart failure when entailed receiving a daily message from a nurse on a telehealth device. They found a statistically significant improvement in blood pressure and improved medication management with a corollary reduction in hospitalizations (Schofield, Kline, Schmalfuss et al, 2005).

Neonatal Intensive Care Unit Graduates

One specific area of transition interest has been on the safe discharge transition of infants from the neonatal intensive care unit (NICU) and the coordination and education needed to prevent readmissions and gain compliance with a first pediatrician visit (Moyer, Singh, Finfel &, Giardino, 2010). Infants being discharged from the Neonatal Intensive Care Unit (NICU) are at risk during transition as their receiving physician has not yet had the opportunity to examine the baby. Often families are frightened and stressed with the responsibilities of equipment or treatments needed for their tiny child. The Agency for Healthcare Research and Quality has developed, through a research grant, the Transitioning newborns from NICU to home: a resource toolkit to assist education development, professional handoffs, and create realistic supports and expectations for parents. Support for these babies has been shown to be effective in reducing readmissions.

First-time parents of normal newborns are also at risk of inappropriate emergency room use or not establishing a first-visit with a medical home. An example of care coordination to impact these families is phone calls to low-income first time mothers by advanced practice nurses. In a study by Hannan (2013), mothers who received calls over an 8 week period had statistically significant levels of lower maternal stress as well as reduced emergency room visits and lower overall cost.

Home Visitation Programs

Home visitation programs provide professional assessment and support at the client's home. Barriers of transportation are nonexistent in home visitation programs although for the case manager there can be missed visits if the client is not home. Seeing an individual function within their own environment typically yields a comprehensive picture of barriers to optimal care and supports a 'safe' place for the client to discuss health issues. The United States Department of Health and Human Services has conducted a program review of home visitation. Evidenced-based Home Visitation Programs as designated by the federal government include:

- Early Head Start-Home Visiting
- Family Check-Up
- Healthy Families
- Healthy Start
- Healthy Steps
- Home Instruction for Parents of Preschool Youngsters (HIPPY)
- Nurse-Family Partnership
- Parents as Teachers
- Public Health Nursing Early Intervention Program (EIP) for Adolescent Mothers
- SafeCare

Case managers work within these programs, visiting families at their residence. An emphasis of these programs ranges across combinations of: positive parenting, safe environments, building resiliency, child abuse prevention, school readiness, and preventive care. An example of nurse case managers delivering a program is Nurse Family Partnership. This program pairs Bachelor's prepared nurses with a caseload of 25 first time, low-income mothers from pregnancy through the child's second birthday. The Health-Start program limits a caseload to 15 women and uses nurses as well as paraprofessionals with training. Parents as Teachers (PAT) is another home visitation program that combines opportunities for group support with home visits and prefers Social Workers in the case management role. Programs differ duration as well as professional background of visitor. The Healthy Families America program, as an example, strives to retain clients over 3-5 years. Each home visitation program is based upon a theoretical framework and has required training and a curriculum.

Adolescent Transition to Adult Care

A specific care coordination area not associated with inpatient discharge is Adolescent Transition. Transition programs as seen in the Adolescent Health Transition Project of the

University of Washington (http://depts.washington.edu/healthtr*) are also expected to be on the rise. The Washington program site provides not only resources and support to families in their area, but offers open source forms, checklists, and processes to families and healthcare professionals in establishing solid transition programs that respect the growing autonomy of the adolescent. A similar resource to support the growing programming recognizing the importance of providing a smooth transition to adult care is the national Center for Health Care Transition Improvement (http://www.gottransition.org/) organization which has resource toolkits for both families and health care providers.* Adolescent transition requires the care coordination team to identify quality providers that will deliver developmentally appropriate services to provide care continuity. The case manager role is to develop an individualized plan to move from pediatric to adult care. Since the active transition ideally occurs between the ages of 18 and 21 years, initial planning begins at age 14 where, as capable, the adolescent begins to become increasingly involved and set expectations for selecting and understanding how to navigate in an adult healthcare environment. Coordinating adolescent transition as a family and healthcare team supports youth as they move to assume adult roles, which includes managing their health (Cooley & Sagerman, 2011).

To assess if your practice is delivering appropriate transition care a good tool to use would be the *Medical Home Health Care Transition Index for Youth Up to Age 18 (*http://www.gottransition.org/UploadedFiles/Files/8_CMHI_HCT_Index_Pediatric_09NOV2011_.pdf)

Finding adult practitioners may not be an easy task. The majority of adult internal medicine providers are not comfortable providing primary care for young adults with chronic illnesses (Okumura, Heisler, Davis, Cabana, Demonner, & Kerr, 2008). Identifying providers willing to provide care for CSHCN, can be initially researched telephonically however, a test of practice style and acceptable communication style and comfort is important. The care coordinator should arrange office visits occurring prior to termination of pediatric care relationships. Efforts to increase familiarity in residency programs with care needs of CSHCN, or creating specialty just-in-time consulting for existing medical homes, are being created to improve practitioner awareness and comfort, and therefore healthcare access for the young adults with complex chronic conditions (Okumura et al., 2008).

Tools and Application

Care coordination uses tools to empower clients in self-management skills. An example of a useful tool is the *Ask Me Three*™ program developed by Partnership for Clear Health Communication at the National Patient Safety Foundation. Encouraging clients to ask their healthcare providers the following three questions an make a difference.

- What is my (child's) main problem? This helps patients and families better understand the diagnosis.
- What do I (child/family) need to do? Helps better understand the plan of care.
- Why is it important for me (child/family) to do this? Helps with internal motivation.

Source: http://www.pfizerhealthliteracy.com/physicians-providers/PchcAskme3.aspx

Answers to these questions have been found to clarify misconceptions which could otherwise lead to error or injury. Case managers are instrumental in coaching patients, caregivers, and family to take an active role in care transitions. Asking questions of healthcare professionals is a great start for families to take an active role in the care coordination team. The University of Texas Health Science Center at San Antonio conducted a study where they evaluated use of Ask Me 3 in a pediatric health center where they found parents felt they had increased understanding of visit recommendations (Mika, Wood, Reiss, Trevino, 2007).

Case Managers can support families in transitions across care setting or practitioners by informing families on choices, providing tools for reminders, and linking families with resources. Motivational interviewing skills lead the case manager to listen and acknowledge the client as the expert of their world. Choices and education are important. The goal is to build competency by engaging the client in their own health care. Providing clients/families with resources, tools, and a timeline (online tool or care binder) can generate self-management to support coordinated, continuous care (Taylor, Lizzi, Marx, Chilkatowsky, Trachtenberg, & Ogle, 2013).

Case managers are most often responsible for transition and should have proficiency in chronic disease management, motivational interviewing, and behavioral change theory to successfully fulfill this role. Home visits to support transition are the most common model of care coordination delivery.

Managed Care and Care Coordination

Managed Care

Case management is an important part of all managed care health plans. Managed care uses predictive modeling to identify individuals for care coordination or referrals from members or health practitioners. Managed care plans perform population management, meaning they assess trends illnesses and costs across the population to make a determination of where to place their efforts. There are three main areas of case management focus in a health plan. The first is catastrophic or high cost cases. These individuals will consume a high amount of health services. An example would be individuals awaiting transplant, persons with a traumatic brain injury or amputation, or individuals who are technology dependent. The second population includes individuals with a chronic illness that requires monitoring and medication or treatment adherence to remain in control. Managed care companies have developed disease management programs that address individuals with conditions such as asthma, diabetes, sickle cell disease, and seizures which provide care coordination and educational outreach to minimize illness exacerbation. The third population covers the general area of health status. This refers to weight management, compliance with immunizations and screening exams. Health plans are judged on their ability to perform, as compared to their peers and against national accreditation standards, in all three of these areas population management. Case managers team with health educators and outreach specialists to improve population health using educational materials, motivational interviewing skills and collaborating with health practitioners. A newer area of case management in managed care is that of embedded case management. Health plans assess the performance and volume of primary care practices. Health plans may embed one of their case manager employees in a practice if that medical home is a busy medical home with many chronic or catastrophically ill patients. The case manager performs coordination activities including assessments, community outreach and links communication between specialists and other care providers to improve patient outcome.

One of the care coordination strategies to keeping individuals out of the emergency room and inpatient environments is the use of advanced nurse practitioners for in-home consultations. The advanced practice perspective of health promotion and partnership adds much to the care coordination team. An example of this concept used with elders was able to significantly reduce acute health events (Imhof, Naef, Wallhagen et al., 2012).

Recommendations and Strategies for the Future

Case management fellowships will appear in academic centers to encourage case managers to enter the care coordination field specific to the special needs child, further developing the discipline. These fellowship opportunities will give case managers a solid foundation in integrated case management. Each state has varying professional continuing education requirements and case management certification adds specific continuing education requirement applicable to the practice of case management. Development of competency-based requirements for positions on the care coordination team will include skill sets for case managers, navigators/community health workers/parent partners. High on that list of competencies will be motivational interviewing and communication skills. Additional required skills include familiarity with legislative, regulatory, and benefit frameworks requirements. Evidenced based practice will continue to grow influenced by continuing research, funding requirements favoring established evidenced-based programming, and protocol development by health plans, professional societies, insurers and advocacy groups partnering to develop efficiencies and quality improvements to meet the requirements for our changing delivery system.

Online training and post graduate degrees are another expanding future opportunity for case management. Currently the University of Alabama offers Case Management/Leadership as a Master's degree nursing program. Undergraduate programs are now including case management into undergraduate curriculums as well as exampled by Idaho State University. The Maternal Child Health Bureau is developing a standardized pediatric care coordination curriculum and other entities such as the Case Management Society of America are developing online curriculum to gain skills in case management practice.

Conclusion

The advance practice nurse interfaces with all aspects of patient care from home care to primary and acute care settings. The ability of the APN to integrate case management and care coordination to clinical practice will ultimately improve patient care and strengthen health care outcomes in new models of care. Development of clinical studies to document outcomes is necessary to prove the role of accountability and quality improvement derived from care coordination programming. Monitoring of cost, care plan effectiveness, and measures of health service utilization are important going forward using analytics to quantify care management activities.

Care coordination is in place to support family centered care that is accessible, coordinated, culturally effective, compassionate and continuous. Case managers are key to the success of care coordination as they practice in clinics, hospitals, managed care companies, and solo practices. Payment, accreditation and certification will be continuing issues to address within the profession. Coordinated care delivery, supported by a professional team of case managers, navigators, parent partners and support staff are poised to deliver patient-centered care to vulnerable populations. Improved care coordination, utilizing technology to enhance communication between all care professionals and the family will transform healthcare to achieve the quality focus consumers are demanding. Case management and care coordination are an integral part of team-based care that is necessary to demonstrate value within newly created models of care. Families need support in managing their conditions and in facilitating communication between healthcare professionals. Case management and care coordination comes to these newer models of care armed with the skills of interprofessional collaboration to support effective team based care.

REFERENCES

Agency for Healthcare Research and Quality. (2007, June).*Closing the Quality Gap: A Critical Analysis of Quality Improvement Strategies: Volume 7—Care Coordination,* Structured Abstract. Publication No. 04(07)-0051-7, Agency for Healthcare Research and Quality, Rockville, MD. Retrieved from http://www.ahrq.gov/clinic/tp/caregaptp.htm.

American Case Management Association. (2013). *Standards of Practice and Scope of Services for Hospital/Health System Case Management.* American Case Management Association, Little Rock, AR. Retrieved from http://www.acmaweb.org/section.asp?sID=22

American Nurses Association. (2012). The Value of Nursing Care Coordination. Whitepaper of the American Nurses Association. Retrieved from http://www.nursingworld.org/carecoordinationwhitepaper

Antonelli, R., McAllister, J., & Popp, J. (2009). *Making Care Coordination a Critical Component of the Pediatric Health System: A Multidisciplinary Framework*, The Commonwealth Fund. Retrieved from http://www.commonwealthfund.org/Publications/Fund-Reports/2009/May/Making-Care-Coordination-a-Critical-Component-of-the-Pediatric-Health-System.aspx#citation

Battersby, M., Harvey, P., Mills, P., Kalucy, E., Pols, R., Frith, P., McDonald, P., Esterman, A., Tsourtos, G., Donato, R., Pearce, R.,& McGowan, C. (2007). SA HealthPlus: A controlled trial of a statewide application of a generic model of chronic illness care. *Milbank Quarterly*, 85(1),37-67. doi: 10.1111/j.1468-0009.2007.00476.x

Bhaumik, U., Norris, K., Gisele, C., Walker, S., Sommer, S., Chan, E., Dickerson, D., Nethersole, S., & Woods, E. (2013, April). A cost analysis for a community-based case management intervention program for pediatric asthma, *Journal of Asthma*, 50(3), 310. doi: 10.3109/02770903.2013.765447

Brandell, J., Ed. (2010). Theory and Practice of Clinical Social Work (2nd edition). Columbia University Press.

Case Management Society of America. (2010). Standards of practice. for case management. Little Rock Arkansas, Case management Society of America.

Center for Disease Control and Prevention. Chronic Disease Calculator. Retrieved from http://www.cdc.gov/chronicdisease/resources/calculator/index.htm

Chase, D. (2012). Patient engagement is the blockbuster drug of the century. Retrieved from http://www.forbes.com/sites/davechase/2012/09/09/patient-engagement-is-the-blockbuster-drug-of-the-century.

Coleman, K., Austin, B., Brach, C., &Wagner, E. (2009). Evidence on the chronic care model in the new millennium. *Health Affairs*, 28(1), 75-85. doi: 10.1377/hlthaff.28.1.75.

Cooley, W., & Sagerman, P. (2011, July). Supporting the health care transition from adolescence to adulthood in the medical home. *Pediatrics,* 128(1), 182-200. doi: 10.1542/peds.2011-0969.

Cousino, M., & Hazen, R. (2013). Parenting Stress Among Caregivers of Children With Chronic Illness: A Systematic Review. *Journal of Pediatric Psychology*, 38(8), 809-828. doi: 10.1093/jpepsy/jst049.

Frie, R. (2013, Sept/Oct). Technological changes can transform medicine by 2020: a conversation with the futurist Jim Carroll. *American Health & Drug Benefits*, 6(8), 510. Retrieved from http://www.ahdbonline.com/issues/2013/september-october-2013-vol-6-no-8/1599-technological-changes-can-transform-medicine-by-2020-a-conversation-with-the-futurist-jim-carroll

Glaser, J. (2013, June). Expanding patients role in their care. *Hospitals and Health Networks*, Retrieved from http://www.hhnmag.com/hhnmag/HHNDaily/HHNDaily Display. dhtml?id=7280003149

Hannan, J. (2013). APN telephone follow up to low-income first time mothers. *Journal of Clinical Nursing*, 22(1-2), 262-270. doi: 10.1111/j.1365-2702.2011.

Imhoff, L. (2012). Effects of an Advanced Practice Nurse In-Home Health Consultation Program for Community-Dwelling Persons Aged 80 and Older.

American Geriatric Society, 60(12), 2223–2231. doi: 10.1111/jgs.12026.

Institute for Healthcare Improvement. *IHI Triple Aim Initiative*. Retrieved from http://www.ihi.org/offerings/Initiatives/TripleAim/Pages/default.aspx

Janvier, A., Farlow, B., & Wilfond, B. (2012). The experience of families of children with trisomy 13 and 18 in social networks. *Pediatrics*, 130: 293-298. doi: 10.1542/peds.2012-0151. Retrieved from http://pediatrics.aappublications.org/content/early/2012/07/18/peds.2012-0151.full.pdf+html

Kathol, R., Perez, R., & Cohen, J. (2010). *The Integrated Case Management Manual.* New York, NY, Springer.

Komisar, H., & Feder, J. (2011, Oct). *Transforming Care for Medicare Beneficiaries with Chronic Conditions and Long-Term Care Needs: Coordinating Care Across All Services.* Georgetown University. Retrieved from http://www.thescanfoundation.org/sites/default/files/Georgetown_Trnsfrming_Care.pdf

Lindeke, L., Anderson, S., Chesney, M., & O'Conner-Von, S. (2010, Nov/Dec). Family-centered Health Care/Medical Home: APN Roles in Shaping New Care Models. Journal of Pediatric Healthcare 24, 413-416. doi:10.1016/j.pedhc.2010.07.009.

Llewellyn, A. (2013, Oct). Case management playing a key role in the advancement of clinical integration. Case in Point, Retrieved from http://www.dorlandhealth.com/cip_weekly/2960.html

McDonald, K., Sundram, V., Bravata, D., Lewis, R., Lin, N., Kraft, S., McKinnon, M., Paguntalan, H., & Owens, D. (2007, June). Care Coordination. *AHRQ Publication No. 04(07)-0051-7.* Rockville, MD: Agency for Healthcare Research and Quality.

Markowitz, A., ed. (2004). *Closing the Quality Gap: A Critical Analysis of Quality Improvement Strategies.* Agency for Healthcare Research and Quality. Retrieved from http://www.ahrq.gov/downloads/pub/evidence/pdf/qualgap2/qualgap2.pdf

Martini, R., & Houston, M, (2013, March). ACO's and CAPs: preparing for the impact of healthcare reform on child and adolescent psychiatry practice. American Academy of Child and Adolescent Psychiatry. Retrieved from: http://www.aacap.org/App_Themes/AACAP/Docs/homepage/2013/preparing_for_healthcare_reform_201303.pdf

Moyer, V., Papile, L., Eichenwalk, E., Profit, J., Guillory, C., Singh, H., Kelly, A., Khan, M., Thomas, E., Magliaro, B., Vega, A., & Collins, E. (2013). Transitioning newborns from NICU to home: a resource toolkit. Agency for Healthcare Research and Quality. Grant # R18HSO17889-01. Retrieved from: http://www.ahrq.gov/professionals/systems/hospital/nicu_toolkit/nicutoolkit.pdf

National Association of Professional Geriatric Care Managers. (2013, Jan). Care Management. Whitepaper of the National Association of Professional Geriatric Care Managers. http://www.caremanager.org/public-policy/position-papers/care-management/

National Center for Medical Home Implementation. (2013.). *A Retrospective Look at Programs and Initiatives Toward Family-Centered Medical Home for Every Child and Youth.* Maternal and Child Health Bureau grant U43MC09134. Retrieved from: http://www.medicalhomeinfo.org/downloads/pdfs/NCMHI%20Retrospective_FINAL_July2013.pdf

National Quality Forum, Prioritization Measures, 2010, Retrieved from: NQF.org

National Committee for Quality Assurance. (2013) 2014 *Standards and Guidelines for the Accreditation of Health Plans.* Washington, D.C. National Committee for Quality Assurance.

Nelson, L. (2012, Jan). Lessons from Medicare's Demonstration Projects on Disease Management and Care Coordination. *Congressional Budget Office Working Paper Series.* 1, 1-2. Retrieved from http://www.cbo.gov/sites/default/files/cbofiles/attachments/WP2012-01_Nelson_Medicare_DMCC_Demonstrations.pdf

Okumura, MJ, Heisler, M., Davis, M.M, Cabana, M., Demonner, S.,& Kerr, E. (2008, Oct) Comfort of general internists and general pediatricians in providing care for young adults with chronic illnesses of childhood Journal of General Internal Medicine, 23(10),1621-7. doi: 10.1007/s11606-008-0716-8.

Patient Protection and Affordable Care Act. (2010). Pub Law No. 111-148. Retrieved from http://www.gpo.gov/fdsys/pkg/PLAW-111publ148/pdf/PLAW-111publ148.pdf

Roussel, L., (2011, 6th edition). *Management and Leadership for Nurse Administrators.* Jones and Bartlett, Burlington, MA.

Santell, J. (2006, Jan) Catching Medication Errors at Admission, Transfer, and Discharge," RN RN, 69 (1), 77.

Schofield, R., Kline, S., Schmalfuss, C., Carever, H., Aranda, J., Pauly, D., Hill, J., Neugaard, B., & Chumbler, N. 92005). Early outcomes of a care coordination enhanced telehome care program for elderly veterans with chronic health failure. Telemed Journal and e-health, 11 (1), 20-7. Retrieved from http://www.ncbi.nlm.nih.gov/pubmed/15785217.

Sebelius, K. (2013). The Department of Health and Human Services 2013 Annual Report on the Quality of Care for Children in Medicaid and CHIP.

Retrieved from http://www.medicaid.gov/Medicaid-CHIP-Program-Information/By-Topics/Quality-of-Care/Downloads/2013-Ann-Sec-Rept.pdf

Shudy, M., Lihinie de Almeida, M., Ly, S., Landon, C., Groft, S., Jenkins, T., & Nicholson, C. (2006, December). Impact of pediatric critical illness and injury on families: a systematic literature review. *Pediatrics*, 118, S203 -S218, doi: 10.1542/peds.2006-0951B

Silow-Carroll, S., & Hagelow, G. (2011). Effective pediatric case management. *Care Management*, 17, 7-13. Retrieved from http://nursing.msu.edu/Images_Docs/CE_Images/CasePresentations/GwenFosse.pdf

Stricker, P. (2013, Aug). Supporting Transitions of Care with Technology. *CMSA Today*. Retrieved from http://www.naylornetwork.com/cmsatoday/articles/index.asp?aid=229952&issueID=30156

Taylor, A., Lizzi, M, Marx, A., Chilkatowsky, M., Trachtenberg, S.,& Ogle, S. (2013). Implementing a care coordination program for children with special healthcare needs: partnering with families and providers. *Journal of Healthcare Quality*, 35(5), 70-77.

Thorpe, J. (2013, April). Needs great evidence lacking. *Partnership to Fight Chronic Disease*. Retrieved from: http://www.scribd.com/doc/137602733/Needs-Great-Evidence-Lacking-White-Paper.

Torio, C., Elixhauser, A., & Andrews, R. (2013). Trends in Potentially Preventable Hospital Admissions among Adults and Children, 2005–2010. Healthcare Cost and Utilization Project, Agency for Healthcare Research and Quality. Statistical Brief #151. Retrieved from: http://www.hcup-us.ahrq.gov/reports/statbriefs/sb151.pdf

Treadwell, J. (2014, March/April) Collaborating for Care: Initial experience of embedded case managers across five medical homes. *Professional Case Management*, 19(2), 1-8.

Wagner, E. (1998). Chronic Disease Management: What Will It Take to Improve Care for Chronic Illness? *Effective Clinical Practice*, 1, 2-4. retrieved from http://www.acponline.org/clinical_information/journals_publications/ecp/augsep98/cdm.pdf

Yell, M. L., Drasgow, E., & Lowrey, K. A. (2005). No Child Left Behind and Students with Autism Spectrum Disorders. *Focus on Autism and Other Developmental Disabilities*, 20 (3), 130-139. doi: 10.1177/10883576050200030101

Part 3: Related Topics to Advanced Practice Nursing

In: Collaboration with the Advanced Practice Nurse ISBN: 978-1-63321-311-1
Editors: E.R. Giardino, R.G. Hanks and A.P. Giardino

Chapter 11

ADVANCING NURSING SCIENCE IN THE ADVANCED PRACTICE NURSING ROLE

Marlene Walden, PhD, RN, NNP-BC, CCNS and Elizabeth C. Elliott, MSN RN NNP-BC
Texas Children's Hospital, Houston TX, US

ABSTRACT

To advance nursing science, advanced practice nurses (APNs) must be versed in and actively engaged in three areas of scholarship: research; evidence-based practice (EBP); and quality improvement (QI). While these three sources of evidence are all systematic approaches to problem solving, each serves a distinct role within healthcare. Research generates new knowledge or validates and refines existing data to influence nursing practice. EBP utilizes existing data from multiple studies to answer vital clinical, education, or administrative questions. QI uses existing knowledge to improve internal organizational processes and outcomes. The APN is in a unique position to use these three approaches in all areas of clinical practice to improve the delivery of healthcare and ensure the best patient outcomes.

INTRODUCTION

For the past two decades, national leaders in healthcare have called for a transformation of the healthcare system in the United States (IOM, 2001). A well-documented gap exists between research and practice (Facchiano & Snyder, 2012; Macellus & Harrison, 2012). Any transformation of the healthcare system will require advanced practice nurses (APNs) to challenge the status quo: “We’ve always done it this way” (Facchiano & Snyder, 2012). Status quo practices are no longer acceptable and further the gap between research and practice, fail to enhance clinical judgment, and does not lead to cost-effective treatment modalities (Facchiano & Snyder, 2012).

The Institute of Medicine (IOM) defines quality healthcare as the “degree to which health services for individuals and populations increase the likelihood of desired health outcomes and are consistent with current professional knowledge" (IOM, 1990; Stevens, 2013, para 3). APNs have the ability to conduct research and engage in evidence-based practice (EBP); skills that are critical to promoting patient safety and improving clinical outcomes. To achieve excellence in clinical practice, APNs must support and promote three areas of scholarship: 1) research; 2) EBP; and, 3) quality improvement (QI) methodology. While these three sources of evidence are all systematic approaches to problem solving, each serves a distinct role within healthcare. Research generates new knowledge or validates and refines existing data to influence nursing practice. EBP utilizes existing data from multiple studies to answer vital clinical, education, or administrative questions. QI uses existing knowledge to improve internal organizational processes and outcomes (i.e., cost, productivity, quality) (Shirey, et al., 2011). APNs that are versed in these methodologies are in a unique position to deliver the highest quality of healthcare and ensure the best patient outcomes.

TAPP Model

The Texas Children's Transformational Advanced Professional Practice (TAPP) Model provides a framework for the role of the APN in research, EBP, and QI. The TAPP Model for APNs was modified from the Strong Model of Advanced Practice (Ackerman, Norsen, Martin, Wiedrich, & Kitzman, 1996) and serves as a conceptual framework to guide professional development for the APN (see Figure 1).

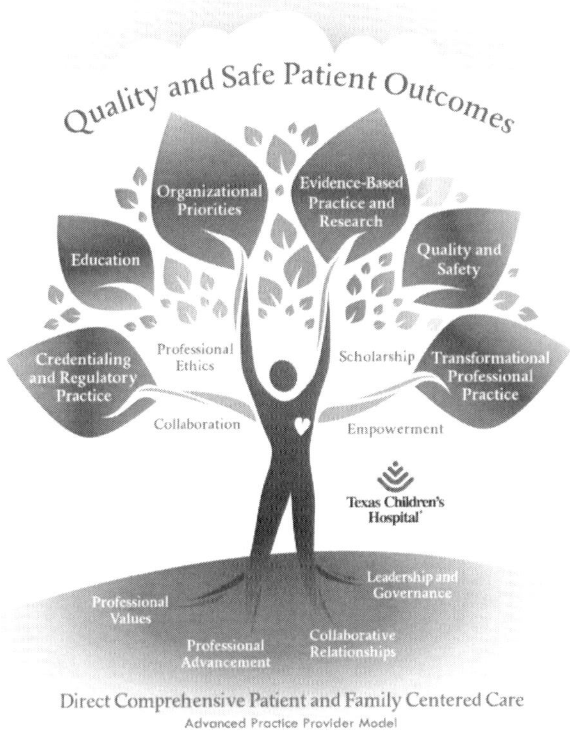

Figure 1. Texas Children's Transformational Advanced Professional Practice Model.

There is congruency between the Strong Model and the TAPP model in the domains of Direct Comprehensive Patient and Family Centered Care, Organizational Priorities, Education, Evidence-Based Practice and Research, and Transformational Professional Practice. With the changes in healthcare reform and attention to accountable care organizations, two additional domains of practice were added to the TAPP model to be more inclusive of the full scope of professional practice of the APN. These domains include Quality and Safety and Credentialing and Regulatory Practice (Elliott and Walden, in press).

The domain of Evidence-Based Practice and Research comprises activities that seek to better patient care through support for the generation of knowledge and the translation of research findings into clinical practice. For example, an entry level APN may identify potential areas of research related to clinical practice or specialty role. As the APN progresses from novice to expert (Benner, 1984), the APN collaborates with others to write and implement a clinical research study (Elliott and Walden, in press).

The domain of Quality and Safety focuses on the IOM's charge to healthcare systems to deliver care that is safe, timely, effective, efficient, equitable, and patient-focused (IOM, 2001). For example, an entry level APN may identify and recommend opportunities for practice improvement while the more experienced APN may evaluate departmental quality and safety initiative data and make further recommendations for practice improvement (Elliott and Walden, in press). The TAPP model serves as a blueprint for establishing the structures and processes to support exemplary advanced practice (Elliott & Walden, in press). This chapter will focus only on advancing nursing science through research, EBP, and QI.

RESEARCH

Research serves two basic purposes: 1) increases the knowledge base of the discipline by discovery of new knowledge; and, 2) increases knowledge as a professional by having the ability to understand and evaluate existing research within one's discipline (Gliner, Morgan, & Leech, 2009).

Definition

Burns and Grove (2009) define nursing research as "a scientific process that validates and refines existing knowledge and generates new knowledge that directly and indirectly influences the delivery of evidence-based practice" (Burns & Grove, 2009, p. 3).

Methodology

Research can be classified into two major categories: 1) quantitative research; and, 2) qualitative research. The APN can choose between these categories based on the question he/she is asking. Burns and Grove (2009) define quantitative research as a "formal, objective, systematic study process to describe and test relationships and to examine cause-and-effect interactions among variables" (p. 717). On the other hand, qualitative research is defined as the "systematic, interactive, subjective approach used to describe life experiences and give them meaning" (Burns & Grove, 2009, p. 717). Quantitative and qualitative methods complement each other because they generate different kinds of knowledge that are useful in nursing practice. For the purposes of this chapter, the steps of the quantitative research process will be discussed.

The quantitative research process involves conceptualizing a research study, designing and implementing that study, and disseminating the findings. An overview of the steps in the research process is presented below (Burns & Grove, 2009; Gliner, Morgan, & Leech, 2009).

- *Step 1*: All studies start with a research problem or research question that addresses what the investigator would like to know. Research questions can arise from various sources including, but not limited to: 1) clinical experiences; 2) QI efforts; 3) review of literature; and, 4) professional organization research priorities (Polit & Beck, 2012).
- *Step 2*: This step involves conducting a literature review to identify what is known about the research problem and what are the gaps in knowledge. The review of literature should focus on the key variables of the study and describe the significance and previous work that supports the need for the proposed study.
- *Step 3*: The APN should develop specific research questions or hypotheses to test the relationships between the key variables in the study. Hypotheses predict relationships among two or more variables and identify the population to be studied; whereas, research questions are used when insufficient knowledge is available to formulate hypotheses.
- *Step 4*: The APN selects a research design for conducting the study that maximizes control over factors that could interfere with the study's desired outcomes. The most commonly used quantitative designs in nursing include descriptive, correlational, quasi-experimental, and experimental. Descriptive research typically explores the discovery of new meaning, describes what exists, determines the frequency with which something occurs, and categorizes information within a particular field of study. Correlational research examines the relationships between or among two or more variables in a single group of individuals. Quasi-experimental research attempts to explain relationships, clarify why certain events happen, and examine causality between selected independent and dependent variables. Quasi-experimental designs attempt to minimize threats to validity as much as possible, but often lack control over random selection of subjects or random assignment to treatment conditions. Experimental designs examine probability and causality among independent and dependent variables for the purpose of predicting phenomena. While an experimental design provides the greatest amount of control over threats to validity, this type of design is often difficult to implement in the clinical setting.
- *Step 5*: In this step, the APN develops a plan for conducting the research including selection of the sample population with inclusion and exclusion criteria specified. The APN also must select instruments to measure each of the variables in the study, paying close attention to issues of validity and reliability. Finally, in this step, the APN must develop a plan for data collection and analysis. The plan should include how and when data will be collected and clearly outline any special data collection

procedures. A power analysis is performed to determine the number of subjects needed for the study. Statistical methods to be used for data analyses should be outlined to answer each research question.

- *Step 6*: The APN must obtain approvals from the human subjects Institutional Review Board (IRB) prior to beginning data collection. The primary purpose of an IRB is to protect the rights of people and animals who are subjects of research projects. In order to approve the research study, an IRB must find that the research meets certain criteria, such as making sure that subjects are selected equitably, have adequate information about the research, and that risks to subjects are minimized. An IRB also ensures that the privacy of subjects is protected and that additional safeguards protect vulnerable populations.
- *Step 7*: The next step in the research process is to collect the data. Data collection usually begins with recruitment of subjects. Most studies will require some aspect of informed consent. During the consenting process, it is important that the subject be informed of the purposes of the research, a description of the procedures to be followed, a description of any benefits or foreseeable risks or discomforts, measures to maintain confidentiality of records, that participation is voluntary, study costs or reimbursements, and plans for dissemination of study findings. During data collection, the APN must also carefully examine collection procedures to ensure consistency and maintenance of controls in order to protect the integrity and validity of the study.
- *Step 8*: Data analyses are conducted to reduce and organize the data. Engaging a research statistician is often helpful in assisting with the inferential statistics chosen to address each research question.
- *Step 9*: In this step, the APN makes inferences and uses the data analyses to give meaning to the data. Study findings are used to accept, support, or reject the study's research hypotheses or questions. Other expected research outcomes include generalization of study findings, implications for nursing, and suggestions for future research.
- *Step 10*: In the final step of the quantitative research process, the APN communicates the study findings through publications and presentations. Dissemination of both significant and nonsignificant study findings are important data to be shared for the purposes of translational research and to direct future research efforts.

The APN is a vital link in the generation of knowledge and the translation of research findings that leads to quality patient outcomes. It is important that the APN be both a *DOER* of research by contributing to the advancement of the nursing profession's knowledge base and a *CONSUMER* of research to improve practice through the use of research findings (Polit & Beck, 2012).

Evidence-Based Practice

APNs must be fully engaged in a culture of clinical inquiry in their professional practice in order to provide competent and quality patient care. Staying up-to-date with the latest evidence, however, can be extremely challenging for the busy APN. Straus and colleagues (2011) suggest that a clinical practitioner would need to read as many as 19 articles every day of the year in order to stay current in their practice (Straus, Glasizou, Richardson, & Haynes, 2011). This translates into 6,688 articles a year! Therefore, the APN must be systematic in their strategy to engage in evidence-informed practice by critically appraising research and applying EBP principles.

Definition

Sackett et al. (1996) defines EBP "as the conscientious, judicious, and explicit use of current best evidence in making decisions about the care of the individual patients" (Sackett, Rosenberg, Gray, Haynes, & Richardson, 1996, p. 71). Melnyk and Fineout-Overholt (2011) further broadens the scope of this definition by also giving consideration to the expertise of the practitioner as well as patient preferences and values when making best practice decisions (Melnyk & Fineout-Overholt, 2011).

Methodology

To achieve excellence in clinical and professional practice, APNs must embrace EBP as the norm. APNs must work in partnership within the organization to promote a spirit of inquiry. APNs that are empowered will be able to challenge traditional clinical practices not supported by best evidence.

To be successful, the organization must embrace EBP in its philosophy and mission and provide the infrastructure to ensure APNs have the resources and freedom necessary to conduct clinical inquiry.

Steps of the EBP Process

Melnyk and Fineout-Overholt (2011) define six critical steps of the EBP process (Melnyk & Fineout-Overholt, 2011).

- *Step 1:* In the first step, the healthcare provider asks a vital clinical question in a specific format that is likely to yield the most relevant and current best evidence. A well-written question will help the APN refine the literature review process to select the relevant literature and ensure the most efficient use of time. To determine a clinical question, a common approach is to use a *PICOT* format to guide the writing of the question (Melnyk & Fineout-Overholt, 2011). The *P* stands for patient population or problem of interest. For example, the APN might consider the age, gender, ethnicity, clinical setting, or client symptoms. The *I* stands for intervention or range of interventions to be considered and includes such examples as therapies, exposure to disease, prognostic factors, or risk behaviors. The *C* represents the comparison intervention or issue of interest. It may include such examples as alternative therapy, placebo, standard of care, absence of disease or risk factors. The *O* stands for outcome of interest and includes examples such as the outcome expected from therapy, risk of disease, accuracy of diagnosis, or rate of occurrence of an adverse outcome. The *T* represents time period such as the time it takes for the intervention to achieve the outcome or the time over which populations are observed for the outcome. The T may not be applicable for all clinical inquiries. Question templates for asking PICOT questions can be found in Table 1.

- *Step 2:* This step involves searching for the most relevant and best evidence to answer the clinical question. Search terms can be generated from the PICOT question and searching should focus on finding the strongest level of evidence on which to base treatment decisions. There are many hierarchies of evidence available in the literature for rating the level of evidence for intervention and treatment questions. Evidence from a systematic review or meta-analysis of all relevant randomized controlled trials produce the highest level of quality data available, whereas expert opinion of authorities and/or reports of expert committees are considered the weakest level of evidence. Although MEDLINE and the Cumulative Index of Nursing & Allied Health Literature (CINAHL) are the best-known comprehensive databases for healthcare literature, other common EBP online databases useful to the APN's practice may include Cochrane Databases, National Guideline Clearinghouse [evidence-based clinical practice guidelines], Excerpta Medica Online (EMBASE) [biomedical and pharmaceutical database], and PsycINFO [psychology, behavioral sciences, and mental health] (Melnyk & Fineout-Overholt, 2011). The APN may also find relevant evidence to answer clinical questions by searching applicable professional organizational websites or using other EBP search engines such as the Joanna Briggs Institute or Turning Research into Practice (TRIP) databases.
- *Step 3:* In this step of the EBP process, the APN should critically appraise the literature and determine if the results of the study are valid, reliable, and applicable to their patient population. *The Crit*ical Appraisal Skills Programme (CASP) has tools that the APN can download and use to assess the validity, reliability, and applicability of published research (http://www.caspinternational.org/?o=1012).
- *Step 4:* The level and quality of the evidence should provide the APN with the confidence to make a recommended change in clinical practice (Melnyk & Fineout-Overholt, 2011). In step four of the EBP process, the APN should incorporate the best evidence from the literature with his/her clinical expertise and patient preferences and values to make the best clinical decision.
- *Step 5:* In this step, the APN should evaluate the effectiveness of the EBP change or clinical decision. Measurement of outcomes is a critical step in order to determine the impact of the EBP change on the quality of healthcare and/or patient outcomes.
- *Step 6:* The final step of the EBP process involves dissemination of the outcomes of the EBP change. Consistent with the domain of Transformational Professional Practice in the TAPP model, it is important that the APN disseminate outcomes of their practice changes through journal publications and podium and poster presentations at local, regional, national, and international conferences (Melnyk & Fineout-Overholt, 2011).

Table 1. Question Templates for Asking PICOT Questions

Type of Question	PICOT Template
Intervention	In _____ (P), how does _____ (I) compared to _____ (C) affect _____ (O) within _____ (T)?
Prognosis/ Prediction	In _____ (P), how does _____ (I) compared to _____ (C) influence/predict _____ (O) over _____ (T)?
Diagnosis Or Diagnostic Test	In _____ (P), are/is _____ (I) compared with _____ (C) more accurate in diagnosing _____ (O)?
Etiology	Are _____ (P), who have _____ (I) compared with those without _____ (C) at _____ risk for/of _____ (O) over _____ (T)?
Meaning	How do _____ (P), with _____ (I) perceive _____ (O) during _____ (T)?

Used with permission from Melnyk, B. M., & Fineout-Overholt, E. (2011). *Evidence-based practice in nursing & Healthcare* (2nd ed.). Philadelphia: Wolters Kluwer Health/Lippincott Williams & Wilkins, p. 31.

Application

A conceptual model is often used in practice to facilitate change efforts. The Iowa Model of Evidence-Based Practice to Promote Quality Care developed by Titler (2001) was designed to support EBP by interdisciplinary teams (Titler, et al., 2001) (see Figure 2). The model is drafted as a clinical algorithm and includes several feedback loops for decision making by the healthcare team. The model has been successfully used by a large number of organizations to promote EBP practice (Melnyk & Fineout-Overholt, 2011).

Quality Improvement

As hospital systems and technologies have become more complex, there is an increasing awareness of the importance of patient safety and need to reduce medical errors. Patient safety has received widespread national attention following the IOM's publication of *To Err is Human* and the follow-up report *Crossing the Quality Chasm* (IOM, 2001; IOM, 2000). While patient safety remains at the forefront of quality, other attributes of clinical quality include care that is patient-centered, timely, effective, efficient, and equitable. Hospitals remain challenged to deliver and evaluate quality of care in a climate of exponential growth in science and technology, changing demographics, and patients who are sicker and more complex (Macellus & Harrison, 2012).

QI is a well recognized process by which hospitals and healthcare providers can provide safe and effective patient care. It is important to remember that QI is process, not simply an end goal (U.S. Department of Health and Human Services, 2011). It is critical that APNs become skillful in the use of tools and information systems that support QI and safe patient outcomes.

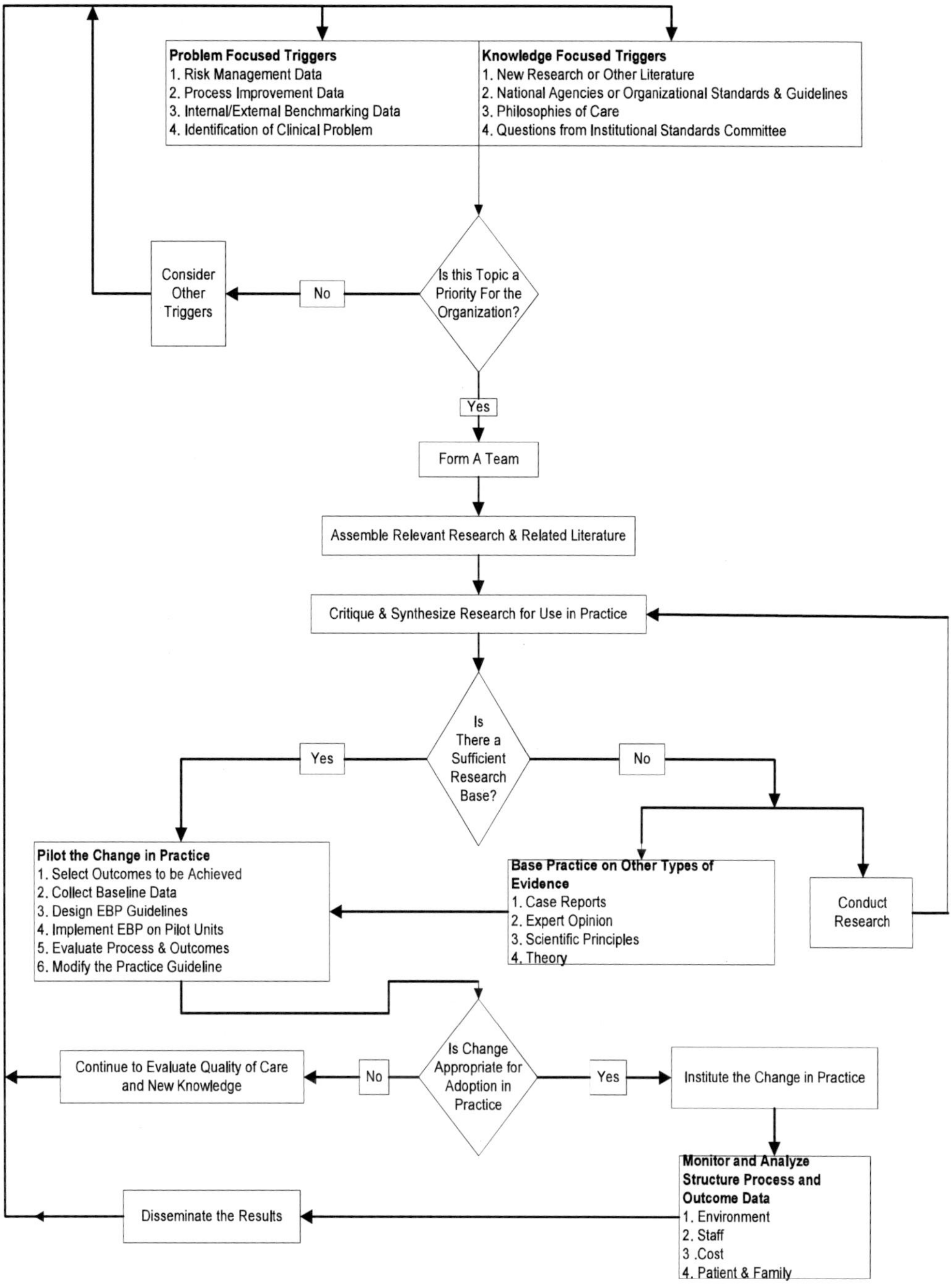

Used with permission from Titler, M. G., Kleiber, C., Rakel, B., Budreau, G., Everett, L. Q., Steelman, V., et al. (2001). The Iowa Model of Evidence-Based Practice to Promote Quality. *Critical Care Nursing Clinics of North America*, *13* (4), 497-509.

Figure 2. The Iowa Model of Evidence-Based Practice to Promote Quality Care.

Definition

QI is defined as a "data-driven systematic approach by which individuals work together to improve specific internal systems, processes, costs, productivity, and quality outcomes within an organization (Shirey, et al., 2011, p. 61).

Principles of QI

A successful QI program always incorporates four principles: 1) QI is the work of systems and processes; 2) QI focuses on patients; 3) QI focuses on teamwork; and, 4) QI focuses on use of data (U.S. Department of Health and Human Services, 2011). In the first principle, an organization must understand its own healthcare delivery systems and processes of care. The Donabedian Model (1980) is the dominant paradigm for assessing the quality of healthcare (Hoenig, Lee, & Stienman, 2010). The APN can use this conceptual model to evaluate quality of care within their clinical practice. According to the model, quality can be examined in terms of structure, process, and outcomes (see Figure 3). Antecedents, assessment of events or incidents, must be in place before the process of QI can begin. For example, prior to evaluating structure, process, and outcomes, the APN must be familiar with the environment in which he/she works and the characteristics of the patient population. The first dimension of care is evaluating the structure which includes all the factors that affect the context in which care is delivered (e.g. physical facility, equipment, and human resources). Process is the next dimension of care and is the sum of all actions that make up healthcare (e.g. interactions between the APN and the patient/family). Finally, outcomes refer to changes in the healthcare of individual patients or populations (e.g. nurse sensitive indicators such as patient falls, central line blood stream infections, pressure ulcers, pain, and patient satisfaction).

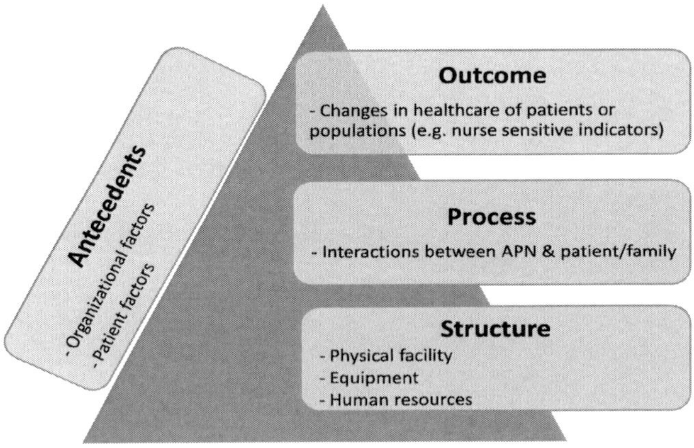

Figure 3. Donabedian's Structure, Process, Outcome Model.

Adapted from Donabedian, A. (1980). *Explorations in Quality Assessment and Monitoring Vol. 1. The Definition of Quality and Approaches to Its Assessment*. Ann Arbor, MI: Health Administration Press.

The second QI principle focuses on patients. This includes the extent to which patients' needs and expectations are met. The Institute for Patient and Family Centered Care and the Institute for Healthcare Improvement are two professional organizations that advocate and support hospitals to partner with patients and families in QI initiatives. Engaging patients in their own healthcare can significantly increase quality, reduce costs, and make the patient safer (IHI, 2014).

The third principle emphasizes that QI is a team process. A team is most effective when the knowledge, skills, experience, and perspectives of each of the team members is listened to and considered when addressing QI initiatives. Organizations that have a formal advanced QI program and infrastructure are better able to support QI teams and facilitate QI initiatives.

The final principle is that QI focuses on the use of data. Focusing on data in a disciplined and methodical way allows an organization to have a laser focus on opportunities for improvement and a mechanism for monitoring performance improvement over time.

Methodology

There are various QI methodologies to evaluate the quality of healthcare delivery. Three of the most commonly used QI methods are the Six Sigma strategy, Lean Design, and the Plan-Do-Study-Act (PDSA) Cycle (Macellus & Harrison, 2012). All three QI methods share common characteristics, yet approach the quality investigation in a slightly different manner. The Six Sigma strategy uses the Define-Measure-Analyze-Improvement Control (DMAIC) technique to reduce process variation by eliminating defects (errors) and waste, thereby improving quality and efficiency (Macellus & Harrison, 2012). For example, Six Sigma might use a Cause and Effect Diagram, commonly called a Fishbone, to brainstorm the various causes for a specific problem such as delays in time to be seen by the APN in the Emergency Department. Lean Design focuses on improving the process flow by cutting out unnecessary and wasteful steps so that only steps that directly add value are taken (Macellus & Harrison, 2012). For example, Lean Design can be used to reduce waiting times in the Emergency Department by mapping out the current steps from admission to time to be seen, standardizing, and eliminating unnecessary steps.

The third commonly used approach, and the focus of this chapter, is the Plan, Do, Study, Act Cycle (also known as the PDSA Cycle) for Improvement. This improvement model begins with three fundamental questions: "1) What are we trying to accomplish?; 2) How will we know that a change is an improvement?; and, 3) What changes can we make that will result in improvement?" (Provost & Murray, 2011, p. 4). To answer the first question, a well-written aim statement should be developed to provide clarity and guidance for the project. The aim statement should be time-specific, measureable, and define the target population (Provost & Murray, 2011). A SMART aim statement would include the following: S (Specific); M (Measurable); A (Attainable); R (Relevant); and T (Time-Bound). For example, an aim statement for reducing wait times in the Emergency Department might be, "To redesign Emergency Department processes to reduce wait times to be seen of patients by greater than 30% before August, 2014".

The second question, "How will we know that a change is an improvement?" involves establishing measures and indicators to determine if a specific change leads to the desired improvement (Provost & Murray, 2011). In the Emergency Department example, the APN might measure the mean or median waiting times of patients presenting to the Department before being seen.

To answer the final question, the APN must select changes that are most likely to result in the desired improvement. In the Emergency Department example, the APN might trial a triage system to identify levels of care based on patient acuity and resource needs.

The next step in the QI process is to test the change using the PDSA cycle. The PDSA cycle is a systematic, rapid cycle, series of four steps to test and implement changes in the clinical setting for process improvement (Provost & Murray, 2011). The first step in the PDSA cycle is Planning. In this step, the APN plans the details of the project and makes predictions regarding expected outcomes. In the Do phase, the APN implements the plan and collects the data. In the Study phase, the APN compares the predictions to the data collected. In the final Act phase, the APN acts upon the results from the analyses of the data. If the change was positive, the APN would build the change into standard practice, but if the change was negative, the APN would refine the plan or start over with a new PDSA cycle. Sequential or simultaneous PDSA cycles may be needed if the previous PDSA cycle suggests a different clinical approach is warranted (Provost & Murray, 2011). In the example on wait times in the Emergency Department, the initial PDSA cycle evaluated the use of a triage system to reduce wait times. Simultaneous PDSA cycles may need to be performed in the acute care areas to identify ways to increase bed capacity and facilitate patient flow from the Emergency Department.

The underpinning of a successful QI program is strong leadership, motivation, and teamwork (Macellus & Harrison, 2012). Following the QI process, it is important that the team share the lessons learned and integrate the successful quality and safety approach in order to "maintain the gain" (Macellus & Harrison, 2012). Furthermore, completed QI projects may be publishable in professional journals and accepted for presentation at local, regional, or national conferences. The focus of knowledge dissemination is usually limited to lessons learned from the local project (Shirey, et al., 2011). Although approval from an institutional research review board is not generally required unless the project exposes patients to risks and burdens, QI projects should have approval from the organization's governance structure prior to external dissemination of results (Shirey, et al., 2011).

The APN implements clinical improvement in collaboration with other people and structures within an organization. Plsek (1999) discusses four habits that are essential in order for healthcare organizations to sustain significant improvement in patient safety and quality patient outcomes. The first habit entails viewing clinical practice as a process; not a rigid, single approach to care delivery. EBP is the second habit that the APN must adopt in order to bring real improvement to clinical practice. The third habit involves collaborative learning and working together in a team to achieve optimal clinical and patient outcomes. The final habit is tolerance for change and having a culture where the entire healthcare team is challenged to engage in the spirit of inquiry to deliver quality patient care. These habits bridge the gap between the art and science of quality healthcare.

CONCLUSION

This chapter presented three approaches in the clinical setting that the APN uses to advance practice and achieve improved patient outcomes: Research, Evidence Based Practice, and Quality Improvement. Shirley et al. (2011) describes the interface of these approaches to knowledge in that "research generates it, EBP translates it, and QI incorporates it" (p. 60). The development of new knowledge then adds to the depth of current clinical, educational, and administrative practice to improve organizational processes. The APN is in a unique position in all areas of clinical practice to apply research, EBP, and QI and then translate research findings into clinical practice to improve the delivery of healthcare and ensure the best patient outcomes.

REFERENCES

Ackerman, M. H., Norsen, L., Martin, B., Wiedrich, J., & Kitzman, H. J. (1996). Development of a model of advanced practice. *American Journal of Critical Care, 5* (1), 68-73.

Benner, P. (1984). *From novice to expert: excellence and power in clinical nursing practice.* Menlo Park, CA: Addison-Wesley Publishing.

Burns, N., & Grove, S. K. (2009). *The practice of nursing research: Appraisal, synthesis, and generation of evidence* (6th ed.). St. Louis: Saunders Elsevier.

Donabedian, A. (1980). *Explorations in Quality Assessment and Monitoring Vol. 1. The Definition of Quality and Approaches to Its Assessment.* Ann Arbor, MI: Health Administration Press.

Elliott, E. C., & Walden, M. (in press). Development of the Transformation Advanced Professional Practice Model. *Journal of the American Association of Nurse Practitioners.*

Facchiano, L., & Snyder, C. H. (2012). Evidence-based practice for the busy nurse practitioner: Part one: Relevance to clinical practice and clinical inquiry process. *Journal of American Academy of Nurse Practitioners, 24*, 579-586.

Gliner, J. A., Morgan, G. A., & Leech, N. L. (2009). *Research methods in applied settings: An integrated approach to design and analysis* (2nd ed.). New York: Taylor & Francis Group.

Hoenig, H., Lee, J., & Stienman, M. (2010). Conceptual overview of frameworks for measuring quality in rehabilitation. *Topics in Stroke Rehabilitation, 17* (4), 239-251.

IHI. (2014). *Improving health and healthcare worldwide.* Retrieved February 18, 2014, from IHI.org: http://www.ihi.org/engage/initiatives/patientfamilycenteredcare/pages/default.aspx.

IOM. (2001, March 1). *Crossing the quality chasm: A new health system for the 21st century. Committee on Quality of Health Care in America, Institute of Medicine.* Retrieved February 18, 2014, from IOM: http://www.iom.edu/Reports/2001/Crossing-the-Quality-Chasm-A-New-Health-System-for-the-21st-Century.aspx.

IOM. (2000). *To err is human: Building a safer health system.*

IOM. (1990). *Medicare: A strategy for quality assurance.* (Lohr, KN, Ed.). Washington, DC: National Academy Press.

Macellus, L., & Harrison, A. (2012). Quality improvement for neonatal nurses, Part I: A framework for advancing the quality and safety of care. *Neonatal Network, 31* (2), 81-88.

Melnyk, B. M., & Fineout-Overholt, E. (2011). *Evidence-based practice in nursing & Healthcare* (2nd ed.). Philadelphia: Wolters Kluwer Health/Lippincott Williams & Wilkins.

Plsek, P. E. (1999). Quality improvement methods in clinical medicine. *Pediatrics, 103* (1), 203-214.

Polit, D. F., & Beck, C. T. (2012). *Nursing Research: Generating and assessing evidence for nursing practice* (9th ed.). Philadelphia: Wolters Kluwer Health/Lippincott Williams & Wilkins.

Provost, L. P., & Murray, S. K. (2011). *The health care data guide: Learning from data for improvement.* San Francisco: Jossey-Bass/John Wiley & Sons.

Sackett, D., Rosenberg, W., Gray, J., Haynes, R., & Richardson, W. (1996). Evidence-based medicine: What it is and what it isn't: It's about integrating individual clinical expertise and the best external evidence. *British Medical Journal, 3* (12), 71-72.

Shirey, M. R., Hauck, S. L., Embree, J. L., Kinner, T. J., Schaar, G. L., Phillips, L. A., et al. (2011). Showcasing differences between quality improvement, evidence-based practice, and research. *The Journal of Continuing Education in Nursing, 42* (2), 57-68.

Stevens, K. R. (2013, May 31). *The Online Journal of Issues in Nursing.* Retrieved February 18, 2014, from nursingworld.org: http://nursingworld.org/MainMenuCategories/ANAMarketplace/ANAPeriodicals/OJIN/TableofContents/Vol-18-2013/No2-May-2013/Impact-of-Evidence-Based-Practice.html.

Straus, S. E., Glasizou, P., Richardson, W. S., & Haynes, R. B. (2011). *Evidence-based medicine: How to practice and teach it* (4th ed.). Edinburgh, London: Churchill Livingstone.

Titler, M. G., Kleiber, C., Rakel, B., Budreau, G., Everett, L. Q., Steelman, V., et al. (2001). The Iowa Model of Evidence-Based Practice to Promote Quality. *Critical Care Nursing Clinics of North America, 13* (4), 497-509.

U.S. Department of Health and Human Services. (2011). *HRSA.gov.* Retrieved February 18, 2014, from Health Information Technology and Quality Improvement: http://www.hrsa.gov/healthit/toolbox/healthITAdoptiontoolbox/qualityimprovement/whatisqi.html.

In: Collaboration with the Advanced Practice Nurse
Editors: E.R. Giardino, R.G. Hanks and A.P. Giardino
ISBN: 978-1-63321-311-1

Chapter 12

ADMINISTRATIVE ASPECTS OF THE DOCTOR OF NURSING PRACTICE

Al Rundio[1], RN, DNP, PhD, APRN, NEA-BC and Eileen R. Giardino[2], PhD, RN, APRN

[1]Drexel University College of Nursing and Health Professions, Philadelphia, PA, US
[2]University of Texas Health Science Center at Houston, School of Nursing, Houston, TX, US

ABSTRACT

The doctor of nursing practice (DNP) advanced practice nurse is prepared to be a leader and administrator in health care settings. The DNP is a practice doctorate with two general categories of preparation within the DNP curriculum. There is the advanced practice registered nurse (APRN) role with a focus on care of individuals, and the role that specializes in practice at an aggregate, systems, or organizational level. This distinction is important as APRNs face different licensure, regulatory, credentialing, liability, and reimbursement issues than those who practice at an aggregate, systems, or organizational level. DNPs are well prepared for leadership and administrative roles. The primary focus of the Essentials for DNP Programs as stated by the American Association of Colleges of Nursing (AACN) is to improve patient care outcomes in all organizational settings (American Association of Colleges of Nursing, 2006). Improvements in all aspects of patient care and organizational development results from the DNP's educational experience, where key concepts of leadership, informatics, statistics, health policy, communication and collaboration, quality improvement, evidence-based practice, translational research, and health outcomes are a strong focus of the DNP curriculum. DNPs are in a pivotal position to effect positive change in organizations through leadership abilities, administrative skills and the application of evidence based practice into clinical settings.

Leadership in Master of Science in Nursing (MSN) and DNP Educational Programs

DNP education is the level at which advanced practice registered nurses (APRNs) learn principles of leadership and organizational management that enables the APRN to become a transformational leader in the healthcare system. The main focus of advanced practice Master of Science in Nursing (MSN) educational programs is to learn how to clinically manage individuals with specific disease processes. Therefore, a primary difference between the masters prepared APRN and the DNP prepared APRN is that the masters prepared APRN is primarily educated to provide medical and nursing care to individuals with illness and disease, while the DNP prepared APRN is educated to address health care delivery at a population based level to improve outcomes and address health policy issues (American Association of Colleges of Nursing, 2006).

A key component of the MSN curriculum is diagnostic reasoning of various disease states with the focus of masters' level course work on the principles of physical assessment, pathophysiology, pharmacology, and medical management of acute or primary care problems. The MSN student completes required clinical practicum hours in specific patient populations such as primary care or acute care setting to prepare the graduate to render care to individual patients in a variety of practice settings, inclusive of outpatient settings and inpatient settings. Although the MSN curriculum may address principles of practice improvement, quality indicators, and administrative aspects of health care, the substance of the curricular content is on the management of diseases and patient care. Consequently, the MSN level of education introduces the NP to population level leadership aspects of the advanced practice role, while DNP education has emerged as the level at which the curriculum focuses clearly on performance improvement and population health (American Association of Colleges of Nursing, 2006).

The DNP graduate is prepared to address quality improvement, outcomes management, and information systems technology, to name a few. DNP educational programs are based on the DNP essentials which are the competencies and curricular elements that must be present in programs conferring the Doctor of Nursing Practice degree (American Association of Colleges of Nursing, 2006). The DNP essentials guide the theory and content that are the hallmark of the DNP degree (Fitzpatrick & Wallace, 2009; (American Association of Colleges of Nursing, 2006). Each of the eight essentials focuses on leadership principles in areas of clinical practice. (Table 1 describes the DNP Essentials). A key component of DNP education is the understanding of evidence-based practice and the translation of scientific evidence into the clinical practice setting with the ultimate goal of improved care outcomes for the patient. Table 1 outlines the DNP Essentials.

Table 1. The DNP Essentials

1	Scientific underpinnings for practice
2	Organizational and systems leadership for quality improvement and systems thinking
3	Clinical scholarship and analytical methods for evidence-based practice
4	Information systems/technology and patient technology for the improvement and transformation of health care

5	Health care policy for advocacy in health care
6	Interprofessional collaboration for improving patient and population health outcome
7	Clinical prevention and population health for improving the nation's health and advanced nursing practice
8	Adapted From: (American Association of Colleges of Nursing (AACN), 2006)

Transformational Leadership

DNP education focuses on building leadership skills that prepare its graduates to understand basic leadership principles and put those principles into action. Transformational leadership is an important skill for advanced practice nurses as it encourages collaboration, risk-taking, and out of the box thinking that ultimately transforms organizations and advances the nursing profession. It is an approach by which leaders encourage positive change by building trust within their teams (Heuston & Wolf, 2011). Transformational leaders lead by example as trustworthy, inspirational, and charismatic role models. They align themselves with tasks and goals to optimize the performance of their team as they team and individual strengths and weaknesses (Bowles & Bowles, 2000). They encourage those they lead to become leaders.

Leadership and the Global Perspective

DNP prepared APRNs are educated to assume more global roles that have an impact on health policy. They are prepared to assume administrative roles in health care systems, such as Chief Nursing Officers (CNOs) of nursing services in a variety of practice settings. The DNP graduate assumes a more global perspective organizationally, locally, nationally and globally. For example, the APRN in a primary care practice will utilize an electronic informatics system for documenting patient care, whereas the APRN in a larger organization may be part of the team that selects the electronic informatics system for clinicians to use.

THE DNP IN HEALTH CARE CHANGES

Health care in the United States (US) is experiencing unprecedented change. The United States of America is the only industrialized nation in the world that does not provide universal health care coverage to its citizens (Vladeck, 2003). As such, DNPs must understand the financial milieu that exists in the health care delivery system. America's health care delivery system is in the process of monumental change from an intervention system to that of a prevention system. An essential part of this change involves reimbursement of health care expenses (Andrulis, 2010; Kaiser Family Foundation, 2014). The US health care reimbursement system is entrepreneurial as evidenced by many different types of insurance products in the marketplace. This phenomenon compares to a country such as Great Britain that has a single payer, governmental paid system of health care. United States' citizens who have health insurance expect treatment in a timely manner. Technological advancements are just one of the factors that have caused a dramatic rise in health care costs. The public demands certain types of procedures and tests without paying attention to the costs. The US health care system is fraught with high costs secondary to abuse of such procedures, tests and treatments. A core concept in ethics is that of futility, which is usually not addressed in the United States health care system.

The DNP is positioned to address the solutions and transformation of the US health care system. The educational focus of DNP education and then subsequent experience in clinical and organizational roles prepares them to be leaders at local, national and global levels of healthcare. There is a need for APRNs, including DNPs, who:

- Think out of the box or "have no box"
- Embrace change
- Enjoy clinical challenges
- Embrace technology and technological advancements
- Challenge the system and individuals and groups within the system
- Think strategically and create new systems of care delivery

APRNs, including DNPs, are essential to helping to orchestrate substantial changes, and are in an optimal position to foster the needed changes in the health care system (Andrulis, 2010). The health care system in the USA is one of the most costly on earth where health care costs continue to rise despite efforts by managed care and the United States government to control such costs [See Figure1]. The increased cost of federally funded health care that began with the initiation of Medicare and Medicaid in 1965 when the federal government became a payer in the health care system, has grown exponentially as those programs continue to insure the elderly, special populations, such as dialysis patients, and those citizens with low incomes. These programs have high costs and relatively poor outcomes. DNPs are positioned to address the needs to improve health intervention outcomes and evaluate the provision of care to both individuals and aggregates. The World Health Organization (WHO, 2000) ranked health care delivery system outcomes by nation and found that the USA ranked number 37 for outcomes among other nations (Murry & Frenk 2010). A major factor in poor healthcare outcomes is that the US health care system is focused on intervention and treatments for diseases, rather than on prevention of disease individuals and populations. The countries with the best health care outcomes have a strong primary care network in place with a focus on prevention and health promotion (WHO 2000, 2013). DNPs can work within the health care system to improve outcomes and influence policy that can address the issues of health care delivery.

HEALTH POLICY

A central core competency of a DNP graduate is that of learning how to influence health policy issues at the local, state levels and national levels (American Association of Colleges of Nursing, 2006). The Institute of Medicine report highlighted that DNP education prepares graduates to influence, and implement health care policies that address all aspects of health care including practice regulation, access to care, safety and quality issues, to name a few {Institute of Medicine;, 2011 62 /id}. An expectation of the DNP graduate is to advocate for high-quality healthcare and play a leadership role in influencing and shaping policies that affect nursing practice (Chism, 2009).

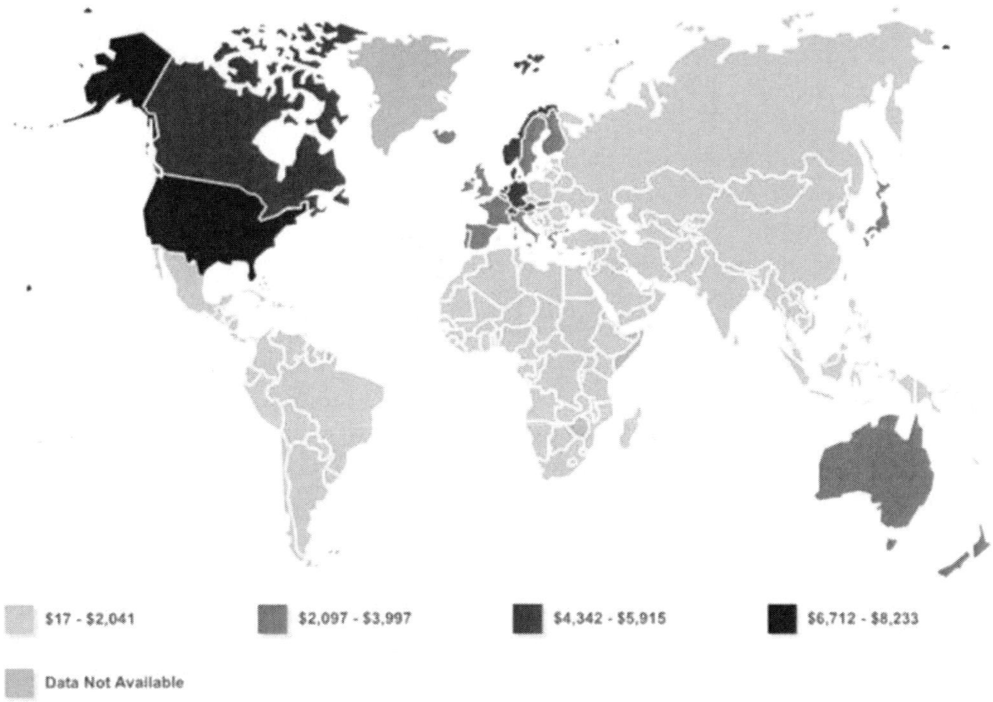

Global Health Facts. The Henry J. Kaiser Family Foundation. Health Expenditure Per Capita (PPP; International $) 2010 timeframe http://kff.org/global-indicator/health-expenditure-per-capita/#.

Figure 1. Health Expenditure Per Capita Internationally.

Nurses have driven health policy from its early beginning in the United States. Consider Margaret Sanger who was jailed for her beliefs and efforts to use birth control for planned pregnancies (Chesler, 2007). Sanger helped to drive health care policy through her efforts to address the issues of women's reproductive rights and health issues in the US and abroad in the early 1900s.

There are 5 areas of policy that DNP practice can impact. These areas are:

- Public Policy
- Social Policy
- Health Policy
- Institutional Policy
- Organizational Policy

THE MAGNET INITIATIVE AND APRN LEADERSHIP

The Magnet initiative provides a way to operationalize the role of the DNP in leadership and administration. Magnet designation is the highest level of recognition that the American Nurses Credentialing Center (ANCC) awards to healthcare organizations. It is the Olympic gold medal of healthcare and recognizes that the health care organization has met the highest standards of expectations for nursing practices. Magnet designation recognizes nursing excellence, and identifies healthcare organizations that epitomize outstanding quality and professionalism. The ANCC stated that magnet organizations serve as the fountain of knowledge and expertise for the delivery of nursing care globally (American Nurses Credentialing Center, 2008; American Nurses Credentialing Center, 2014). The ANCC developed The Magnet Recognition Program® to recognize healthcare organizations that provide excellence in all aspects of nursing. The program provides a way to disseminate successful nursing practices and strategies into healthcare organizations. The process to become a magnet organization involves the appraisal of qualitative factors in nursing.

DNPs are positioned to lead healthcare delivery system reforms as advanced practice nursing care is inclusive of the patient, family and community, and embraces quality care that meets standards of practice and measures outcomes. Magnet Organizations are recognized as incorporating the highest standards of knowledge and expertise in the delivery of nursing care. Magnet status implies that the organization stands by Magnet principles, strives towards innovative practices, and is a leader in health care reformation, and care of the patient, family, and community (American Nurses Credentialing Center, 2014). The strong corollary between the principles of the Magnet recognition program and that of the leadership and administrative role of the doctor of nursing practice is that DNPs focus on the delivery of nursing care at the local, national and global levels, flexibility, cost effective, and embrace discovery and innovation. DNPs strive to improve healthcare delivery to the patients they serve, and set the bar high reaching for the Olympic gold medal.

Table 2. Describes specifics about each type of policy

Policy	Policy Specifics
Public policy	Goal of policy is to benefit and protect the general public Based by Congress at the federal or state level. Origin of policy is from the government. Example: legislation that mandates auto drivers and passengers to wear a seat belt when in a motor vehicle based on research that showed that seat belts save lives in motor vehicle accidents.
Social policy	Goal: Promotes general welfare of society Example: labels on alcohol advising that pregnant women should not drink alcohol while they are pregnant because of alcohol effect on the fetus
Health policy	Goal: Promotes the health of individual citizens. Example: mandatory vaccination for certain illnesses such as being vaccinated against the polio virus.
Institutional policies	Goal: Regulate what employees can do and not Policy established by an institution and for the institution. Example: health care facility may mandate that every employee must have an annual physical examination or specific vaccinations.
Organizational policy	Goal: Serves as a form of internal organizational control Governs organizational entity (Such as a state nursing association or a specialty nursing organization). Example: a nursing organization may have policy that bans alcohol at meetings.

Table 3. Leadership Qualities of the DNP

Leadership Qualities	Examples
Effective communication	Communicates across disciplines or teams
Assume leadership Roles	Model transformational leadership principles to affect change
Boldness	Identify needed changes in healthcare system and assume the lead in making those changes
Advocate	Advocate for patients and colleagues
Problem Solver	Able to evaluate situations and develop strategies to change the environment

Adapted from (Chism, 2009).

Table 3 shows some of the leadership qualities that DNP advanced Practice Nurses exhibit in clinical and administrative practice settings.

The Magnet Recognition Program configures five Magnet Model Components. Each component in the model reflects a focus on measuring outcomes, and allows for more streamlined documentation (American Nurses Credentialing Center, 2008; American Nurses Credentialing Center, 2014). Each component is described in terms of how the DNP is prepared to address the Magnet components in an administrative capacity.

Model Component 1: Transformational Leadership

The Transformational Leadership component addresses quality of nursing leadership. The magnet program embraces the concept of transformational leadership that enables people to transform the culture of organizations or systems of care to where it needs to be to meet changing needs. A transformational leader allows risk taking and works collaboratively with others to transform care. DNPs are able to apply transformational leadership principles that can in turn transform healthcare delivery. As profound changes to health care delivery will be implemented in this decade as a result of the Affordable Care Act of 2010, advanced practice nurses will be key stakeholders in transforming the United States healthcare delivery system.

Model Component 2: Structural Empowerment

Influential leadership within an organization develops infrastructure and processes to form an innovative environment that supports professional practice and achieves determined outcomes that in turn strengthen the organization (American Nurses Credentialing Center, 2014). The DNP is positioned to develop structures that implement cost effective health care and ensure judicious use of resources as the health care delivery system goes through reform. The DNP is positioned to work with staff to develop their skills and empower them to achieve organizational goals and desired outcomes. The DNP has the ability to evaluate health care interventions such as diagnostic testing and medical interventions to determine ways to improve the delivery of health care services, and then recommend ways to streamline services and decrease overall costs to the system. In a system where unnecessary testing procedures need to be controlled, the DNP can affect such positive change.

Model Component 3: Exemplary Professional Practice

Component 3 addresses professional practice models and exemplary professional practice. In order to provide competent and successful patient care at all levels of practice in the future, there needs to be a redesign of current clinical practices within health care delivery systems. There is a need to develop new models of care, develop new evidence for clinical practices, and apply existing evidence that contributes to the science of nursing (American Nurses Credentialing Center, 2008). It is questionable that the current model of primary care is adequate to carry nursing into the future within a reformed healthcare delivery system. The DNP is positioned to be the trendsetter for new models of care delivery in all practice settings and has the knowledge and education to be a part of such innovation. Implementation of middle range theoretical models that enhance and improve nursing practice should be coupled with new models of practice.

In a Magnet organization, the DNP is positioned to develop the exemplary professional nursing practice that is a hallmark of Magnet organizations (American Nurses Credentialing Center, 2014). Exemplary practice demonstrates an understanding of what nursing does and applies those principles to patients, families, communities, and interdisciplinary teams. The DNP can strengthen the role of the APRN within healthcare organizations and establish strong professional practice principles within organizations.

DNPs are positioned to be role models for exemplary practice. Such practice requires critical, analytical thinking and communication skills. Such skill can be incorporated into any practice setting by the DNP. The elements of exemplary professional practice include: Scientific underpinnings for practice, organizational and systems leadership for quality improvement, systems thinking, clinical scholarship and analytical methods for evidence-based practice, information systems/technology and patient technology for the improvement and transformation of health care, health care policy for advocacy in health care, interprofessional collaboration for improving patient and population health outcomes, and clinical prevention and population health for improving the nation's health (American Association of Colleges of Nursing, 2006).

Model Component 4: New Knowledge, Innovations & Improvements

Magnet Component four addresses research and evidence-based practice, the development of new knowledge, the translation of knowledge into practice to improve patient care outcomes, and development of innovation initiatives. The DNP serves as a consultant to research and evidence-based practice issues within healthcare organizations to evaluate synthesize and translate clinical evidence to improve patient care outcomes. The DNP educates and mentors staff to apply evidence-based practice to improve care and works collaboratively with other disciplines to achieve these goals.

MODEL COMPONENT 5: EMPIRICAL OUTCOMES

Empirical outcomes centers on outcomes research and management, empirical quality indicators and outcomes to improve quality of care. A magnet organization tries to evaluate what are the differences are that have been made when the organization implements innovative initiatives. Such information comes when an organization determines clinical outcomes that evaluate workforce issues, patient concerns and organizational improvements. Critical to the magnet process is the improvement of patient care in the monitoring of quality outcomes. The DNP is educated to design systems for the collection and analysis of such data, and is in a position to establish initiatives that determine quantitative benchmarks that can demonstrate excellence.

CONCLUSION

The DNP graduate is prepared for leadership and administrative roles in all areas of healthcare, from clinical practice positions to leaders of healthcare organizations. The DNP graduate has the ability to become a transformational leader in the healthcare system to improve health care from patient care outcomes to changes in systems that decrease healthcare costs. The DNP promotes scholarship, technology information systems and practice innovations to influence policy changes that transform healthcare and improve outcomes in all aspects of healthcare.

REFERENCES

American Association of Colleges of Nursing. (2006). The essentials of doctoral education for advanced nursing practice. American Association of Colleges of Nursing [On-line]. Available: http://www.aacn.nche.edu

American Association of Colleges of Nursing (AACN). (2006). The essentials of doctoral education for advanced nursing practice. American Association of Colleges of Nursing [On-line]. Available: http://www.aacn.nche.edu

American Nurses Credentialing Center. (2008). A New Model for ANCC's Magnet Recognition Program. American Nurses Credentialing Center [On-line]. Available: http://www.va.gov/nursing/docs/ANCC_NewMagnetModel.pdf

American Nurses Credentialing Center. (2014). Magnet Recognition Program® Model. American Nurses Credentialing Center [On-line]. Available: http://www.nursecredentialing.org/Magnet/ProgramOverview/New-Magnet-Model?css=print

Andrulis, D. (2010). *Patient Protection and Affordable Care Act of 2010: Advancing health equity for racially and ethnically diverse populations*. Joint Center for Political and Economic Studies.

Bowles, A. & Bowles, N. B. (2000). A comparative study of transformational leadership in nursing development units and conventional clinical settings. *Journal of Nursing Management*, *8*, 69-76.

Chesler, E. (2007). *Woman of valor: Margaret Sanger and the birth control movement in America*. New Youk: Simon and Schuster.

Chism, L. A. (2009). Toward clarification of the doctor of nursing practice degree. *Advanced emergency nursing journal*, *31*, 287-297.

Fitzpatrick, J. J. & Wallace, M. (Eds.). (2009). The doctor of nursing practice and clinical nurse leader: Essentials of program development and implementation for clinical practice. New York, NY: Springer Publishing Company

Global Health Facts. (2010). The Henry J. Kaiser Family Foundation. Health Expenditure Per Capita (PPP; International $) timeframe http://kff.org/global-indicator/health-expenditure -per-capita/#

Heuston, M. & Wolf, G. (2011). Leadership Development. Transformational Leadership Skills of Successful Nurse Managers. *Journal Of Nursing Administration*, *41*, 248-251.

Institute of Medicine (US). (2011). *The Future of Nursing: Leading Change, Advancing Health* The National Academies Press.

Kaiser Family Foundation. (2014). Summary of the Affordable Care Act. Kaiser Family Foundation [On-line]. Available: http://kff.org/health-reform/fact-sheet/summary-of-new-health-reform-law/

Vladeck, B. (2003). Universal Health Insurance in the United States: Reflections on the Past, the Present, and the Future. *American Journal of Public Health*, *93*, 16-19.

World Health Organization. (2000). World Health Organization's ranking of the world's health systems accessed at http://www.who.int/whr/2000/media_centre/press_release/en/ on 2-23-2014.

World HealthOrganization. (2013). World Health Statistics accessed at: http://www.who.int/gho/publications/world_health_statistics/EN_WHS2013_Full.pdf?ua=1

In: Collaboration with the Advanced Practice Nurse ISBN: 978-1-63321-311-1
Editors: E.R. Giardino, R.G. Hanks and A.P. Giardino

Chapter 13

Advanced Nursing Practice Environments: Considerations for Practice

Mary Pat Hildebrand[1], DNP, RN, CPNP and Eileen R. Giardino[2] PhD, RN, APRN
[1]University of Texas Health Science Center at Houston, School of Medicine,TX, US
[2]University of Texas Health Science Center at Houston, School of Nursing, TX, US

Abstract

The clinical settings of advanced practice nurse practitioners (APNP) practice are diverse and their scope of practice parameters are determined by state rules and regulations. While some states allow APNP's to work independently of physician oversight, other states require APNP's to have a collaborative agreement with physicians stipulating prescriptive authority and the specifications of patient care delivery. Although The Institute of Medicine (IOM) and National Council of State Boards of Nursing (NCSBN) support full practice agreements, there are states permitting only reduced or restrictive practices. Consequently, APNP licensure and scope of practice are specific to each state and have a direct impact on the type of collaborative agreement allowed. In states requiring collaborative practice, the APNP has the opportunity to work in a variety of settings from a physician owned and managed practices to nurse practitioner owned and managed practices. In either case, the APNP needs to consider the type of preferred practice setting and the practice and legal implications of any practice site. This chapter addresses types of practices an APNP's may choose as well as guidelines that will facilitate the decision making process.

Introduction

Advanced practice nurse practitioners (APNPs) practice in a variety of clinical settings. Whether the clinical setting is in academia, private office or in an independently owned APNP practice, APNP's must be compliant with certain state and federal requirements governing the scope of practice and practice settings.

It is important that the APNP understand the implications of different practice settings before entering into any contractual agreement with a physicians or a practice employing nurse practitioners. In order to make a wise practice decision, the APNP needs to analyze all aspects of a practice setting from a business and medical practice perspective. The APNP should follow a sequential and structured format that considers the job description, compensated and uncompensated salary and benefits, potential for advancement, and the culture of the organization (Glasgow & Donnelly, 2011). This chapter provides information about types of clinical practice and provides a format by which the APNP can ask questions concerning job options using the *Doctorate of Nursing Practice Essentials* to make wise careers choices.

Basic Practice Requirements for Nurse Practitioners

Each state board of nursing mandates APNP's to meet certain requirements prior to granting licensure to practice in the state of employment. State requirements dictate the APNP to be a graduate of an accredited Masters of Nursing Program, attain national board certification in a designated advanced practice role and population focus area, and meet individual state licensure requirements (National Council of State Boards of Nursing & National Council of State Boards of Nursing, 2008). Once the APNP meets national and state board requirements, there are varied practice options in a wide range of settings available. For example, the APNP who has trained as a family nurse practitioner may coordinate care, manage chronic care patients and provide wellness and preventive care in an accessible and cost effective manner (Stanley, Werner & Apple, 2009).

Nurse Practitioner: MSN or DNP

There can be confusion among professionals and consumers alike as to who is an advanced practice nurse practitioner and what degree is required to practice as an APNP. At the present time, APNP's have earned a master's degree from an accredited nursing program. The program of study is in a in a specific role such as a family nurse practitioner, adult nurse practitioner or pediatric nurse practitioner, to name a few. Most states grant nurses the privilege to practice as an advanced practice nurse when they have met all qualifications for licensure as a registered nurse, hold current specialty certification by a board-approved credentialing organization, and have earned a master's or DNP degree from an accredited college or university.

In 2004 the American Association of Colleges of Nursing (AACN) endorsed a position statement recommending to move the educational preparation level for advanced nursing practice from the master's degree to the doctoral level by the year 2015 (AANP, 2014, APNR Joint Dialogue Group Report, 2008, AACN, 2004). Nursing organizations are advocating for the DNP to be the terminal degree for all who enter a nurse practitioner program (AANP, 2014; Chism, 2009; American Association of Colleges of Nursing, 2006). The 2015 time frame for doctoral degree has not yet been implemented for nurse practitioners. The DNP is still an option for prospective nurse practitioners, not a requirement. But for those nurses who choose a post baccalaureate to DNP program to become a nurse practitioner or those who continued education at the DNP level, they are certified as a nurse practitioner. However, the AACN position statement strives to require doctoral degrees for APNPs who desire educational positions and top leadership/organizational roles in nursing and healthcare. DNP education provides the APNP with a more intense and expanded knowledge of the multifaceted integration of scientific, psychosocial science and business management theories. Dennison, Payne and Farrell (2012a) implied the DNP's knowledge of the integration of these theories prepares a DNP to have a firmer grasp of strategies to improve present practice settings. Also, the AACN recommendation places the requirement for advanced practice nursing at the same educational level as medicine, physical therapy, and pharmacy.

Types of Practice for Nurse Practitioners: Full or Collaborative Practice

State boards of nursing have provided well defined expectations and legal parameters as to whether an APNP can practice independently of physician oversight or in collaboration with a supervising physician (American Nurses Association, 2012; New York State Nursing Board Office, 2013). It is important to understand the practice considerations for a collaborative practice as well as what constitutes independent practice.

Collaborative Practice

Many state boards of nursing require the APRN to work in collaboration with and under the supervision of a licensed physician in order to perform delegated medical acts. A collaborative practice is a formal relationship that is supported by a legal document or written protocols between a nurse practitioner or a group of nurse practitioners with a physician who provides oversight of their advanced practice role (New York State Nursing Board Office, 2013; North Carolina Board of Nursing, 2014). It is important to note that collaborative practices must adhere to the rules and regulation of the state board of nursing in the state of practice or in some states both the state board of nursing and board of medical examiners. In most states, an APNP working in a collaborative practice does not need direct or on-site supervision but must have the resources to contact physician either electronically or by phone. It is also, important for both parties to engage in chart reviews and discuss referrals or consultations with other professionals.

Both physician and nurse practitioner need to be cognizant that a collaborative practice is more than a legal relationship or a list of written protocols. For a collaborative practice to be successful, there must be a shared mutual respect, open communication to overcome barriers, candid exchange of clinical knowledge and expertise and if needed consultation to improve patient outcomes (Bridges, 2013).

There are some states have rules and regulation that reduce or restrict the ability of nurse practitioners to engage in at least one element of APNP practice. Reduced practice states requires a regulated collaborative agreement with an outside health discipline in order for the APNP to provide patient care while restricted practice states requires that APNPs have supervision, delegation or team-management by an outside health discipline in order to provide patient care (AANP, 2013a).

Full Practice or Independent Practice

As of 2013, there are 17 states along with the District of Columbia allowing full practice for APNP's (Vestal, 2013). The *Institute of Medicine and National Council of State Boards of Nursing* (Institute of Medicine (US), 2011) recommends the full practice model that allows APNP' to practice by the licensure authority of the state board of nursing alone. In this model, there are no state regulations requiring the APNP to work collaboratively with a physician. The state practice and licensure laws allow nurse practitioners to evaluate patients, diagnose, order and interpret diagnostic tests, initiate and manage treatments, and prescribe medications without the need of a collaborating physician (AANP, 2013a).

The AANP identifies 17 states that allow full autonomous practice for APNPs (AANP, 2013). The National Institute of Medicine includes two other states in that category that do not yet meet the AANP definition of autonomous practice (Maryland and Utah). There is a discrepancy in the precise language in laws outlining the APNPs needed association with the physician (Vestal, 2013).

Collaborative Practice Agreement

As a requisite to practice, an APNP may need to have a written collaborative practice agreement (CPA) with a physician that states the specific practice considerations required for physician and nurse practitioner to practice together. The CPA is a legal document addressing the provision of care services between an APNP and a collaborating physician. In states requiring a CPA, the CPA must comply with the state board of nursing and medical board's rules and administrative codes. Many agreements define the availability of the physician to the nurse practitioner, as well as details of the supervision, consultation, collaboration, referral, and evaluation of care provided by the nurse practitioner The CPA may further define the exact stipulations required of both the collaborating physician and the nurse practitioner. Some of the most important stipulations addressed are prescriptive authority, patient management guidelines, designation of the collaborating physician's responsibilities, the nature and scope of the nurse practitioner's practice regarding practice complexities, delineation of patients with complex comorbidities, and the exact stipulation of what services can be provided by an APNP within institutional policies and procedures (Trilla & Patterson, 1998). From a risk management perspective, the CPA is an effective tool protecting the working relationship between the nurse practitioner and the collaborating physician. Table 1 shows content that is appropriate to include in a collaborative practice agreement.

Nurse Practitioner Owned Practices

In reduced or restrictive practice states that require the nurse practitioner to practice in collaboration with a physician, APNPs can establish private practices and own their own clinical practice. In this scenario, the APNP establishes a collaborative agreement with a physician in accordance with state rules and regulations. The APNP maintains the scope of practice afforded by state board of nursing licensure and certification, as there are no federal laws or standards regarding APNP practices (Furlow, 2011a).

There are challenges with a nurse practitioner owned practice because the APNP may experience less autonomy than physicians in private practice. Issues such as obtaining hospital privileges, third party reimbursement, Medicare and Medicaid enrollment, and prescriptive authority vary from state to state (Furlow, 2011b). The APNP owned practice is responsible for liability and malpractice insurance, health insurance and employee salaries. If a collaborating physician severs the practice agreement for any reason, the APNP cannot continue to see patients until a new collaborating physician is legally in place.

Considerations for Appropriate Practice Site

The APNP who is organized and structured in the search process for the right type of practice site that is compatible with professional goals and values has a better chance of finding the right position (Barnes, 2007). Soelberg's outlines a four phase process in making a career choice. The process is:

1. Identification of the perfect job
2. Creating a strategy to attain the job
3. Initiation of the strategy
4. Making a decision regarding the choices

There are two steps within the four phases. Step one is search and step two is choice. Personal ambitions and goals influence both steps of the process (Power & Aldag, 1985). Screening and gathering of criteria important to a job seeker is the first step when seeking a position and while the second step is confirming or making a decision (Osborne, 1990).

In order to screen for the appropriate professional practice, it is important to determine what type of practice is most desirable. There are medical, businesses and legal practice issues that may differ when working in a physician run practice or organizationally owned practice versus a practice owned by the nurse practitioner.

Table 1. Sample template of a Collaborative agreement

Advanced Practitioner Information (licensure and certification data)
Collaborating Physician information (licensure and certification data)
Practice Site - details
Purpose of the agreement: In accordance with licensing state rules and regulation
Scope of Practice
Collaboration,Consultation & Referral
Prescriptive Authority
Coverage for emergency absences of either APNP or collaborating physician
Clinical Practice Evaluation Methodology
Signatures

The DNP Essentials

An APNP's need to be cognizant of the implications and impact they will have on practice decisions. The *Consensus Model* standardization to APNP scope of practice and the *Doctorate of Nursing Practice* will more readily prepare the APNP to deal with medical, legal and financial complexities of providing care to individuals or populations.

Considerations for the Choice of Practice: Using the DNP Essentials

The DNP Essentials outline curricular elements and competencies present in programs that confer the Doctor of Nursing Practice degree. The essentials are foundational to all advanced nursing practice roles. The DNP Essentials are used as a framework to provide an organized process to consider what type of a practice setting an APNP wants to consider. The eight foundational DNP Essentials provide a framework or template for the APNP to evaluate a practice setting and determine if that setting is a good fit for a practice site. The framework includes a description of the DNP Essential and its relationship to practice considerations (American Association of Colleges of Nursing (AACN), 2006). In comparing the educational focus of the masters prepared nurse practitioner to the DNP prepared APNP, the difference is in the focus of the MSN is on clinical diagnosis and treatment whereas the DNP graduate has a more focused and stronger background in outcomes assessment.

Even though, the *American Association of Colleges of Nurses (2006b)* recommended all nurses entering a nurse practitioner program should enter a DNP program, by the 2015, this recommendation has not been operationalized. This requirement provides the APNP with a more intense and expanded knowledge of the multifaceted integration of scientific, psychosocial science and business management theories. Dennison, Payne and Farrell (2012b) implied the DNP's knowledge of the integration of these theories prepares a DNP to have a firmer grasp on the strategies to make changes in her present practice setting, realize she has to make a change, or establish an independent practice.

Essential I: Scientific Underpinnings for Practice

Unique to every practice domain are the scientific underpinnings that provide a foundation for practice. The determinants outlined in *Essential I* identify and emphasize the need for APNP's to be well grounded in philosophical, scientific and organizational theories to deal with the multifarious challenges of nursing practice (American Association of Colleges of Nursing, 2006c). The consideration for a practice site is determined by the type of practice it is, whether it be a private practice that serves an insurance population where resources are plentiful and ability to pay for needed care is not an issue, or a community health based that serves underserved population. The challenges of providing care are different in each type of practice and the APNP should understand what is needed from a philosophical and organizational perspective to work in a specific practice.

Essential II: Organizational Systems Leadership for Quality Improvement and System Thinking

Essential II addresses the clinician's ability to be a leader in improving the quality of clinical care and clinical outcomes in practice settings. When considering a practice, the APNP should ask questions about what a practice does to evaluate clinical outcomes and improve them. The DNP should be able to address conceptual and practical strategies for balancing productivity with quality care. This includes strategies to promote optimal health and safety and steps to reduce healthcare gaps.

An APNP must be mindful that the Institute of Medicine directs all practices to have quality improvement structures in place to assess, improve and report healthcare outcomes (Institute of Medicine (US), 2011). It is important to consider that reimbursement from federal and state sources may be tied to these quality improvement systems (Farquhar, 2008).

Essential III: Clinical Scholarship and Analytical Methods for Evidence–Based Practice

A master's level APNP has the competencies to initiate evidence based practices within an organizational setting while the DNP nurse practitioner has the background and ability to lead practice initiatives, and manage and evaluate the process of dissemination into practice (Hamric, Spross & Hanson, 2009). The DNP has the knowledge delineated *in Essential III* to answer questions pertaining to the process of design, implementation and evaluation of evidence based practices to improve patient outcomes. Spector (2005) reported that DNP nurses using evidence based practices provide a pathway to deliver quality health that is efficient and cost effective, and allows nurses to be innovative and resourceful.

Essential IV: Information Systems/Technology and Patient Care Technology for the Improvement and Transformation of Health Care

An important precepts for the APNP to ascertain from *Essential IV* is the ability understand and apply budget and productivity tools, practice information systems and decisions supports, and web-based learning or intervention tools to support and improve patient care" (AACN, 2006d). Nursing informatics helps to improve and transform healthcare by enhancing work flow, supporting patient safety, and assisting health care providers to deliver enhanced care using the current evidence based practice guidelines (Shuler, 2011). When considering a practice site, the APNP may evaluate the type of information technology that a practice has in place. It is important to consider what type of electronic health care system is in place. Essential IV gives a framework for understanding that the information systems and technology at a practice is essential in supporting the provision and monitoring of care and healthcare outcomes, handling administrative functions, and aid in the delivery of educational material and support research (Staggers & Thompson, 2002).

Essential V: Health Care Policy for Advocacy

Ward stated (2011) that the advocacy determinants of *Essential V* enable the DNP to recognize key political issues affecting vulnerable populations, and be a agent to initiate social justice reforms at all levels of government. The *Essential V* competencies enable the DNP to translate health care policy into practice (Cronenwett, Dracup, Grey, McCauley, Meleis, & Salmon, 2011). When considering a practice setting, a site usually has an underlying value that dictates the population served. An ACNP may want to provide care to vulnerable populations or practice with a less vulnerable and insured group of patients. As such, it is important to evaluate what the mission of a site is, and how that mission translates into the provision of care for specific types of populations.

Essential VI: Inter Professional Collaboration for Improving Patient and Population Health Outcomes

In the article *Doctorate of Nursing Practice: Blueprint for Excellence,* Sperhac and Clinton (2008a) affirmed the American Association of Colleges of Nursing program of study for the DNP. A key concept the authors implied was that a DNP graduate has been mentored in the theories and strategies needed to work inter professionally to better patient and population outcomes. This mentoring with leaders in business, policy and healthcare reform and clinical practice allows the DNP student to be exposed to a plethora of knowledge needed to resolve complex healthcare problems. DNP's collaborating and communicating with professionals outside the realm of nursing can critique and evaluate the various facets of healthcare needed to improve patient and population outcomes. They are equipped not only to improve mortality and morbidity but also quality of life measures (Magyary, Whitney and Brown, 2006).

Essential VII: Clinical Prevention and Population Health for Improving the Nation's Health

The competencies outlined in Essential VII enable the DNP to first identify gaps in the health care system and address them by determining ways to improve access to health care and initiate preventive models of care. Evaluating a practice's commitment to addressing prevention of disease in a patient population can be an important consideration Preventive care is an important aspect of on is a for it is important for the DNP to recognize that she can be a leader in changing the healthcare system to improve the nation's health (Chism, 2009).

Essential VIII: Advanced Nursing Practice for Improving the Delivery of Patient Care

To err is human: Building a safer health system and *Crossing the quality chasm: a new health system for the 21st century* sent a message to healthcare providers that changes need to be made to meet future healthcare needs (Institute of Medicine (US), 2001). The AACN responded to this message by proposing the entry level for advanced nursing to be the DNP. As DNP's are now graduating and are beginning to make their presence known, they need to be cognizant that the roles they are assuming have implications for future DNP graduates. As a result, DNP's become leaders of change in the health care system. They need to provide evidence that their competencies and leadership are needed and valued and do reflect a positive change for the health care system.

Career Considerations: Evaluation of Practice Site Options

There are a number of questions the APNP should consider when evaluating a potential practice site or career opportunity. Table 2 provides questions to consider when evaluating a potential practice site or career opportunity.

Table 2. Questions to ask when evaluating a practice site or setting

Organizational Mission	• Does the mission statement of the practice reflect sound principles? • Does the mission statement reflect my personal goals and values?
Knowledge Base	• Do I have the theoretical knowledge and clinical skills needed for this practice? • How will this practice enhance my get more experience?
Quality Care/Patient Outcomes	• What is the current approach in the practice to improving patient outcomes? • How does this practice setting balance productivity with quality care?
Evidence based Practice	• In what ways does this practice support the implementation of evidence based practice? • What are the opportunities to ensure that evidence based protocols meet state and federal rules and regulations?
Informatics	• What does the practice offer regarding information technology to support clinical practice and delivery of care? • What are the strengths and weaknesses of the informatics systems in place? • In what ways does the practice informatics enhance patient flow from patient scheduling to monitoring outcomes or effectiveness of care?
Health care policy for advocacy	• Does this practice support participation in healthcare policy reform at the state or federal level?
Health care initiatives	• Does the practice support a formal role to develop programs and care initiatives for diverse populations? • What initiatives has the practice implemented to improve outcomes and patient care? • What preventive models of care are in place in the practice? • How will my role at this practice promote positive change?

Conclusion

This chapter provided an overview of the types of practice environment that individual states support for advanced practice nurse practitioners. It explained the practice options of collaborative and independent practice and implications of how APNPs work in each type of practice. Collaborative practice agreements were discussed in the context of what the essential components are for the agreement. The DNP Essentials provide a framework to determine what type of a practice setting an APNP wants to consider. The framework helps the APNPs create a well- organized plan of the pro and cons of each setting and in turn make a wise career choice.

References

AACN. (2004). AACN position statement on the practice doctorate in nursing. American Association of Colleges of Nursing [On-line]. Available: http://www.aacn.nche.edu/publications/position/DAPNPpositionstatement.pdf

AACN. (2004b). AACN position statement on the practice doctorate in nursing. American Association of Colleges of Nursing [On-line]. Available: http://www.aacn.nche.edu/publications/position/DAPNPpositionstatement.pdf

AACN. (2014a). DNP Fact Sheet: The Doctor of Nursing Practice (DNP). American Association of Colleges of Nursing [On-line]. Available: http://www.aacn.nche.edu/media-relations/fact-sheets/dAPNP

AACN. (2014b). DNP Fact Sheet: The Doctor of Nursing Practice (DNP). American Association of Colleges of Nursing [On-line]. Available: http://www.aacn.nche.edu/media-relations/fact-sheets/dAPNP

AANP. (2013a). State Practice Environment. American Association of Nurse Practitioners [On-line]. Available: https://www.aaAPNP.org/legislation-regulation/state-legislation-regulation/state-practice-environment

AANP. (2013b). State Practice Environment. American Association of Nurse Practitioners [On-line]. Available: https://www.aaAPNP.org/legislation-regulation/state-legislation-regulation/state-practice-environment

AANP. (2013c). State Practice Environment. American Association of Nurse Practitioners [On-line]. Available: https://www.aaAPNP.org/legislation-regulation/state-legislation-regulation/state-practice-environment

AANP Consensus Work Group, (2008). *Consensus model for AANP regulation: Licensure, accreditation, certification & education.*

American Association of Colleges of Nursing. (AACN). (2006). *The Essentials of Doctoral Education for Advanced Nursing Practice.* Retrieved. December 17, 2013 from http://www.aacn.nche.edu/DAPNP/pdf/Essentials.pdf.

APRN Joint Dialogue Group Report. (2008). *Consensus Model for APNP Regulation: Licensure, Accreditation, Certification & Education* APNP Joint Dialogue Group Report.

Barnes, S. (2007) On the market: strategies for a successful academic job search.

Bridges, S. (2013) Exploration of the concept of collaboration within the context of nurse practitioner-physician collaborative practice. *Journal of the American Association of Nurse Practitioners. 00*, 1-9.

Brown, M. A. & Crabtree, K. (2013). The development of practice scholarship in DNP programs: a paradigm shift. *Journal of Professional Nursing*, *29*, 330-337.

Buyens, D., De Witte, K. & Martens, G. (2001). Building a conceptual framework on the exploratory job search. www.feb.ugent.be/nl/Ondz/wp/Papers/wp_01_108.pdf

Chism, L. A. (2009a). *The doctor of nursing practice: a guidebook for role development and professional issue*. Sudbury, MA: Jones and Bartlett.

Chism, L. A. (2009b). Toward clarification of the doctor of nursing practice degree. *Advanced Emergency Nursing Journal*, *31*, 287-297.

Cronenwett, L. Dracup, K., Grey, M., McCauley, L., Meleis, A. & Salmon, M. (2011). The doctor of nursing practice: a national workforce perspective. *Nursing Outlook*, *59*, 9-17.

Dennison, R., Payne, C. & Farrell, K. (2012). The doctorate in nursing practice: moving advanced practice nursing even closer to excellence. *Nursing Clinic of North American*, *47*, 225-240.

Farquhar, M. (2008). AHRQ Quality Indicators. In Hughes RG (Ed.), *Patient Safety and Quality: An Evidence-Based Handbook for Nurses* (Rockville (MD): Agency for Healthcare Research and Quality (US).

Furlow, B. (2011). Business advice for nurse practitioners considering private practice. Clinical Advisor [On-line]. Available: http://www.clinicaladvisor.com/business-advice-for-nurse-practitioners-considering-private-practice/article/203953/

Furlow, B. (2011b). Business advice for nurse practitioners considering private practice. Clinical Advisor [On-line]. Available: http://www.clinicaladvisor.com/business-advice-for-nurse-practitioners-considering-private-practice/article/203953/

Glasgow, M. & Donnelly, G. (2011) A new level of advocacy for nurses in the doctoral advance nursing practice role. In. H.M. Dreher & M.Smith Glasgow, *Role development for doctoral advanced nursing practice*, (231-241). New York, NY: Springer Publishing.

Hamric, A., Spross, J. & Hanson, C. (2009). Advanced practice nursing an integrative approach (4th ed). St. Louis: Saunders Elsevier.

Institute of Medicine (US). (2011). *The future of nursing: Leading change, advancing health.* National Academies Press

Magyary, D., Whitney, J. & Brown, M. (2006a). Advancing practice inquiry: research foundations of the practice doctorate in nursing. *Nursing Outlook*, *54*, 139-151.

Montgomery, K. & Byrne, S. (2011). A new level of advocacy for nurses in the doctoral advance nursing practice role. In. H.M. Dreher & M. Smith Glasgow, *Role development for doctoral advanced nursing practice*, (99-113). New York, NY: Springer Publishing.

Osborne, D. (1990). A reexamination of the organization choice process. *Journal of Vocational Behavior*, *36*, 45-60.

Power, D. & Aldag, R. (1985). Soelberg's job search and choice model: a clarification, review, and critique. *Academy of Management Review*, *10*(1), 48-58.

Rounds, L. R., Zych, J. J. & Mallary, L. L. (2013). The consensus model for regulation of APRNs: Implications for nurse practitioners. Journal of the American Academy of Nurse Practitioners, 25: 180–185. doi: 10.1111/j.1745-7599.2013.00812.x

Shuler, G. (2011) Role of nursing informatics for leadership. Retrieved January 15, 2014 from http: //nursing.advancwe.com/Columns/Nursing-Informatics/Role-Nursing-Informatics

Snyder, M. (2014). Emancipatory knowing: empowering nursing students toward reflection and action. *Journal of Nursing Education*, *53*, DOI: 10.3928/01484834-20140107-01

Spector, N. (2005) Evidence-based health care in nursing regulation. https://www.ncsbn.org/Evidence_based_HC_Nsg_Regulation_updated_5.

Sperhac, A. & Clinton. P. (2008). Doctorate of nursing practice: blueprint for excellence. *Journal of Pediatic Health Care*, *22*(3), 146-151.

Sperhac, A. & Clinton. P. (2008). Doctorate of nursing practice: blueprint for excellence. *Journal of Pediatic Health Care*, *22*(3), 146-151

Stagger, N. & Thompson, C. (2002). The evolution of definitions for nursing informatics: a critical analysis and revised definition. *Journal of the American Medical Informatics*, *9*, 255-261.

Stanley, J. M., Werner, K. E. & Apple, K. (2009). Positioning advanced practice registered nurses for health care reform: Consensus on APRN regulation. *Journal of Professional Nursing*, *25*(6), 340-348.

Trilla, F. & Patterson, A. (1998). Physicians and nurse practitioners in collaborative practice. In.

Vestal, C. (2013). Nurse Practitioners Slowly Gain Autonomy. Kaiser Health News [On-line]. Available: http://www.kaiserhealthnews.org/stories/2013/july/19/stateline-nurse-practitioners- scope-of-practice.aspx

Ward, L. (2011). A new level of advocacy for nurses in the doctoral advance nursing practice role. In. H.M. Dreher & M. Smith Glasgow, *Role development for doctoral advanced nursing practice*, (357-367). New York, NY: Springer Publishing

In: Collaboration with the Advanced Practice Nurse ISBN: 978-1-63321-311-1
Editors: E.R. Giardino, R.G. Hanks and A.P. Giardino

Chapter 14

LOOKING TOWARD THE FUTURE: WORK FORCE PROJECTIONS AND HEALTH CARE REFORM

Eileen R. Giardino[1], PhD, RN, APRN and Angelo P. Giardino[2], MD, PhD
[1]The University of Texas Health Science Center School of Nursing at Houston
[2]Baylor College of Medicine, Texas Children's Health Plan, Texas Children's Hospital, US

ABSTRACT

Advanced practice registered nurses (APRNs) are positioned to play a major role in the health care delivery in the 21st century. The numbers of certified nurse practitioners (CNP), certified registered nurse anesthetists (CRNA), certified nurse-midwifes (CNM), and clinical nurse specialists (CNS) are increasing and are able to help to meet the demands for medical care services (APRN Consensus Work Group & National Council of State Boards of Nursing APRN Advisory Committee, 2008). With the changes that are expected to take place as a result of the Affordable Care Act, APRNs are there to provide the services across the lifespan and across acuity needs from primary to acute care. This chapter discusses current workforce projections for physicians and advanced practice nurses based on authoritative reports from the Health Resources and Services Administration (HRSA) and a brief description of the ACA reforms that will likely impact work force projects and especially the roles and responsibilities for advanced practice nurses. Advanced practice nurses who provide care for the full range of patient populations and across all care settings have proven their value and ability to meet the growing need for health care providers in acute and primary care areas (Institute of Medicine (IOM), 2011). There is discussion about key projection models that forecast work force needs and what the future might hold in terms of workforce projections.

INTRODUCTION

There is a growing need for competent and knowledgeable health care providers to meet the health care needs of the growing number of people who have received access to care due to the recent health care reform efforts. In 2012, the Center for Workforce Studies (Association of American Medical Colleges, 2012) at the Association of American Medical Colleges (AAMC) summarized 33 state reports of physician shortages, 22 reports of specialty practice shortages and 6 national studies on physician workforce issues. An August of 2013, US Government Accountability Office (GAO) report to Congress stated that "a well-trained and diverse health care workforce is essential for providing Americans with access to quality health care services." (GAO, August, 2013, pg 1). Another GAO report, issued in September of 2013 described that governmental, academic and health professions' organizations have been projecting national shortages for physicians, nurse practitioners and physician assistants (GAO, September 2013). Both lay and professional groups have raised concerns that the shortages of key health care professionals, particularly physicians and nurse practitioners, could jeopardize the nation's ability to meet the primary and specialty patient care needs of the US population. In January of 2014, Dr. Danielle Ofri writing for the New York Times wrote that patients and health care systems are facing challenges related to the mal-distribution of medical services which routinely leads to long wait times for patients and families seeking care.

In 2010, the Robert Wood Johnson Foundation (RWJF) and the Institute of Medicine (IOM) wrote the report entitled *The Future of Nursing: Leading Change, Advancing Health* that addressed the health care work force projections from the perspective of what registered nurses and advance practice registered nurses (APRNs) could contribute both at and as advanced practice nurses who can practice across the full range of care settings and patient populations (Institute of Medicine [IOM], 2011). The Future of Nursing report recommends that nurses practice to the fullest extent of their education and roles to provide health care services and improve patient care outcomes. The nursing profession and advance practice nurses can help to close the projected gaps for primary and specialty care health services in the future (Institute of Medicine [IOM], 2011).

The 2010 passing of the Patient Protection and Affordable Care Act (PPACA) or more simply stated as the Affordable Care Act (ACA) by the US Congress set in motion sweeping reforms for the health care system in the US. The ACA envisioned a number of health care reforms geared to enable US residents to obtain insurance coverage with a goal of near universal coverage. These reforms focus on providing preventive care to decrease disease, changes in reimbursement, and improvement in the quality of care delivery. The ACA directed reforms are intended to promote massive structure and process changes in the US health care system that will have potentially large impacts on the health care professions that provide that care, and on the patients who receive the care. The ACA aims to substantially strengthen the provision of primary care to a large number of people who were without access to health care while stressing the need to bring down the cost of health care coverage (as Enacted, 2010) (Institute of Medicine (IOM), 2011). To that end, advanced practice nurses have a number of opportunities to be a part of the coverage of the new and larger number of people who can now access the health care system. Initiatives and programs that involve advanced practice nurses can be developed to meet the demand for health care providers and can bridge the gap between insurance coverage and access to care.

WORK FORCE PROJECTIONS

Background

To determine if there is currently an adequate work force and to project if the supply is adequate to meet future national needs a number of factors must be considered. These factors are complex and despite dire predictions on the one hand that project shortages, other analyses temper these projections with information about increased provider productivity and use of technology which serve to mitigate the potential short fall (GAO, Sept 2013). Predicting the future is difficult, so robust forecasting methodologies are called for.

Workforce projections in health care tend to measure both 1) the supply of the needed health care professionals and 2) the demand for their services in a given period of time typically a "base year". The projections then predict how the supply and demand is likely to change in the future as expected changes come into play. In the parlance of workforce projects, the supply aspect of the equation uses "stock and flow" models, and for the demand aspect, a utilization-based model is employed (GAO, September, 2013). The stock and flow models typically begin with the current number of health care professionals, add new entrants to the workforce, and then subtract providers who will likely leave the workforce, e.g. those who retire, are disable or who die. See Figure 1 for projecting primary care physician supply.

A number of factors affect the supply of health care providers such as physicians, nurse practitioners and physician assistants, and include the ability of educational programs to train new health care professionals, and expected attrition rates from the training programs and the profession itself. Utilization models measure current utilization rates for health care services as well as projected patterns of future utilization factoring in adjustments expected to occur because practice patterns change over time. These projection efforts are complex and factors that may affect demand include economic conditions, population growth, and applicable demographic changes such as an aging population or increases or decreases in a population's insurance coverage (GAO, September 2013). Among the most important reports that inform this work force projection discussion are two from the federal government, one undertaken and released prior to the ACA and the other after the ACA passage. These will be discussed below in that order.

Projections Pre-ACA: 2008 HRSA Report

The Health Resources and Services Administration (HRSA) (GAO, September 2013) is the Federal agency with responsibility for the monitoring of both the supply of and demand for health care professionals and HRSA is expected to disseminate workforce projects to inform policymakers and the public. To be clear, another Federal agency, the Bureau of Labor Statistics within the Department of Labor also produces national 10-year projections for particular occupations. These Bureau of Labor projections are different from HRSA's in a material way in that they count the number of jobs rather than the number of people and are not dynamic in that they do not assess demand for the services so they do not project if there will be a shortage or surplus. HRSA issued a 2008 a workforce report containing national supply and demand projections for physicians from 18 medical specialties. Surprisingly physician's assistants and advanced practice nurses projects are absent in this report. Table 1 lists the key finding and associated details for the HRSA 2008 workforce report.

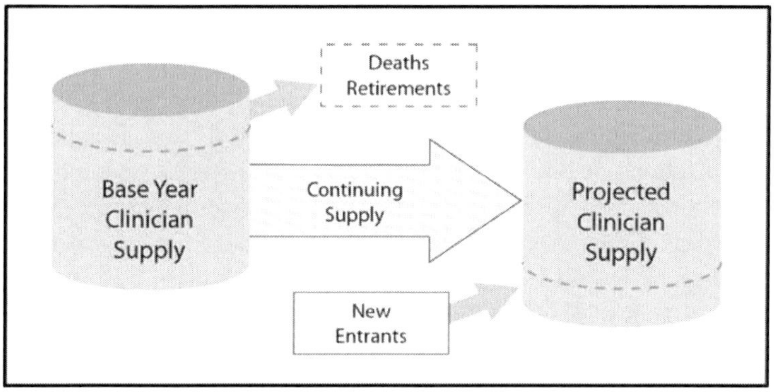

U.S. Department of Health and Human Services, Health Resources and Services Administration, National Center for Health Workforce Analysis. (2013) Projecting the Supply and Demand for Primary Care Practitioners Through 2020. Rockville, Maryland: U.S. Department of Health and Human Services. http://bhpr.hrsa.gov/healthworkforce/supplydemand/usworkforce/primarycare/

Figure 1. Projecting Primary Care Provider Supply.

Table 1. HRSA 2008 Workforce Report: Key Finding and Associated Details

Key finding	Associated details
The baseline projections assume that over the next 1 to 2 decades factors affecting physician supply, health care utilization patterns, and health care delivery patterns will continue largely unchanged	• Physician supply will increase from current levels of approximately 817,000 active physicians under age 75 in 2005 to approximately 952,000 active physicians by 2020. The increasing proportion of physicians who are women and are older, and who typically work fewer hours per year compared to their younger male colleagues, suggests that total hours of physician services provided is increasing less rapidly than the number of licensed physicians (13 percent versus 16 percent between 2005 and 2020).The growth and aging of the population will contribute to a 22 percent increase in demand for physician services between 2005 and 2020. Growth in demand will be highest among specialties that predominantly serve the elderly (e.g., cardiology, internal medicine, and most surgical specialties).Growing public expectations and the ability to pay for higher levels of care through economic growth could increase demand substantially above the baseline projections. Factors that may offset the growth in demand for physicians include improvements in physician productivity such that each physician can care for a larger population, scientific advances that can contribute to improved health, and increased use of non-physician clinicians.

U.S. Department of Heath and Human Services, Health Resources and Services Administration. (December 2008) The Physician Workforce: Projections and Research into Current Issues Affecting Supply and Demand. Health Resources and Services Administration. http://bhpr.hrsa.gov/healthworkforce/reports/physwfissues.pdf.

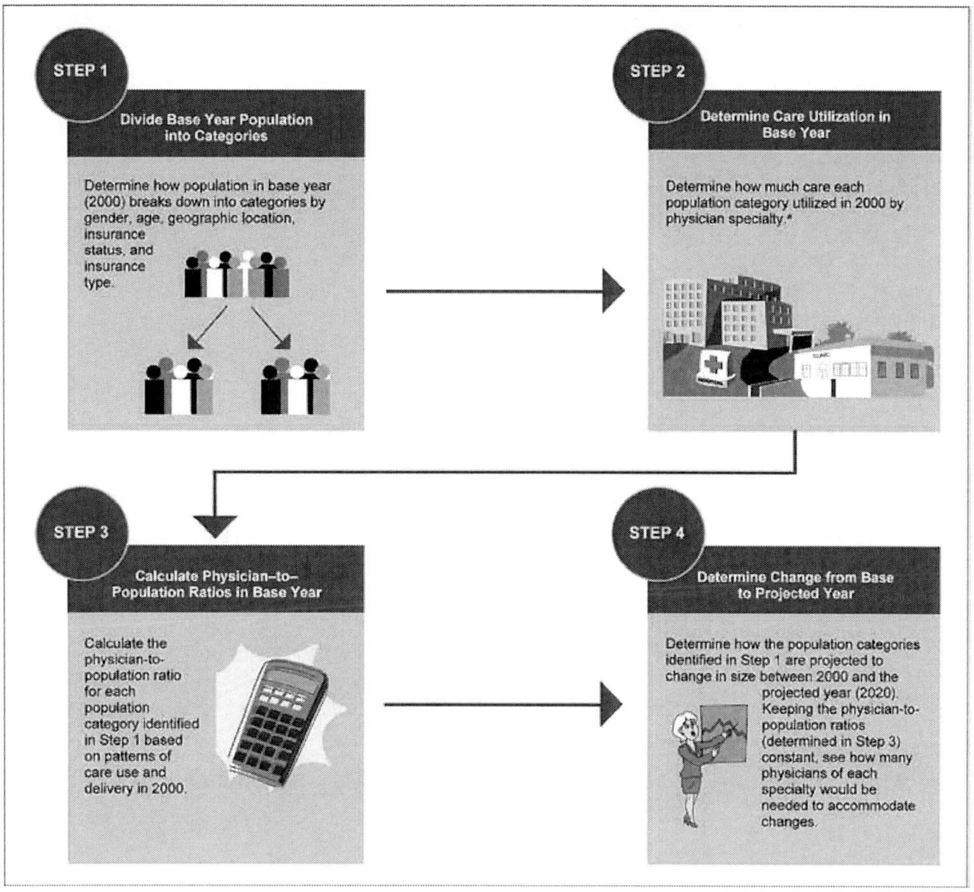

Sources: GAO analysis of HRSA information; Art Explosion (images).

[a]HRSA examined health care utilization patterns by population category using national survey data from 1999 to 2001.

U. S. Government Accountability Office (GAO). (September 2013). Health Care Workforce. HRSA Action Needed to Publish Timely National Supply and Demand Projections. (GAO-13-806). http://www.gao.gov/products/GAO-13-806.

Figure 2. Process for Determining Physician Requirements in the HRSA 2008 Report Based on its Physician Requirements Model.

The 2008 HRSA report used a work force model using the Physician Supply Model (PSM) and Physician Requirements Model (PRM). The PSM was a stock and flow model and as such took the number of physicians in the base year, 2000, added expected new entrants and subtracted the number of physicians leaving practice from retirement, disability and death. The effective number of full time equivalent (FTE) physicians used the average number of hours worked for physicians in each specialty by age and gender. The PRM model was used to determine demand and is a utilization-based approach to project future physician requirements using current use patterns of physician services and expected trends in U.S. demographics, insurance coverage, and patterns of care delivery. These use patterns are expressed as physician-to-population ratios for each specialty and population segment defined by age, sex, metropolitan/non-metropolitan location, and insurance type. Figure 2 shows how the GAO has pictorially described the steps that were used to construct the workforce projections by HRSA in 2008.

Table 2. HRSA 2013 Workforce Report: Key Findings and Associated Details

Key Findings	Associated details
Demand for primary care services is projected to grow, mostly due to population aging and growth.	• Aging and population growth are projected to account for 81 percent of the change in demand between 2010 and 2020. • The remainder of the projected change in demand is associated with the estimated expansion of health insurance coverage under full implementation of the Affordable Care Act, including an assumption that all states expand Medicaid.
Based on current utilization patterns, demand for primary care physicians is projected to grow more rapidly than physician supply.	• The number of primary care physicians is projected to increase from 205,000 FTEs in 2010 to 220,800 FTEs in 2020, an 8-percent increase. • The total demand for primary care physicians is projected to grow by 28,700, from 212,500 FTEs in 2010 to 241,200 FTEs in 2020, a 14-percent increase. • Without changes to how primary care is delivered, the growth in primary care physician supply will not be adequate to meet demand in 2020, with a projected shortage of 20,400 physicians. While this deficit is not as large as has been found in prior studies, the projected shortage of primary care physicians is still significant.
The primary care NP and PA workforces are projected to grow far more rapidly than the physician supply.	• The supply of primary care NPs is projected to increase by 30 percent, from 55,400 in 2010 to 72,100 in 2020. The supply of primary care PAs is projected to increase by 58 percent, from 27,700 to 43,900 over the same period. • Assuming that NPs and PAs provide the same proportion of services in 2020 that they did in 2010, the combined demand for NPs and PAs would increase by only 17 percent. If NPs and PAs are used to provide a greater proportion of primary care services, their projected demand will be higher.
Increased use of NPs and PAs could somewhat alleviate the projected primary care physician shortage if they are effectively integrated into the health care delivery system.	• Under a scenario in which the rapidly growing NP and PA supply can effectively be integrated, the shortage of 20,400 physicians in 2020 could be reduced to 6,400 PCPs.[1] • If fully utilized, the percent of primary care services provided by NPs and PAs will grow from 23 percent in 2010 to 28 percent in 2020. Physicians would remain the dominant providers of primary care, only decreasing from 77 percent of the primary care services in 2010 to 72 percent in 2020.

U.S. Department of Health and Human Services, Health Resources and Services Administration, National Center for Health Workforce Analysis. (2013) Projecting the Supply and Demand for Primary Care Practitioners Through 2020. Rockville, Maryland: U.S. Department of Health and Human Services. http://bhpr.hrsa.gov/healthworkforce/supplydemand/usworkforce/primarycare/

Based on this work force model, HRSA in 2008 projected a shortfall of approximately 49,000 FTE physicians by 2020. This number includes both primary care and specialty care physicians. The 2008 projections from HRSA need to be updated as a result of actual practice pattern changes that have occurred from 2000 to now in 2014, and also to account for the expected changes emanating from the evolving health care landscape, due to the implementation of the ACA as well. The Congressional Budget Office for example estimated that the ACA would likely extend health insurance coverage to an additional 25 million uninsured individuals beginning in 2014. In November 2013, HRSA issued its long awaited report on the supply and demand for primary care practitioners projected through 2020. This updated report limited itself to primary care.

PROJECTIONS POST ACA: 2013 HRSA REPORT

In response to a growing demand for updated health care professional workforce forecasting data, HRSA, in November 2013, released a study that examined the adequacy of primary care practitioners (PCPs). This study was more inclusive of health care professionals trained and able to deliver primary care than was the 2008 HRSA report, it used 2010 as its base year and it projected supply and demand in 2020 for physicians, nurse practitioners (NPs), and physician assistants (PAs). An effort was made to build as robust a model as possible so demand was adjusted for PCP shortages in Health Professional Shortage Areas and assumptions were made around utilization trends, practice patterns, and productivity. Since this report is viewed as an authoritative source for important future discussions and policy initiatives its key findings are listed below:

The supply calculation for the physicians, nurse practitioners and physician assistants who could be counted on to deliver primary care was straightforward and used the stock and flow approach described above. The supply of clinically active nurse practitioners was estimated using data from the 2008 National Sample Survey of Registered Nurses and then projecting forward to the expectation for the base year in 2010. Using this approach, it is estimated that there were approximately a total of 110,800 clinically active nurse practitioners in 2010, with half of these, or 55,400, practicing primary care. The numbers of nurse practitioners graduating at the Master's and post-Master's levels are expected to increase as well. Figure 3 shows the increase from 2002 thru 2012 going from 6,979 to 14,409. The total supply of nurse practitioners delivering primary care is projected to increase by 30 percent going from 55,400 in 2010 to 72, 100 in 2020 resulting in an increase of 16,700 PCPs.

The supply of clinically active physician's assistants was estimated using data from the 2008 American Academy of Physician Assistants Census and then projecting forward to the expectation for the base year in 2010. Using this approach it is estimated that there were approximately 84,000 clinically active physician assistants in 2010 and about a third of these, or 27,700, who practiced primary care. Numbers of physician assistants graduating from 2010 to 2020 is expected to increase as well going from 6,000 to 8,800 and approximately one-third of physician assistants are anticipated to practice in the primary care arena. In the report, an effort was made to determine the practitioner-to-population ratio for full time equivalent (FTE) practitioners per 100,000 persons in different age groups. Nurse practitioners in this analysis have large connections to populations at both extremes of the age continuum with 35 FTE's per 100,000 people 0-5 years of age and 35 and 28 FTE's per 100,000 respectively for people 65 to 74 and above 75 years of age respectively. See figure 4 for comparison of physician primary specialties, nurse practitioners and physician assistants FTEs per 100,000 persons within each age group.

While the 2013 HRSA primary care workforce report did not address the other types of advance practice nurses, namely clinical specialists, certified nurse anesthetists and nurse midwives, a different report on the nurse workforce issued in April of 2013 did provide some information on the increase in numbers of nurse anesthetists and nurse midwives comparing the growth in these professions from 2001 to 2011 (US Department of Health and Human Services, April 2013). Figure 5a and 5b present that information for completeness. Unfortunately, projections for these other types of advanced practice nursing were not provided as they were for primary care.

The 2013 HRSA report incorporated a number of factors as it moved beyond PCP supply and worked to estimate the demand for primary care services. The report describes population needs, economic factors around cost and price, technological innovations, system induced demands as well as public perceptions and expectations. Based on the structure of the model being used, the demand for nurse practitioners available for primary care in 2010 was set as the supply number available that year, namely 55,400 and the same for the demand for physician assistants available for primary care in 2010 was set as the supply, namely 27,700. In contrast, using physician short fall data from Health Professional Shortage Areas (U.S. Department of Health and Human Services, 2013), it was estimated that in 2010, 205,000 primary care physicians were available but the demand was for 212,500 physicians in primary care in 2010 leading to a shortfall in primary care physicians of 7,500 in that base year.

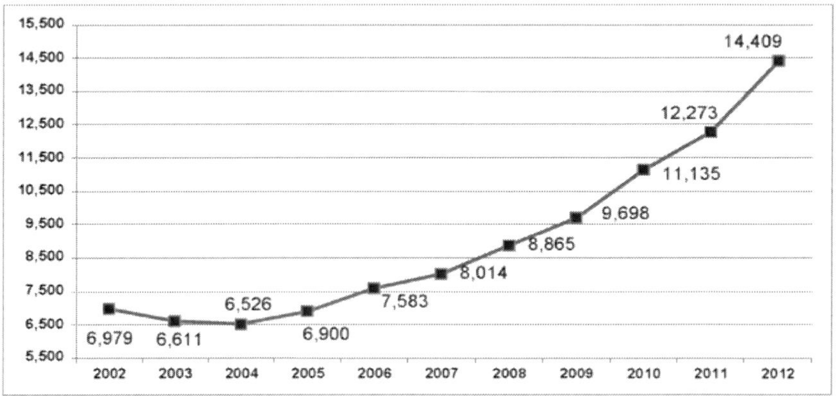

Data Source: HRSA compilation of data from the AACN Annual Survey (in collaboration with the National Organization of Nurse Practitioner Faculties for collection of nurse practitioner data). Note: Counts include master's and post-master's degree NP and NP/clinical nurse specialist graduates as well as bachelor's-to-doctorate of nursing practice graduates.

U.S. Department of Health and Human Services, Health Resources and Services Administration, National Center for Health Workforce Analysis. (2013) Projecting the Supply and Demand for Primary Care Practitioners Through 2020. Rockville, Maryland: U.S. Department of Health and Human Services. http://bhpr.hrsa.gov/healthworkforce/supplydemand/usworkforce/primarycare/

Figure 3. Annual number of Graduates from NP Programs: Master's and Post-Master's Graduates, 2002 through 2012.

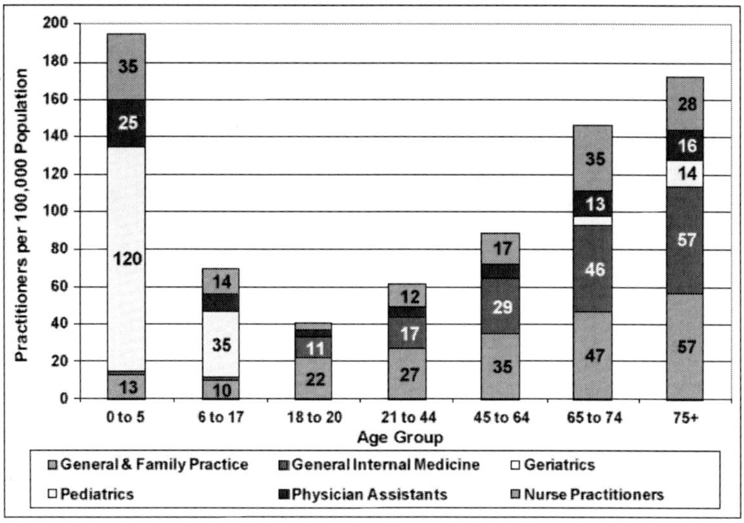

Data Source: Analysis of the multiple sources of data outlined in this report on patient utilization by setting (e.g., the NAMCS, NHAMCS, and NIS) and those on physician time allocation across settings of care.

U.S. Department of Health and Human Services, Health Resources and Services Administration, National Center for Health Workforce Analysis. (2013) Projecting the Supply and Demand for Primary Care Practitioners Through 2020. Rockville, Maryland: U.S. Department of Health and Human Services. http://bhpr.hrsa.gov/healthworkforce/supplydemand/usworkforce/primarycare/

Figure 4. Estimated Use of PCPs (FTEs) per 100,000 Persons Within Each Age Group, 2012.

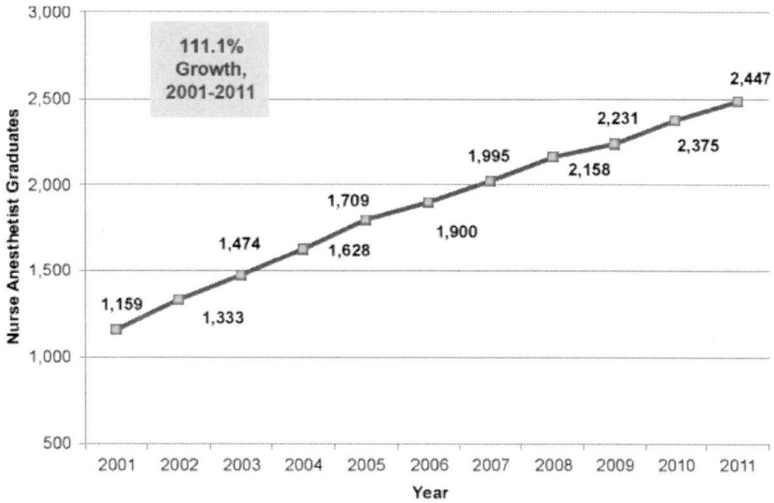

Data Source: National Board of Certification and Recertification for Nurse Anesthetists

Figure 5a. Nurse Anesthetist Graduates, 2001-2011.

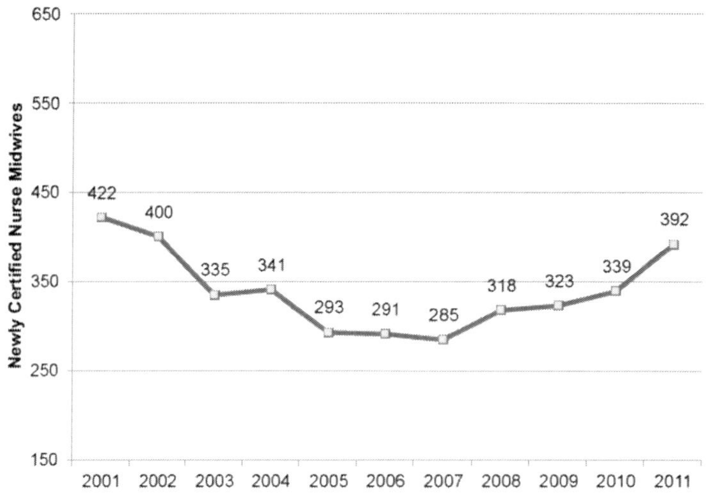

Data Source: HRSA compilation of data from the AMCB, 2010 and 2011 Annual Reports

U.S. Department of Health and Human Services, Health Resources and Services Administration, Bureau of Health Professionals, National Center for Health Workforce Analysis. (April 2013) The U.S. Nursing workforce: Trends in Supply and Education. Rockville, Maryland: U.S. Department of Health and Human Services. http://bhpr.hrsa.gov/healthworkforce/reports/nursingworkforce/nursingworkforcefullreport.pdf.

Figure 5b. Newly Certified Nurse Midwives, 2001-2011.

Four drivers were identified to project forward for future demand of primary care providers. The drivers are the growth of the population overall, the growth of the aging population specifically, changes in health insurance landscape, and, finally, disease risk factors particularly around rising obesity rates in the population. The majority of the increased PCP demands, or 81%, of the increased demand is projected to arise from the growth in the population, to aging of the population and to disease risk factors, and the remaining 19% increase in demand is attributable to the full implementation of the ACA.

Finally, the 2013 HRSA report provides projections for adequacy of the PCP work force for 2020. Looking at physician supply, the report finds that between 2010 and 2020 the total supply of primary care physicians grows more slowly than needed to meet the projected needs and as such, there will be a shortage of 20,400 primary care physicians. On the other hand, the supply of nurse practitioners and physician assistants will grow faster. Assuming that nurse practitioners and physician assistants provide the same proportion of services in 2020 that they did in 2010, the combined demand for them would increase by 17 %. The projected 17% could be higher if nurse practitioners and physician assistants provide a greater share of primary care services in the future which would make their effective demand even higher.

Table 3 below lists the supply and demand statistics for physicians and Table 4 does so for nurse practitioners and physician assistants for 2010 and 2020.

Finally, the 2013 HRSA report concludes with the observation that physicians will continue to be the dominant primary care provider in 2020, and recognizes that nurse practitioners and physician assistants can make a significant contribution to meeting the anticipated PCP demands expected in 2020. Using historic productivity weightings for nurse practitioners and physicians assistants relative to primary care physicians, a scenario emerges where the shortage of 20,400 primary care physicians could be reduced to 6,400 PCPs, with physicians going from providing 77% of primary care services in 2010 to 72% in 2020 and nurse practitioners and physician assistants growing from providing 23% of primary care in 2010 to 28% in 2020.

Table 3. Projected Demand for Primary Care Physicians.

	2010	2020
Total primary care physician demand (FTE)	212,500[a]	241,200[c]
General[b]	164,400	187,300
Pediatrics	44,800	49,600
Geriatrics	3,300	4,300
Primary care physician supply	205,000	220,800
Supply and demand	(7,500)	(20,400)

[a] National demand projections presented in this report assume that in 2010 the national supply of primary care physicians was adequate except for the approximately 7,500 FTEs needed to de-designate the primary care HPSAs.

[b] This category includes general and family practice, and general internal medicine.

[c] Assumes all states expand Medicaid.

U.S. Department of Health and Human Services, Health Resources and Services Administration, National Center for Health Workforce Analysis. (2013) Projecting the Supply and Demand for Primary Care Practitioners Through 2020. Rockville, Maryland: U.S. Department of Health and Human Services. http://bhpr.hrsa.gov/healthworkforce/supplydemand/usworkforce/primarycare/

If NPs and PAs provide a greater share of primary care services, their effective demand would be higher.

Table 4. Projected Supply and Demand for Primary Care NPs and PAs

Provider Type/Specialty	2010	2020
Supply		
Nurse Practitioners	55,400	72,100
Physician Assistants	27,700	43,900
Demand		
Nurse Practitioners	55,400	64,700
Physician Assistants	27,700	32,700
Supply and Demand		
Nurse Practitioners	*	7,400
Physician Assistants	*	11,200

*There were no data available for estimating if there were base year shortages of NPs and PAs. Note: Counts of NPs and PAs are not adjusted for productivity.

U.S. Department of Health and Human Services, Health Resources and Services Administration, National Center for Health Workforce Analysis. (2013) Projecting the Supply and Demand for Primary Care Practitioners Through 2020. Rockville, Maryland: U.S. Department of Health and Human Services. http://bhpr.hrsa.gov/healthworkforce/supplydemand/usworkforce/primarycare/

As with any complex analysis, one must recognize the limitations of these projections. The projections could be significantly modified if team-based models of care become more efficient, or if technology permits additional provider productivity, but, they are stating point and clearly show how advanced practice nursing, in almost any scenario, is part of an overall and comprehensive solution to the balancing of the supply and demand for health care services in the USA. The report specifically calls attention to the study by Dill and colleagues (2013) which found strong acceptance of care by nurse practitioners and physician assistants especially by those patients who had prior direct experience with them. Thus, the projections above are likely to be met and surpassed in terms of advanced practice nurses providing health care services to increasing numbers of patients.

Health Care Reform: What Will the Likely Impact Be of the ACA?

The ACA health care law is positioned to give health care providers in general and advanced practice nurses specifically an unprecedented opportunity to improve the health of countless numbers of Americans through the offering of preventive care, wellness efforts and medical intervention when needed. Advanced practice nurses can be at the forefront of health care reforms and interventions to those who now have access to care that they did not have before. According to the Administration statements issued from the White House, the ACA should open up opportunities to increase access to prevention and wellness efforts/measures, primary care providers, and improved care coordination, and in turn enable advanced practice nurses to provide every aspect of the new care opportunities (The White House, 2013).

The Effects of the ACA and the Recovery Act on nursing related interventions/ innovations (The White House, 2013):

- Between 2009 and 2011, a threefold increase in the number of National Health Service Corps primary care providers supporting greater than 1,900 certified nurse midwives and nurse practitioners.
- Community health centers have added more than 3,000 nursing positions (approximately 800 in advanced practice) since 2009
- An investment in Nurse Managed Clinics that are anticipated to help to train more than 900 nurses and serve 94,000 patients.
- Additional supports for the training of 600 new nurse practitioners and nurse midwives by 2015

Demand

The passage of the ACA in March 2010 set in a motion of number of delivery system reforms that are likely to have an impact on the workforce projects discussed above. First, there is the aspect of demand in the reforms. According to the GAO (September 2013), the ACA will establish new delivery of care models such as accountable care organizations

(ACO) and patient-centered medical homes (PCMH). The new care models will most likely increase the need for comprehensive team based care paradigms. Such models of care will most likely require the utilization of advance practice nurses, particularly at the primary care level. The impetus for the ACO model primarily emerged from analysis of health care practice patterns demonstrating that fee-for-service payment was a major contributor to escalating medical expenditures within a fragmented health care system (Fisher, Staiger, Bynum, Gottlieb, 2007; Meyer, 2012). An ACO is defined as a group of providers who work together to assume the responsibility and cost of care for the patient population they serve, sharing in savings achieved if predefined quality metrics are achieved. (Fisher, Staiger, Bynum, Gottlieb, 2007) ACOs will incentivize providers across practice settings to improve quality and reduce or slow down spending (Lowell & Bertko, 2010; Crosson, 2009; Berwick, 2012). Under the ACO model, payers establish quality benchmarks and risk-adjusted spending targets for patients served by providers in an ACO. If the ACO meets its benchmarks, it shares in the savings achieved below the specified spending target (Fisher, Staiger, Bynum, Gottlieb, 2007; Crosson, 2011; Berwickm 2012). In some models, the entity is at risk for a portion of any spending exceeding the target. Across all models, organizations build the capacity to achieve their goals through multiple mechanisms: disease management programs, use of non-physician providers, establishment of medical homes, pay for performance, and information technology (Burns, Pauly, 2010). At this point it is not clear if the adoption of new health care delivery models such as the ACO and the PCMH will allow physicians to care for larger numbers of patients because the models allow for delegation to non-physician providers, or whether these models will require additional physicians and other non-physician providers because additional services such as care coordination and patient education will be offered remains an open question (Green, Savin, Lu, 2010). As cited in the 2013 HRSA report, when primary care physicians were asked in an AAMC survey how they would meet significant provider demands from innovations such as the ACA many practices would respond by hiring additional staff (52.7%), additional physicians (46.5%), nurse practitioners (43.7%) and physician assistants (33.6%) (HRSA 2013, pp. 29).

Even before passage of the ACA, data on ACOs already existed from a number of demonstration projects. The Medicare Physician Group Practice demonstration serves as one of the sentinel demonstration projects assessing the benefits of an ACO model (Congressional Budget Office, 2012; Centers for Medicare and Medicaid, 2011; Colla, Wennberg, Meara, et al., 2012, pp. 11-13). This large-scale demonstration project was implemented during 2005-2010 in 10 large practices comprising 5000 physicians and 224,000 Medicare fee-for-service beneficiaries. Sine nearly all organizations achieved quality benchmarks, except for cost savings, the dollars shared back to the practices to offset the cost necessary to achieve the quality improvements were variable (Table 5). Since the Physician Group Practice demonstration project, ACO experiments by Blue Cross Blue Shield (Chernew, Mechanic, Landon, Safran, 2011; Song, Safran, landon, et al., 2012) and Cigna (Salmon, Sanderson, Walters, Kennedy, et al., 2012) have also shown substantial quality improvement and variable cost savings. Over the past 4 years, implementation of ACOs has rapidly increased in response to promising results from demonstration projects but the return on investment remains in question. Such models are likely to continue to encourage shifting care provision to non-physician providers such as advance practice nurses, potentially decreasing the need for additional physicians.

Table 5. Physician Group Practice Demonstration: Performance Year (PY) 1 to Preliminary Performance year 5 Summary Results

	Quality Percentage					Shared Savings Payments				
	PY1	PY2	PY3	PY4	PY5	PY1	PY2	PY3	PY4	PY5
Billings	90.91%	97.78%	98.11%	92.45%	100.00%	$—	$—	$—	$—	$—
Dartmouth	95.45%	97.78%	92.45%	94.34%	96.23%	$—	$6 689 879	$3 570 173	$328 798	$—
Everett	86.36%	95.56%	94.34%	94.34%	100.00%	$—	$129 268	$—	$—	$—
Forsyth	100.00%	100.00%	96.23%	96.23%	100.00%	$—	$—	$—	$—	$—
Geisinger	72.73%	100.00%	100.00%	100.00%	100.00%	$—	$—	$1 950 649	$1 788 196	$—
Marshfield	81.82%	100.00%	98.11%	100.00%	98.11%	$4 565 327	$5 781 573	$13 816 922	$16 154 242	$15 832 603
Middlesex	86.36%	95.56%	92.45%	94.34%	100.00%	$—	$—	$—	$—	$—
Park Nicollet	95.45%	97.78%	100.00%	100.00%	100.00%	$—	$—	$—	$—	$5 673 177
St John's	100.00%	100.00%	96.23%	98.11%	100.00%	$—	$—	$3 143 044	$8 185 757	$2 598 859
Michigan	95.45%	100.00%	94.34%	96.23%	98.11%	$2 758 370	$1 239 294	$2 798 005	$5 222 852	$5 329 967

Source: Research Triangle Institute International; Center for Medicare and Medicaid Services; Shared Savings Payments; Physician Group Practice Demonstration; Performance Year 1 to Preliminary Performance Year 5 Summary. http://www.cms.gov/Medicare/Demonstration-Projects/DemoProjectsEvalRpts/downloads/PGP_Summary_Results.pdf.

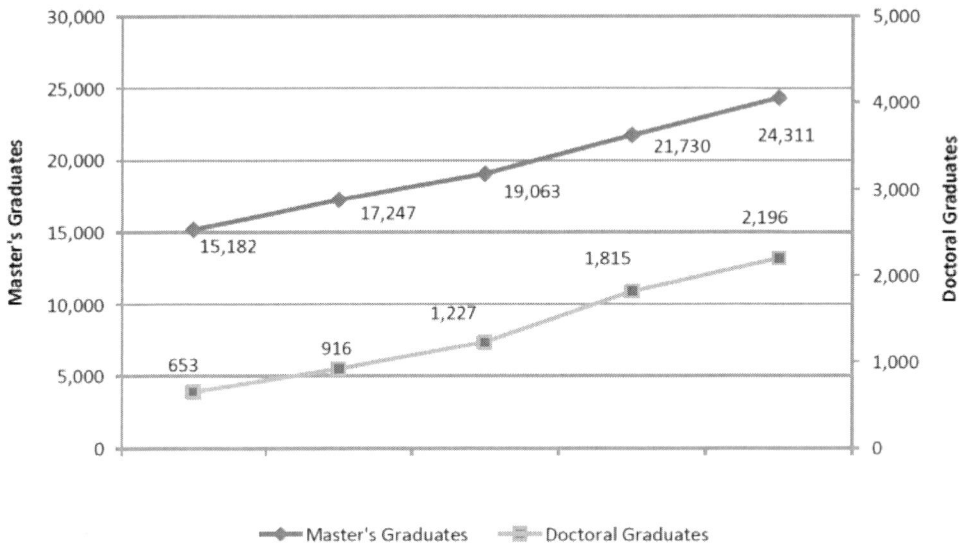

Data Source: HRSA compilation of data from the AACN Research and Data Center, 2012

U.S. Department of Health and Human Services, Health Resources and Services Administration, Bureau of Health Professionals, National Center for Health Workforce Analysis. (April 2013) The U.S. Nursing workforce: Trends in Supply and Education. Rockville, Maryland: U.S. Department of Health and Human Services. http://bhpr.hrsa.gov/healthworkforce/reports/nursingworkforce/nursingworkforcefullreport.pdf.

Figure 6. Master's and Doctoral Graduates, 2007-2011.

Beyond the ACO and PCMH, the ACA also promotes health care marketplace reform which is likely to impact work force planning for advance practice nursing as well. First, according to the GAO report (Sept 2013), the expansion of public and private health insurance coverage via the individual mandate may increase the number of non-elderly Americans with health insurance by approximately 25 million. The individual mandate requirement requires a move towards everyone having a route towards insurance coverage either by expanded Medicaid coverage, coverage through the insurance exchanges, or coverage via employer based benefits,

The ACA also established a national quality strategy focused on a move towards promoting prevention services, the provision of coordinated care, quality-based payments for health care providers, transparency around improved information on provider quality, and enhanced data collection to address health care disparities. These performance or quality improvement areas are areas of activity in which nursing leaders excel. Many of the nursing leaders are advance practice nurses at either the master's or doctoral level.

Supply of Workforce

From a supply perspective, the ACA includes provisions meant to increase the focus on workforce planning at both the federal and state levels. The National Health Workforce Commission is established to evaluate and make recommendations about the health care workforce. Previously, there are some who contend that the lack of coordinated workforce planning contributed to the projected primary care workforce shortage projected for 2020 (CRS, 2013).

Specifically, around the additional training of advanced practice nurses, in addition to the White House statements above, the ACA's Public Health, Workforce, Quality, and Related Provisions include efforts designed to increase the primary care workforce and promote preventive services. *The ACA specifically addresses existing health workforce programs authorized under the sections of health professions (*Title VII) and nursing (Title VIII) of the Public Health Service Act (PHSA). There are a number of programs under PHSA Title VIII to support the development of the advanced practice nursing workforce. The programs include funding for grant and scholarship programs for graduate nursing education including workforce diversity, cultural competency, advanced education nurses, and nurse faculty. These efforts are underway now and evaluation data on the impact of these provisions will be closely monitored in the coming years as more and more attention is focused on tracking and impacting the development of the health care workforce necessary to meet the needs of the US population. The trends from 2007 to 2011 thus far in terms of Master's and Doctoral preparation for nursing professionals certainly is cause for optimism that additional advance practice nurses will be available to meet the primary and specialty care needs of the growing US population (U.S. Department of Health and Human Resources, April 2013). Figure 6 shows a graphic representation of the rising numbers of Master's and Doctorally prepared nursing professionals from 2007 to 2011.

Conclusion

Workforce projections for advanced practice registered nurses (APRNs) indicate that APRNs are positioned to play a major role in health care delivery in the 21st century. The ACA health care law has given advanced practice nurses the opportunity to be on the forefront of efforts to improve health through preventive care, wellness efforts and medical interventions.

HRSA reports on workforce projections for physicians and advanced practice nurses show a likely increase in the need for advanced practice nurses to provide care for the full range of patient populations and across all care settings. APRNs have proven their value and ability to meet the growing need for health care providers in acute and primary care areas (Institute of Medicine (IOM), 2011).

REFERENCES

Association of American Medical Colleges. Center for Workforce Studies. (October 2012). Recent Studies and Reports on Physician Shortages in the US. https://www.aamc.org/download/100598/data/

Berwick, D. M. (2012). ACOs: promise, not panacea. *JAMA.*, *308*,1038-1039.

Berwick, D. M. (2011). Making good on ACOs' promise: the final rule for the Medicare shared savings program. *New England Journal of Medicine*, *365*, 1753-1756.

Burns, L. R. & Pauly, M. V. (2012). Accountable care organizations may have difficulty avoiding the failures of integrated delivery networks of the 1990s. *Health Affairs* (Millwood). *31*, 2407-2416.

Centers for Medicare and Medicaid Services. (2011). Medicare Physician Group Practice Demonstration. Baltimore, MD: CMS, http://www.cms.gov/DemoProjectsEvalRpts/downloads/PGP_Fact_Sheet.pdf. Accessed March 1, 2013.

Chernew, M. E., Mechanic, R. E., Landon, B. E. & Safran, D. G. (2011). Private-payer innovation in Massachusetts: the "alternative quality contract." *Health Affairs* (Millwood)., *30*, 51-61.

Colla, C. H., Wennberg, D. E., Meara, E., et al. (2012). Spending differences associated with the Medicare Physician Group Practice Demonstration. *JAMA*, *308*,1015-1023.

Congressional Budget Office. (2012). Lessons From Medicare's Demonstration Projects on Disease Management, Care Coordination, and Value-Based Payment (Issue Brief). Washington, DC: CBO.

Crosson, F. J. (2009). 21st-Century health care: the case for integrated delivery systems. *New England Journal of Medicine*, *361*, 1324-1325.

Dill, M., Pankow, S., Erikson, C. & Shipman, S. (2013). Survey shows consumers open to a greater role for physician assistants and nurse practitioners. *Health Affairs*, *32*(6), 1135–1142.

Fisher, E. S., Staiger, D. O., Bynum, J. P. & Gottlieb, D. J. (2007). Creating accountable care organizations: the extended hospital medical staff. *Health Affairs* (Millwood), *26*, w44-w57.

Green, L. V., Savin, S. & Lu, Y. (2010) "Primary Care Physician Shortages Could Be Eliminated."; R. J. Reid et al., "The Group Health Medical Home at Year Two: Cost Savings, Higher Patient Satisfaction, and Less Burnout for Providers," *Health Affairs*, vol. *29*, no. 5.

Heisler, E. J. (January 15, 2013). *Physician Supply and the Affordable Care Act*. Congressional Research Service. http://op.bna.com/hl.nsf/id/myon-93zpre/$File/crsdoctor.pdf

Isaacs, S. & Jellinek, P. (2012). Accept No Substitute: A Report on Scope of Practice. The Physicians Foundation: Empowering Physicians, Improving Healthcare. http://www.physiciansfoundation.org/uploads/default/A_Report_on_Scope_of_Practice.pdf

Lowell, K. H. & Bertko, J. (2010). The accountable care organization (ACO) model: building blocks for success. *Journal of Ambulatory Care Management*. *33*, 81-88.

Ofri. D. (January 16, 2014). *Lots of New Patients, Too Few Doctors*. The New York Times. https://www.aamc.org/download/100598/data/

Research Triangle Institute International; Center for Medicare and Medicaid Services; Shared Savings Payments; Physician Group Practice Demonstration; Performance Year 1 to Preliminary Performance Year 5 Summary. http://www.cms.gov/Medicare/Demonstration-Projects/DemoProjectsEvalRpts/downloads/PGP_Summary_Results.pdf.

Salmon, R. B., Sanderson, M. I., Walters, B. A., Kennedy, K., Flores, R. C. & Muney, A. M. (2012). A collaborative accountable care model in three practices showed promising early results on costs and quality of care. *Health Affairs* (Millwood),*1*, 2379-2387.

Schwartz, M. D. (2011). Health Care Reform and the Primary Care Workforce Bottleneck. *Journal of General Internal Medicine*, *27*(4), 469-472.

Schwartz, M. D. (2011)/ The US Primary Care Workforce and Graduate Medical Education Policy. *Journal of the American Medical Association*, *308*. 21, 2252-2253.

Song, Z., Safran, D. G., Landon, B. E., et al. (2012). Health care spending and quality in year 1 of the alternative quality contract. *New England Jounal of Medicine*, *365*, 909-918.

The White House. (2013). The Obama administration's record on supporting the nursing workforce. The Obama Administration’s Record on Supporting the Nursing Workforce Posted on Tuesday May 28, 2013. http://www.whitehouse.gov/sites/default/files/docs/nurses_report.pdf.

U.S. Department of Heath and Human Services, Health Resources and Services Administration. (December 2008). The Physician Workforce: Projections and Research into Current Issues Affecting Supply and Demand. Health Resources and Services Administration. http://bhpr.hrsa.gov/healthworkforce/reports/physwfissues.pdf.

U.S. Department of Health and Human Services, Health Resources and Services Administration, National Center for Health Workforce Analysis. (2013). Projecting the Supply and Demand for Primary Care Practitioners Through 2020. Rockville, Maryland: U.S. Department of Health and Human Services. http://bhpr.hrsa.gov/healthworkforce/supplydemand/usworkforce/primarycare/

U.S. Department of Health and Human Services, Health Resources and Services Administration, Bureau of Health Professionals, National Center for Health Workforce Analysis. (April 2013) The U.S. Nursing workforce: Trends in Supply and Education. Rockville, Maryland: U.S. Department of Health and Human Services. http://bhpr.hrsa.gov/healthworkforce/reports/nursingworkforce/nursingworkforcefullreport.pdf.

U.S. Government Accountability Office (GAO). (August 15, 2013). Health Care Workforce: Federally Funded Training Programs in Fiscal Year 2012. (GAO-13-709R) Health Care Workforce Training Programs. http://www.gao.gov/assets/660/656960.pdf.

U. S. Government Accountability Office (GAO). (September 2013). Health Care Workforce. HRSA Action Needed to Publish Timely National Supply and Demand Projections. (GAO-13-806). http://www.gao.gov/products/GAO-13-806.

INDEX

B

C

D

E

F

I

J

K

L

M

N

O

P

Q

R

S

T

U

V

W

Y